Martha E. Rogers: Her Life and Her Work

Violet M. Malinski, RN; PhD
Associate Professor and Graduate Specialization Coordinator
Psychiatric-Mental Health Nursing
Hunter-Bellevue School of Nursing
Hunter College
City University of New York
New York, New York

Private Practice, Health Patterning for Individuals and Families

Elizabeth Ann Manhart Barrett, RN; PhD; FAAN
Professor and Coordinator
Center for Nursing Research
Hunter-Bellevue School of Nursing
Hunter College
City University of New York
New York, New York

Private Practice, Health Patterning

With special contributions by
John R. Phillips, RN; PhD
Associate Professor and Coordinator of Doctoral Studies
Division of Nursing
New York University
New York, New York

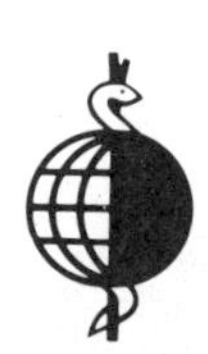

F. A. Davis Company • Philadelphia

F. A. Davis Company
1915 Arch Street
Philadelphia, PA 19103

Printed in the United States of America

Last digit indicates print number: 10 9 8 7 6 5 4 3 2 1

Publisher: Robert G. Martone
Nursing Editor: Alan Sorkowitz
Production Editor: Marianne Fithian
Cover Design: Donald B. Freggens, Jr.

Library of Congress Cataloging-in-Publication Data

Rogers, Martha E.
Martha E. Rogers : her life and her work / [edited by] Violet M. Malinski, Elizabeth Ann Manhart Barrett.
p. cm.
Contains articles reprinted from various sources.
Includes bibliographical references and index.
ISBN 0-8036-5807-9
1. Nursing—Philosophy. 2. Rogers, Martha E. I. Malinski, Violet M. II. Barrett, Elizabeth Ann Manhart. III. Title.
[DNLM: 1. Rogers, Martha E. 2. Nursing Theory—collected works. 3. Education, Nursing—collected works. 4. Philosophy, Nursing—collected works. WY 7 R728m 1994]
RT84.5.R644 1994
610.73'092—dc20
[B]
DNLM/DLC
for Library of Congress

94-6137
CIP

To Martha E. Rogers, 1914–1994

For her creativity, courage, conviction, and compassion, with our thanks for the lasting legacy she has left this nursing generation and generations to come.

Publisher's Note

As this book was being prepared for press, we received word of the death of Martha Rogers. This news was received here with great sorrow because Martha Rogers and the F. A. Davis Company had enjoyed a warm working relationship reaching back more than thirty years. The following is a tribute to Martha from our Publisher, who worked with her during all that time.

> I climbed aboard her spacecraft a long time ago. It wasn't made of metal or plastic, and it had no rigid form. It was the web of the mind that carries us beyond our expectations. She brought a Slinky along to demonstrate "The Spiral of Life."
>
> I cannot visualize Martha at rest. She is out there somewhere discovering, developing, and nurturing ideas to challenge us when next we meet.

Robert H. Craven, Sr.
Publisher

Foreword

Martha E. Rogers. The power of the name: advocate, charisma, commitment, creator, visionary. Imagine that your creative visions are so controversial that you shock and upset people, stir feelings of anger, argument, and confrontation. Imagine that your critics call you the "crazy space nurse," along with various unprintable words. How would you like to experience negative reactions as you articulate your views of nursing and reality? Martha Rogers endured all of that and even more during her professional career. Yet, she did not reject those people but, rather, spun them into the design of her vision. By doing so, the negative reactions dwindled over the years.

Today, the name Martha E. Rogers signifies compassion, love, respect, reverence, and nursing. Many nurses, nursing students, and people in the general public stand in awe of her accomplishments, courage, and convictions. There is wonderment of how she transcended various challenges and adversities to continue to enlarge her love and commitment for nursing and the betterment of humankind. One imagines the "dark secrets" that gave energy and meaning to her life and her work, what her family and family life were like, and the nature of her energy flow with people. *Martha E. Rogers: Her Life and Her Work* chronicles her living presence in nursing.

The editors show how some of the major threads of the fabric of Rogers' life were woven, both personal and professional. One prominent thread is how a family of love helped to create a woman of love. The content shows her family as an active participant in the evolution of the beauty of her human field. Needless to say, however, there was a resonance in her receiving and giving love during her youth and throughout her life, so she too, can lay claim to her unfolding beauty as a human being, especially as a nurse and a humanistic scientist.

There is no question her family fostered a deep and longing sense of respect of self and others. It was from her family and colleagues that she obtained the fortitude to face problems and issues in her life. It was her intense love for learning and nursing and the desire to express her ideas that played an important role in the whole course of her life. As such, Rogers is an active participant in the unfolding of the potentials of scholars through her expressions of love and humanness and her giving of knowledge.

The diversity of the thread of her love for knowledge and nursing encompasses what one might call her family of the universe. She engenders in innumerable people the love of learning, acceptance of new ideas, different ways of viewing reality, and the desire to fertilize the potentials of their life that lay dormant. Faculty members document how they were able to see beyond her avowed administrative skills to understand her contributions to nursing. The many significant awards that faculties have bestowed upon her further attest their love of Rogers and for her contributions to the universe of knowledge.

History confirms visionary people are frequently misunderstood and have difficulty entering the "inner circle." This was especially true for Rogers in her unswerving commitment to nursing education. The various chapters on education show Rogers was not always accepted since she is known to question the "right" rules of the profession of nursing on education. However, recall what Governor Clinton said in accepting the Democratic nomination for the U.S. presidency: "For where there is no vision, the people perish" (*Text of Address,* 1992, p. A15).

Nursing has survived in part due to Rogers' enduring voice for nursing education, especially through her ardent stance against antieducationism in nursing. Unfortunately, much of this antieducationism came from within the ranks of nursing, including some nurses considered to be leaders in nursing. Her vision was, in part, an attempt to go beyond the confines of the deadwood educators in nursing. As you digest Rogers' writings, note how she advocated change aimed toward a *Reveille in Nursing,* so nursing could grow both as a profession and as a science. Those who understood her saw hope for the advancement of nursing, while those who did not hung tenaciously to what they felt was secure, the proven "truths" of the past, the visionless people. Thus, another controversial thread in the weaving of the changing fabric of Rogers' life was her advocacy for and commitment to nursing education.

One frequently hears of the antics of Rogers and the turmoil she created as she advocated for substantive nursing knowledge. Some of these are quite humorous, as illustrated in this book, which again signify her humanness and joy of life. One wonders what a "reading of her lips" would have been then. Today, there is no question it would be: "Yes, I did help transform nursing from a prescience to a science."

Can you imagine a dean of a school of nursing refusing monies? Rogers did. The money was for nursing educational programs that were contrary to her beliefs about nursing and nursing education. Some of the programs based upon such monies did not survive, and in some cases the educational concepts they were built on are no longer accepted. Do we have such strong-willed nursing administrators and educators today, or do we have those who write all kinds of grant proposals or create diverse programs primarily to obtain money and students, frequently with little vision for their school or the nursing profession? Let's recall again what Clinton said, "Where there is no vision, the people perish" (p. A15). Will such nursing programs and administrators and educators survive as testaments to the profession of nursing?

The editors have chosen wisely examples of early writings of Rogers on education. As you read these writings, notice how her ideas overshadow today's current thinking about nursing education. In fact, some of these writings were so visionary, they are still applicable to the ongoing needs of nursing education. Specifically, the articles published in the *Journal of Professional Nursing* in 1985 were written some 20 years ago. The juxtaposition of these views with her ideas about nursing in space certainly gives a futuristic view of nursing that is creative and diverse. Rogers believes that as we educate nurses about nursing in space, which will eventually involve schools of nursing in space, we must go beyond the current processes of education and health care.

The book confirms Rogers lived a powerful vision of nursing education. This is especially true when you examine how Rogers' participation in professional and political issues and activities relates to education. Today, some of the things for which she was damned are being advocated by other nurses. For example, look at her views on "a nurse is a nurse is a nurse." As you read about this, you will see that no more needs to be said.

Synthesize Rogers' writings on education and what people have said and written about them. These writings confirm Rogers is a living legend besides being a creator and visionary person. As you read the book, keep asking yourself, what was it like to be "a lone voice in the wilderness" for such a long period of time? This is one of those "dark secrets" of Rogers we may never fully know or understand. This may remain one of the "legendary" aspects of Rogers: a person who has "a special status as a result of possessing or being held to possess extraordinary qualities . . ." (Webster's, 1981, p. 1291).

Rogers' life has not always been structured and well-ordered. She certainly had chaotic deviations from the traditional stream of thinking. This is evident in her vision of the science of nursing, where she set her course to explore the unchartered territory of the infinite nature of reality. Many nurses did not believe such a reality existed. This belief still exists today, over 20 years after *An Introduction to the Theoretical Basis of Nursing* was published. While reading selections drawn from the book, see if you agree Rogers is a scientific rebel, even revolutionary, in that she gave nurses something new they had never experienced before. Actually, she created a science that never existed before (Land & Jarman, 1992). It was nurses' unfamiliarity with this unknown reality that made them uncomfortable, especially since their traditional ideas and ways of thinking were challenged.

Fortunately, Rogers' Science of Unitary Human Beings, as it is called today, resonated with experiences and feelings of many nurses who were unable to express themselves fully in a scientific way. These nurses realized that nursing, nursing science, and reality were more than they were able to put into words. Rogers was able to articulate in a succinct way those things they could not express. Equally as important was the large, vociferous group that challenged Rogers' ideas and dubbed her the "crazy space nurse." These supports and challenges participated in refinement of her ideas as the Science of Unitary Human Beings evolved. This new science dissolved boundaries to knowledge and broke old rules that no longer worked in a new reality (Land & Jarman, 1992).

The editors show that Rogers assumed an awesome responsibility for the evolution of nursing science. She quickened nurses' sense of wholeness and transcendence to give new meaning to nursing and life. Through her Science of Unitary Human Beings, Rogers showed the integral nature of all life and revolutionized the way change was viewed. She helped to optimize the potentials of individuals, groups, and the world, especially the profession of nursing. This responsibility was difficult to fulfill at times. One can only speculate how this relates to her "dark secrets." This is indicated in Rogers comment to me: "There were times I wondered if I were right, now I know I was."

Fortunately, the power of Rogers' vision pulled the future into nursing, the relative present. We are no longer mired in past truths, but are creating truths congruent with a new reality. As you read this book, look for the new truths and the truths that are needed to accelerate the advancement of our profession and the people we can be. Let us revel in the glorious unfolding of nursing knowledge and human potentials. Realize, too, that Rogers' Science of Unitary Human Beings overturns assumptions people hold dear to life. The fact is, we can no longer deceive ourselves through narrow, concrete, cause-and-effect thinking.

Be assured. Many people use the Science of Unitary Human Beings to give meaning to changes in their lives and the accelerating changes occurring in nursing and the world today. Document these changes through scientific and other creative forms of communication and share them.

Why should you feel assured? In the history of nursing, Rogers, like Nightingale, gives us a vision that changes the whole development of the science of nursing. Let us conspire with Rogers "to breathe together" so as to have "an intimate joining" (Ferguson, 1980, p. 19). Let's make Rogers' Science of Unitary Human Beings the hundredth monkey (Watson, 1980). Yes, there is need for an overwhelming power for the betterment of humankind. We can do this by being willing to "breathe" the all-consuming passion Rogers has for nursing and life. The continued evolution of this passion is up to us, the reader.

Look at the photographs of Rogers before reading the book. Pay particular attention to those of the oil and holographic portraits and the bronze bust. Look intently. Do you experience more than you can perceive with your five senses? Are there clues to the "dark secrets" of Rogers' life? Recall Leonardo da Vinci's *Mona Lisa.* Wallace (1966), in discussing the *Mona Lisa,* states, "Leonardo far transcended portraiture to make his subject not only a woman, but Woman; in his hands the individual and the symbolic became one" (p. 27). People have for centuries "looked at her with delight, with puzzlement, or with something approaching dread" (p. 127). The content of the book confirms that Rogers is not only a nurse, but Nurse for the profession of nursing.

The enigma of Rogers' love for life and nursing can be understood better through an understanding of her portraits and bronze bust. They "speak" of what can be found in Lewis Carroll's (1981) *Through the Looking-glass.* "You don't know how to manage Looking-glass cakes . . . hand it round first, and cut it afterwards. . . ." (pp. 184–185). A similar feeling is present when we consider how much there is still to know about the Science of Unitary Human Beings and its potentials for nursing.

Let us seize the golden opportunity to experience the fragrance of life Rogers offers to us. Let Rogers "induce us to be a little more than we are by 'seeing' us just a bit in the future" (Josselson, 1992, p. 111), her relative present. There is no question that Rogers "represents for us what may be possible, what we might strive toward" (p. 128). Indeed, let Rogers free us from the past so we can experience the dynamic ever-changing universe.

John R. Phillips, RN; PhD
Division of Nursing
New York University
New York, New York

References

Carroll, L. (1981). *Alice's adventures in wonderland & through the looking-glass.* New York: Bantam.

Ferguson, M. (1980). *The aquarian conspiracy: Personal and social transformation in the 1980s.* Los Angeles: Tarcher.

Josselson, R. (1992). *The space between us: Exploring the dimensions of human relationships.* San Francisco: Jossey-Bass.

Land, G., & Jarman, B. (1992). *Breakpoint and beyond: Mastering the future—today.* New York: HarperBusiness.
Text of address by Clinton accepting the Democratic nomination. (1992, July 17). *The New York Times,* pp. A14–A15.
Wallace, R. (1966). *The world of Leonardo: 1452–1519.* New York: Time Incorporated.
Watson, L. (1980). Lifetide: The biology of consciousness. New York: Simon & Schuster.
Webster's third new international dictionary of the English language unabridged. (1981). Springfield, MA: Merriam.

Preface

The written contributions of Martha E. Rogers to the profession and discipline of nursing deserve to be lastingly memorialized. As with many great leaders, thinkers, poets, artists, and scientists, the full extent of her accomplishments and the profound ways they have changed nursing science, nursing education, and nursing practice will probably not be known for some time to come. We invite present and future generations to search for new recognitions of her contributions and to celebrate the ways Rogers' legacy will enrich the continuing revolution in nursing science.

Sometime during the 1960s Rogers made a quantum leap from the road toward nursing science that the profession was traveling to a road less traveled. Indeed, this road she began building continues to make quantum jumps into the next millenium. The earlier path of science "for" nursing maintained that knowledge from the biological, physical, and social sciences assumed "its own unique configuration" and was applied for social ends (We Believe, 1959, p. 1). The new direction on the road built by Rogers, where no other nurses were traveling at the time, was a basic science "of" nursing. A new product of knowledge different from other sciences emerged (Rogers, 1970). Her vision of nursing; her hopes, dreams, ideas, and convictions; and the science she created have undoubtedly led the profession and discipline in a direction different from what might have been achieved without her. This book is an acknowledgement of the seminal contributions Martha E. Rogers has made to nursing and to humankind.

For the first time, Rogers' major writings and presentations have been collected in one volume. The sections are organized chronologically according to her interests and activities. The 1950s and 1960s represented the height of her work on nursing education. In two books, various articles, and numerous presentations at conferences across the country, Rogers presented her ideas about the importance of a "valid" baccalaureate degree in nursing, possible only in a 5-year program, and outlined what that program would encompass. She offered her ideas regarding graduate and doctoral education as well as the role of nursing faculty in each program. She identified areas for nursing research.

The decade of the 1970s witnessed the height of Rogers' participation in and concern with professional and political issues as well as the early development of nursing science. She helped draft and obtain legislative passage of the revised New York Nurse Practice Act and addressed issues such as the need for separate licensure for baccalaureate nurses, different from associate degree/ diploma nurses, and her opposition to the burgeoning nurse-practitioner movement.

The 1980s marked an acceleration in the continuous development and refinement of the Science of Unitary Human Beings as well as an increased emphasis on space. Although references to intergalactic travel and space living can be found in Rogers' earliest writings, she has been most prolific on this subject in later years.

Each of these topics is addressed in a section of the book. Dr. Rogers granted the editors access to her filing cabinets at New York University, Division of Nursing, to begin the process of reading through all her documents and selecting the ones to be used in this book. Dr. Rogers graciously allowed us to visit her at her home in Pigeon Forge, Tennessee, where she invited various members of her family to meet with us. Family members were kind enough to share their recollections of Martha as sister and as aunt. The editors wish to thank Dr. Rogers for graciously opening both her files and her family to us.

During these preliminary stages, Dr. John Phillips, Associate Professor in the Division of Nursing, New York University, was the third editor. He participated in the selection process, helping to choose the materials that appear in the sections on nursing science and education and research, and assisted in writing the draft of the proposal submitted to F. A. Davis. Unfortunately, Dr. Phillips had to cease participation in the project due to other commitments. We wish to acknowledge and thank him for his contributions.

Rogers' major ideas and seminal publications are collected in this book. Although she has over 200 publications and presentations to her credit, many of them are variations on a theme. The editors chose those that best reflect her ideas on each theme represented in the book. Readers will find some repetition of ideas. This was done deliberately to ensure that each section would be complete on its own. Some papers were partially edited to reduce unnecessary repetition. Although the themes are recurring ones, some new idea appears in each and every selection. Equally important, Rogers' teaching style was to reinforce through reiteration. The book reflects this.

Each section is introduced by an overview chapter written by one or both editors. These chapters are designed to guide the reader in synthesizing the wealth of ideas on each topic. Drawing from material reprinted in the section as well as other works of Rogers, we also aimed to share insights concerning main currents of Rogerian thought. Finally, we hope to convey to the reader a personal sense of Martha E. Rogers as a truly remarkable human being.

Section One presents the "Historical Perspective: Rogers' Role in the Development of Nursing Science and the Influences that Shaped Her Life." Here the reader will find recollections from Dr. Rogers' family and the contributions from her earliest books, *Educational Revolution in Nursing* (1961) and *Reveille in Nursing* (1964). Section Two, "Education and Research," presents Rogers' ideas on the structure of nursing education, baccalaureate through doctoral programs, and necessary changes in licensure and practice, as well as her views on nursing research. Section Three, "Professional and Political Issues," establishes Rogers' position as an eloquent and effective political statesperson for nursing. Also discussed is the organization she helped to found, SAIN (Society for Advancement in Nursing). Section Four, "Nursing Science: Evolution of the Science of Unitary Human Beings," traces the development of nursing science from its earliest expression in the 1960s through the 1970 publication of her classic book, *An Introduction to the Theoretical Basis of Nursing,* to the refinements of the early 1990s. Section Five, "Futuristic Visions," presents Rogers' contributions to nursing in space, showing how the Science of Unitary Human Beings makes a signal contribution to facilitating health and well-being for people in space as well as on earth. Section Six, "A Historical Salute to Martha E. Rogers," contains the five papers presented at the historical salute to Martha E. Rogers on her 75th birthday, co-sponsored by the Society of Rogerian Scholars and the Division of Nursing, New York University, in June 1989.

Three other people deserve recognition and thanks. Dr. Jacqueline Fawcett, RN; PhD; FAAN, University of Pennsylvania School of Nursing, generously shared her expertise in conducting computer searches and provided regular updates from her continuing search for publications related to the Science of Unitary Human Beings. Robert G. Martone, Nursing Publisher at F. A. Davis Company, was instrumental in successfully guiding the proposal for this book through F. A. Davis. Alan Sorkowitz, Nursing Editor at F. A. Davis Company, was extremely helpful to us as we compiled the manuscript for this book. Marianne Fithian, Production Editor, lent her expertise to the final editing of the manuscript. We thank them all.

The editors hope that readers will enjoy reading the book as much as we enjoyed putting it together. We thank Dr. Rogers for the privilege. It was a labor of love.

Violet M. Malinski
Elizabeth Ann Manhart Barrett

References

Rogers, M. E. (1970). *An introduction to the theoretical basis of nursing.* Philadelphia: F. A. Davis.

We believe. (1959, May). *League line: New York State League for Nursing,* pp. 1, 3, 6.

Acknowledgments

In addition to the individuals acknowledged in the Preface we offer sincere thanks to the following:

Martha E. Rogers, for granting us persmission to reproduce the text of previously unpublished speeches that she has given across the country over the years and for the photograph of her portrait.

Laura Wilhite, for furnishing the beautiful family photographs.

Jane Coleman, for organizing and collecting the family reminiscences.

John R. Phillips, for the photographs of the portrait sculpture and hologram.

Gean Mathwig for the photo of Martha Rogers and other nurses lobbying in Albany for passage of the revised New York State Nurse Practice Act.

Martha Bramlett, for the photograph of Martha Rogers, "Just Visiting."

Donna Brian, Patricia Dunn, Joan Frizzell, Adrienne McDonnell, Beth Ann Swan, and Jacqueline Fawcett, for reviewing the first draft of the manuscript and providing excellent suggestions for the book's development.

List of Contributors

Elizabeth Ann Manhart Barrett, RN; PhD; FAAN
Professor and Coordinator
Center for Nursing Research
Hunter-Bellevue School of Nursing
Hunter College/City University of New York
Private Practice, Health Patterning
New York, New York

Joyce J. Fitzpatrick, RN; PhD; FAAN
Professor and Dean of Nursing
Elizabeth Brooks Ford Professor of Nursing
Frances Payne Bolton School of Nursing
Case Western Reserve University
Cleveland, Ohio

Lynne M. Hektor, RN; PhD
University of Miami
Coral Gables, Florida

Violet M. Malinski, RN; PhD
Associate Professor and Graduate Specialization Coordinator
Psychiatric-Mental Health Nursing
Hunter-Bellevue School of Nursing
Hunter College/City University of New York
New York, New York
Private Practice, Health Patterning for Individuals and Families
Yonkers, New York

Patricia Moccia, RN; PhD; FAAN
Executive Vice President
National League for Nursing
New York, New York

J. Mae Pepper, RN; PhD
Chairperson, Department of Nursing
Mercy College
Dobbs Ferry, New York

John R. Phillips, RN; PhD
Associate Professor and Coordinator of Doctoral Studies
Division of Nursing
New York University
New York, New York

Francelyn Reeder, RN; PhD; RSM; CNM
Associate Professor and Faculty Associate of the Center for Human Caring
School of Nursing
University of Colorado Health Sciences Center
Denver, Colorado

Martha E. Rogers, RN; ScD; FAAN
Professor Emerita
New York University
New York, New York

Contents

Foreword v

Preface x

Acknowledgments xiii

List of Contributors xiv

Section One: Rogers' Role in the Development of Nursing Science and the Influences That Shaped Her Life 1

Section Editor: Violet M. Malinski

Chapter 1: A Family of Strong-Willed Women 3
Violet M. Malinski

Chapter 2: Martha E. Rogers: A Life History 10
Lynne M. Hektor

Chapter 3: Rogers' Early Views: An Ever-Expanding Vision of Nursing 28
Violet M. Malinski

Section Two: Education and Research 35

Section Editors: Elizabeth Ann Manhart Barrett and Violet M. Malinski

Chapter 4: Revolution and Reveille in Nursing Education and Research 37
Elizabeth Ann Manhart Barrett and Violet M. Malinski

Chapter 5: Untitled 48
Martha E. Rogers, 1962

Chapter 6: Nursing Charts Her Course 54
Martha E. Rogers, 1962

Chapter 7: Editorial 59
Martha E. Rogers, 1963

Chapter 8: Educating the Nurse for the Future 61
Martha E. Rogers, 1963

Chapter 9: Editorial 69
Martha E. Rogers, 1963

Chapter 10: Editorial—Professional Standards: Whose Responsibility? 74
Martha E. Rogers, 1964

Chapter 11: Editorial 76
Martha E. Rogers, 1964

Chapter 12: Editorial 78
Martha E. Rogers, 1964

Chapter 13: For Public Safety: Higher Education's Responsibility for Professional Education in Nursing **80**
Martha E. Rogers, 1969

Chapter 14: Graduate Education in Nursing at New York University **89**
Martha E. Rogers, 1970

Chapter 15: Ph.D. in Nursing **97**
Martha E. Rogers, 1971

Chapter 16: Nursing Education: Preparing for the Future **103**
Martha E. Rogers, 1985

Chapter 17: Nursing Science: Research and Researchers **107**
Martha E. Rogers, 1968

Chapter 18: Nursing Research in the Future **114**
Martha E. Rogers, 1987

Section Three: Professional and Political Issues **117**
Section Editor: Elizabeth Ann Manhart Barrett

Chapter 19: Rogers' Professional Politics **119**
Elizabeth Ann Manhart Barrett

Chapter 20: Excellence Is Where You Find It **126**
Martha E. Rogers, 1959

Chapter 21: Accountability **128**
Martha E. Rogers, 1971

Chapter 22: Nursing's Expanding Role and Other Euphemisms **133**
Martha E. Rogers, 1972

Chapter 23: Nursing: To Be or Not to Be? **140**
Martha E. Rogers, 1972

Chapter 24: Nursing Is Coming of Age . . . Through the Practitioner Movement, Con (Position) **147**
Martha E. Rogers, 1975

Chapter 25: Euphemisms in Nursing's Future **155**
Martha E. Rogers, 1975

Chapter 26: Legislative and Licensing Problems in Health Care **163**
Martha E. Rogers, 1978

Chapter 27: Peer Review: A 1985 Dissent **170**
Martha E. Rogers, 1978

Chapter 28: The Umbrella That Isn't! **173**
Martha E. Rogers, 1980

Chapter 29: Unification: SAIN [Society for Advancement in Nursing] Model Myth Versus Reality: An Overview **175**
Martha E. Rogers, 1981

Chapter 30: Obsolescence Revisited: The Doing Syndrome **179**
Martha E. Rogers, 1980

Chapter 31: Resolution on Licensure for Entry Levels to Practice in Nursing 181
Governing Council of the Society for Advancement in Nursing, 1982

Chapter 32: SAIN [Society for Advancement in Nursing] Perspective 182
Governing Council of the Society for Advancement in Nursing, 1977

Chapter 33: Proposed Act to Amend the Education Law in Relation to Requirements for Independent, Registered, and Practical Nursing in New York State 185
Governing Council of the Society for Advancement in Nursing, 1983

Chapter 34: The Need for Legislation for Licensure to Practice Professional Nursing 192
Martha E. Rogers, 1985

Section Four: Nursing Science: Evolution of the Science of Unitary Human Beings 195
Section Editor: Violet M. Malinski

Chapter 35: Highlights in the Evolution of Nursing Science: Emergence of the Science of Unitary Human Beings 197
Violet M. Malinski

Chapter 36: The Aims of Nursing Science 205
Martha E. Rogers, 1970

Chapter 37: Nursing's Conceptual Model 210
Martha E. Rogers, 1970

Chapter 38: Homeodynamics: Principles of Nursing Science 214
Martha E. Rogers, 1970

Chapter 39: The Theoretical Basis of Nursing 220
Martha E. Rogers, 1971

Chapter 40: Nursing: A Science of Unitary Man 225
Martha E. Rogers, 1980

Chapter 41: Science of Unitary Human Beings 233
Martha E. Rogers, 1986

Chapter 42: Nursing Science and Art: A Prospective 239
Martha E. Rogers, 1988

Chapter 43: Nursing: Science of Unitary, Irreducible, Human Beings: Update 1990 244
Martha E. Rogers, 1990

Chapter 44: Space-Age Paradigm for New Frontiers in Nursing 250
Martha E. Rogers, 1990

Chapter 45: Nursing Science and the Space Age 256
Martha E. Rogers, 1992

Section Five: Futuristic Visions 269
Section Editor: Elizabeth Ann Manhart Barrett

Chapter 46: On the Threshold of Tomorrow 271
Elizabeth Ann Manhart Barrett

Chapter 47: The Future of Nursing 276
Martha E. Rogers, 1980

Chapter 48: A Scenario for Nursing in 2001 A.D. 280
Martha E. Rogers, 1982

Chapter 49: Beyond the Horizon 282
Martha E. Rogers, 1983

Chapter 50: High Touch in a High-Tech Future 288
Martha E. Rogers, 1985

Chapter 51: Dimensions of Health: A View from Space 292
Martha E. Rogers, 1986

Chapter 52: A Conversation with Martha E. Rogers on Nursing in Space 296
Martha E. Rogers, Maureen B. Doyle, Angela Racolin, and Patricia C. Walsh, 1990

Section Six: A Historical Salute to Martha E. Rogers on the Occasion of Her 75th Birthday 307
Section Editors: Violet M. Malinski and Elizabeth Ann Manhart Barrett

Chapter 53: The Social Context Within Which Martha E. Rogers Developed Her Ideas 309
Patricia Moccia

Chapter 54: The Nursing Context Within Which Martha E. Rogers Developed Her Ideas 313
J. Mae Pepper

Chapter 55: The Philosophical Context Within Which Martha E. Rogers Developed Her Ideas 317
Francelyn Reeder

Chapter 56: Rogers' Contribution to the Development of Nursing as a Science 322
Joyce J. Fitzpatrick

Chapter 57: Rogers' Contribution to Science at Large 330
John R. Phillips

Epilogue 337

Bibliography 339

Glossary 352

Appendix A: Genealogy as Provided by Laura Wilhite, Family Historian 353

Appendix B: Selecting Your Career in Nursing 355

Index 357

SECTION ONE

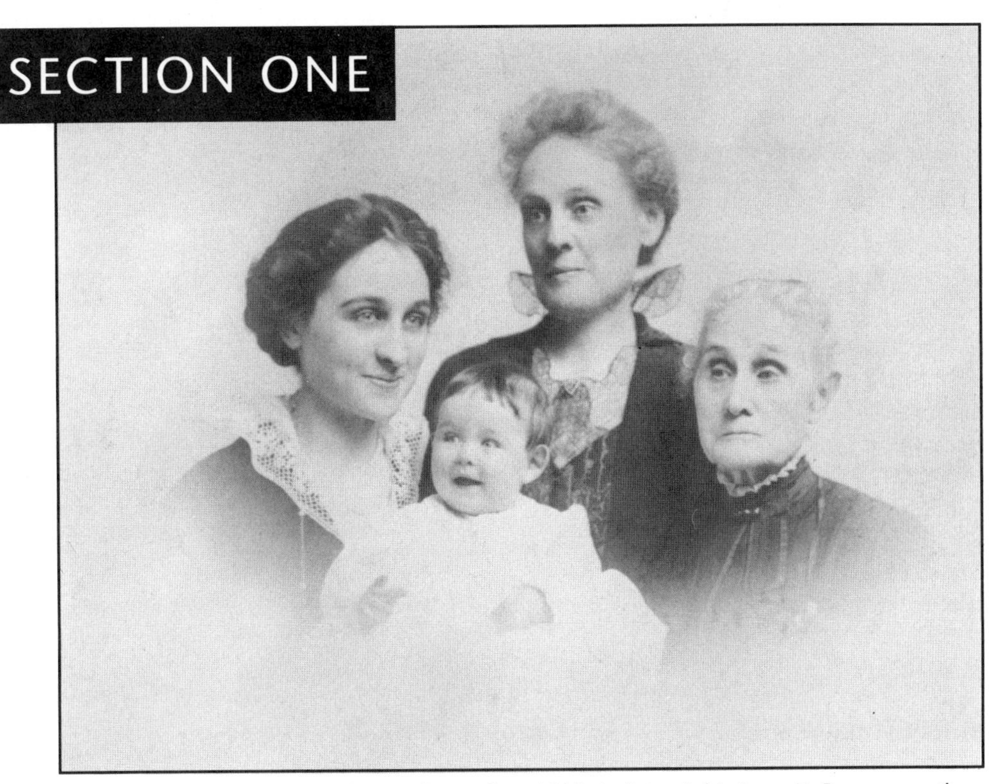

Four Generations, circa 1913. Left to right: Lucy K. Rogers, mother; Martha E. Rogers; Laura B. Keener, grandmother; Lucy M. Brownlee, great-grandmother.

Rogers' Role in the Development of Nursing Science and the Influences That Shaped Her Life

Section Editor
Violet M. Malinski

CHAPTER 1

A Family of Strong-Willed Women

Violet M. Malinski

Although it is possible to examine the Science of Unitary Human Beings from a purely theoretical perspective, it helps immeasurably to gain an understanding of the person behind the ideas. As Laudan (1977) and Capra (1982) have argued, science is not a value-neutral product of objective observation; rather, it is a process deeply marked by the values and thoughts of the person putting forth the ideas. Therefore, this chapter seeks to illuminate the life process and experiences of the person who synthesized the Science of Unitary Human Beings, Martha E. Rogers. Interviews have been conducted with Rogers over the years, appearing in print in a number of publications. Notable among these are the works by Safier (1977), Sarter (1988), and Hektor (1989). The latter, representing the latest interview to appear in print, is reprinted in this book. What has not appeared before are recollections from those who have known Rogers within the intimate circle of family, nuclear and extended, who have their own unique insights and remembrances to share. These include her sisters, Laura Wilhite and Jane Coleman (Fig. 1–1); two of her nieces, the Reverend Nancy J. Wilhite and Katherine Lundy; and two of her nephews, Mel B. Wilhite and James Wilhite. They were kind enough to share their recollections of Martha E. Rogers as sister and aunt rather than as educator, theorist, researcher, or politician.

Family Portrait

Martha Elizabeth Rogers was born May 12, 1914, to Bruce Taylor Rogers and Lucy Mulholland Keener Rogers. Martha was the oldest of four siblings, three girls and one boy. She was named after her paternal grandmother, Martha Elizabeth Luttrell Rogers, on whose side the family traces its lineage to Sir Geoffrey Luttrell, who died circa 1216. The Luttrells inhabited Dunster Castle in Somerset, England. Laura Wilhite, the family historian, provided information on the family tree (see Appendix A).

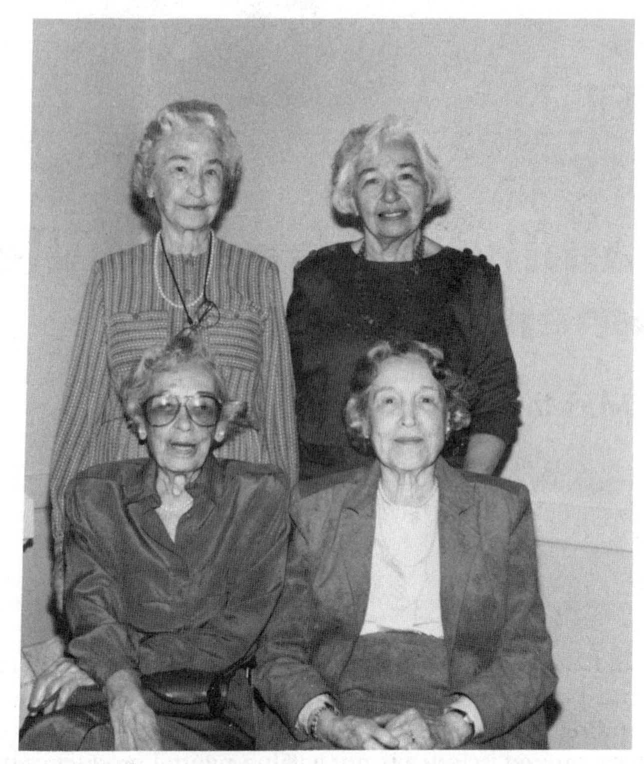

Figure 1–1. Top row: Laura Rogers Wilhite and Jane Rogers Coleman, Martha Rogers' sisters. Bottom row: Martha Rogers and her aunt, Laura Keener Brakebill, April 1991.

Mel B. Wilhite provided what is perhaps the best description of the important role Aunt Martha played in the lives of her many nieces and nephews:

Martha has always been a worthy advocate of education and life experiences for all her family, and she has always been more than generous with her time and money and in sharing her encouragement with each of us to see that we made the most of our lives in whichever field of endeavor we chose to follow.

Trips west were always fun family times and educational experiences as well. We traveled literally from border to border, saw places and things and shared adventures that otherwise might have been learned about only in books.

Each of Martha's seven nieces and nephews (Melvin, Nancy, James, and Bruce Wilhite and Martha Ann, Kathy, and John Coleman) received a trip to Europe and England upon graduating from high school. I (being the eldest) was the first to receive this wonderful opportunity. Three weeks on the continent and in England! Martha's love and generosity made it all possible. But she has gone beyond the original seven, as *our* children have been fortunate enough to travel with her, as well.

Martha Rogers can be a very hard, driven woman when she needs to be and feels it is necessary, but on the other hand, she has always been loving and so very generous to each member of her family and, if truth be known, to countless others as well.

Following are other family descriptions of Martha E. Rogers.

Laura Wilhite, Martha's sister, remembers back when with Martha:

Martha was always a "fresh air fiend." Regardless of how hot or how cold it was the year round, she wanted windows open wide (also doors if possible). And so it was that I awoke one cold morning in the 1930s (we were sharing the same bed) with snow on everything from the window to the bed. During the night the temperature had dropped, the window screen had disappeared, and a breeze had quietly but surely carried snow into our room. Needless to say, I snuggled deeper under the covers, but Martha was elated. Even today this love of fresh air continues. More than once I have arrived at her mountain cottage and found her enjoying a log fire with windows wide open.

In the late 1940s Martha worked in Phoenix. From the first moment she set foot on Arizona soil, she was "hooked," and her love for the desert country and climate has never wavered. She bought property and put down "roots." Though she left there a few years later, she would return each summer, taking with her a car full of relatives. Our brother Sam (nicknamed Kenner), a World War II veteran, returned to Phoenix and lived in her home. In 1958 my husband "Buck," our two youngest sons, and I planned to go west with her. We had loads of fun planning the itinerary, etc. Then my husband became ill and was hospitalized for 6 weeks. About a month before our departure date, Buck and I knew there was no way we could finance such a trip. I wrote Martha that it was time we faced reality and to be truthful—we could not make it past the city limits. In return mail she wrote—"Will pick you up at the city limits," and we all had an outstanding vacation.

In 1963 we made another trip west with Martha. This time we included our mother—wheelchair and all. This trip we took a northern route and spent 2 weeks or more getting to Phoenix. We included numerous national monuments, forests, and parks. The scenery was magnificent and breathtaking. As we were going through Glacier National Park, I remarked about the beauty, how fantastic it was, hoping that someday we would be able to return and perhaps include the International Peace Park, Calgary, Lake Louise, and other points of interest. Martha said, "Well, what's wrong with now?" And so we did, even having lunch at the lovely Grand Hotel at Lake Louise—wonderful! Martha is truly a person who helps make one's dreams come true.

Jane Rogers Coleman's memories of her sister include the following:

Martha Elizabeth Rogers . . . What a woman! What a treasure! And sometimes what a frustration. . . . For instance: Martha turned 8 years old just 1 month before her youngest sibling (me) was born. Since mother had invited only her mother and teenage sister to celebrate the occasion, little Martha quickly made additional plans. Promptly at 2:00 a stream of young children wearing party clothes and bearing gifts began to arrive. Martha admitted she had invited them. "But don't worry! I've made a lollipop pie for refreshments." She proudly displayed a pie pan covered with a round of brown paper marked with a crayon to resemble a pie crust. Inside were 15 or so suckers bought with pennies from her piggy bank. While Auntie directed games, Grannie tripped to a nearby grocery store for ice cream and cake to go with the "pie." It must have been wild and wonderful—and surprising.

Martha was our parents' first child and our maternal grandparents' first grandchild. Several young aunts and uncles lived nearby. All gave Martha their attention and adoration. By the time younger siblings and cousins arrived, Martha's position was secure. She was sometimes challenged but seldom upstaged. Martha was well suited for the position of leadership: smart, pretty, confident. Mother recognized Martha's precocity almost from the cradle: "It was scary."

My brother and sisters always treated me quite well. As children, we played the usual games and rode tricycles, bicycles, and skates. There were always plenty of neighborhood children to play with. Martha sometimes made up plays for her siblings to act out. I was only 2 or 3 when we did the one on "Nutrition and Health." I remember it well. Brother got sick and never ate carrots again!

Martha and Laura always seemed to have plenty of beaux when they were in high school and college. I am sure Martha considered one young man quite seriously. In my snooping about, I came across a paper she had written. The headings were "Reasons I should marry Mr. X" and "Reasons I shouldn't marry Mr. X." The second list was longer.

I was 12 or 13 when Martha left home for nursing school, college, and career. She visited when possible—often unannounced and after everyone was sound asleep. But no matter—she sometimes brought gifts and always, excitement. Phone and doorbell rang often and parties just happened.

As Martha acquired an R.N. and college degree she became a font of health information for all the family. Over the years she has also become the reservoir of a million secrets (which will surely follow her to the grave).

Our brother, Sam, knew Martha about as well as anyone. After his discharge from the army following World War II, he went to Phoenix to visit Martha. He liked it so well he stayed. He went to college and then went to work. Sam found Martha a welcome source of strength at a difficult time of readjustment to civilian life. Martha moved back east, but Sam lived out his life in Phoenix (1919–1987). His home became a summer vacation spot for Martha and other family members.

I, and sometimes my husband and children, have visited Martha in most of the places she has lived across the country; she has visited us as well. Whether hostess or guest, she has been fun to be with—generous, energetic, challenging, and humorous.

Martha's record shows that she has exhibited many characteristics. She has been brilliant, knowledgeable, hardworking, willing to sacrifice (when necessary), committed with a sense of priorities, and visionary. Perhaps it is *vision* which has set her apart from the crowd.

Mel B. Wilhite shared other fond memories of growing up as Rogers' nephew:

From as early an age as I can remember, everyone in our family has looked up to Aunt Martha with great respect and admiration, either for what she *had* accomplished, *was* in the process of accomplishing, or was *about to* accomplish. She was the member of the family who traveled, even then, to far-off mysterious places and then returned, eager to share her latest adventure. As I look back, I suspect it was not the purpose of the trip that got the attention of us kids but rather the miniature imprinted bars of soap, sugar, and matches that proved she had been where she said she had been. Hotels, restaurants, airlines, and railroads kept us kids sweet and clean for many summers while we were growing up.

However, like all of us, she was guilty of an infrequent mess-up and we all loved to "catch" her when she slipped. One incident comes readily to mind. It occurred over 40 years ago—I believe I was 6 or 7 years old—and involved one of Martha's favorite foods, potato salad. The entire family had gathered to prepare a picnic lunch to take to the Great Smoky Mountains, approximately 1 hour's drive from Knoxville. I (for some reason) distinctly remember Martha making quite a fuss over her potato salad, and justifiably so. I think she was trying a new recipe and was quite excited about it. This was to be the *best ever!* Pickles, eggs, celery, potatoes cooked just right, mayonnaise, mustard, salt, and pepper—it all had to be just right. Finally, after much taste-testing, it was declared ready. After deciding who would be riding in whose car, we were off. On arrival at the picnic grounds (I believe it was at the "Chimneys," halfway up Highway 441 between Gatlinburg and Newfound Gap), the proper table was selected, and we began to unpack the cars and to spread our meal. The more we unpacked, the more a look of consternation crossed Aunt Martha's face. Finally we realized that everything was on the table except for one thing. That "perfect potato salad" had been overlooked in packing and had been left at home.

For years Aunt Martha would, on completing the school year in Baltimore or New York, come through Johnson City and Knoxville and collect a carload of nieces, nephews, cousins, etc.—really, anyone who wanted to go—and head for Phoenix, Arizona, her "home away from home." I, being the eldest of seven nieces and nephews, was the first of my generation chosen to make this exciting and challenging trip.

I was 12 years old at the time and more than once wondered if I would survive to see my 13th birthday. Uncle Keener, Aunt Martha, Grandmother Rogers, Aunt Mary Shanton—and me. What an entourage. Four adults and me in a two-door, 1954 Plymouth Plaza. What a way to go!

Ah, but those were certainly *good* times together, family times, and like families everywhere we laugh together as warm remembrances wash over us again . . . and we shed a tear for those who shared those experiences but are no longer with us to share in the remembering.

Nephew James Wilhite shared some of the family's love of humor and jest in his recollections:

I went to visit Aunt Martha in New York for 3 weeks and ended up staying with her for 12 years. We both liked to laugh, so we shared jokes and funny stories. I remember Aunt Martha was trimming my mustache one day when she asked me what I would do if she cut my mouth. "I will get you for 'female' practice," I said. We both roared with laughter.

Another time Aunt Martha and I were going to Knoxville from Johnson City. I told Aunt Martha to go to the corner and make one turn to the right. Instead she turned left and ended up back at the Colemans' house. Like Aunt Martha, the car had a mind of its own.

The Reverend Nancy J. Wilhite shared her reminiscences about Aunt Martha:

About the age of 12 I read the book *Auntie Mame* by Patrick Dennis. From that time on I knew that Aunt Martha was the Auntie Mame of all her nieces and nephews! I was never quite sure she *totally* appreciated the nickname. . . . Certainly the education she gave us was not quite as liberal as Mame's, but she did show us the world—quite literally—and she taught us that we could do anything we wanted to do!

As she had learned to do, she taught us to dream. No dream was impossible! At the same time she managed to keep us somewhat realistic by teaching us also that in achieving those dreams we would have to make choices. It was all up to us. And then, she was there . . . to listen to those dreams . . . and to encourage . . . and to give sound guidance along the way.

As the older nieces and nephews had the job of breaking the adults into the system of summer adoption by Aunt Martha, we did not make quite as many trips west as the younger ones did. Consequently, we did not get to see everything that the younger ones did—like when they went from Knoxville, Tennessee, to Phoenix, Arizona, by way of Lake Louise, Canada, or Honolulu, Hawaii. A few years ago when I was driving with her to San Francisco for a week's seminar she was doing, we were reminiscing about the various trips. We were only a couple of hours outside of Denver when she asked me if I had ever gotten to Yellowstone National Park. When I responded that we had not traveled north on any of my trips, she immediately pulled out her atlas. After a couple of minutes' study, she informed me that when we got to Denver, we were heading north. It would take only one extra day to take in this unique site. Yellowstone was fabulous, and the drive back south through the state of Idaho is one of my most treasured memories! That's just the kind of person Aunt Martha is . . . totally unselfish . . . always giving . . . and always making each person feel special.

Katherine Lundy's reflections include the following:

As a child there were the ubiquitous books—gifts to encourage nieces and nephews to read, but less appreciated than the accompanying monetary gift. The books were always didactic in nature, usually of the "All About" genre. She has continued this practice with great-nieces and -nephews, giving my daughter Lara books on world geography, space, and Sally Ride.

My earliest recollection of Martha is of her visiting my house when I was very young, and she got down on the floor and played with us (me and my two siblings). She played the horse as all three of us mounted her back and rode her all over the living room.

When I graduated from high school, Martha's congratulatory sentiment was expressed in the card she sent—a world map, with the message, "The world is your oyster." A proper accompaniment to her graduation gift of a trip to Europe.

Then there was the time I flunked out of nursing school my senior year. I was working as a desk clerk at a low-rent hotel, trying to regain my compass, when Martha visited. "Well," she said, having commandeered me for breakfast, "everybody is entitled to one mistake, but you'd sure better not make the same mistake twice." Her point was well taken. In a similar vein, Martha often said with respect to her own style, "You can get away with anything once!"

I lived with Martha for several months early in my New York career. She contributed money when I was short, an occasional theater ticket, and frequent dinners out. Most importantly, she nurtured, nudged, and baby-sat with my young daughter. I will never forget coming home one night to hear her telling Lara a story—Little Red Riding Hood, gone to the moon.

Martha is a gracious hostess, and this extends to my friends, whom she embraces as if they were family. Visitors to the apartment, whether my fellow doctoral students or some more exotic breed, quickly learned to call her "Aunt Martha." Withal, she is a charming, delightful companion, recounting stories of her life and travels and conjuring visions of the future (space travel, rapid transit, evolving potentialities). She is engaged with her company as well, encouraging them to talk and share, listening heartily.

For years, for most of her adult life, she rose at 5:00 or 5:30 A.M. and read—her intention being to read at least five books a week. And that in addition to her Agatha Christies. She read serious books, obscure books, Hofstadter, Capra, Bohm, Bronowski, Laing. She protested the depressing nature of *100 Years of Solitude,* which I gave her, but acknowledged it was one of the best statements of the human condition she had ever read.

Finally, I have seen Martha to be a person of absolute determination and unwavering optimism. She brooks no weakness in herself or any other person. She overcame her motor vehicle accident to resume a demanding schedule of world travel, conferences, and lectures. She focuses herself and her energy toward life, and she modulates her activities such that she remains one of the most productive people I have ever seen. She has great sympathy for and patience with those who are perceived as different. Ever unorthodox, she promulgates the view that schizophrenics are evolutionary emergents, preparing the species for life in a new dimension.

Her intellectual honesty and personal honesty are also noteworthy. She was *never* one to support the status quo; rather she derived great pleasure from deflating egos, mocking pretensions, and disabusing institutions and individuals of their illusions (and in some cases, delusions).

I will close with an interchange I had with her some years ago which I think is instructive. I was lamenting some professional insult I had received and told her, "It's a dog-eat-dog world out there." To which she replied, "So you've got to learn to eat dogs and like it!"

Rogers' Evolving Life Process

To further illuminate the person behind the ideas, Chapter 2 presents Rogers' own recollections of her childhood and early education, the years of work and study followed by her tenure at New York University, and her life beyond the university as told to Lynne M. Hektor. Chapter 3 summarizes Rogers' early views as expressed in her first two books, published in the early 1960s, that served as a catalyst for the work for which she has since become famous, the continuing delineation of Rogerian nursing science, the Science of Unitary Human Beings. Also included in Chapter 3 is a summary of Rogers' contributions as editor of the journal *Nursing Science.*

References

Capra, F. (1982). *The turning point: Science, society and the rising culture.* New York: Simon & Schuster.

Hektor, L. M. (1989). Martha E. Rogers: A life history. *Nursing Science Quarterly, 2,* 63–73.

Laudan, L. (1977). *Progress and its problems: Toward a theory of scientific growth.* Berkeley: University of California Press.

Safier, G. (1977). *Contemporary American leaders in nursing.* New York: McGraw-Hill.

Sarter, B. (1988). *The stream of becoming: A study of Martha Rogers' theory.* New York: National League for Nursing.

CHAPTER 2

Martha E. Rogers: A Life History

Lynne M. Hektor, M.S.N.

This is an age of theory development in nursing. Since the 1960's, there has been a deliberate effort on the part of the profession to define a theoretical base. The process and context of theory development, who it emerges from, when, how, and why, are all essential elements of a comprehensive understanding of theory. Thus, it seems a logical progression to travel the path of a contemporary nurse theorist. It was natural and appropriate to select Martha E. Rogers as the theorist upon whom to focus. Author of the seminal text *An Introduction to the Theoretical Basis of Nursing* (1970), Rogers, like Nightingale, is nothing if not original, controversial, and independent. They share the same birthday, May 12, as well as the attribute of basic intellectual prowess.

Many describe Rogers' thought as "radical" (Malinski, 1986, p. xiii). Indeed, the freshness, depth, and breadth of Rogers' ideas yielded and continue to yield important changes in the perspective of the discipline of nursing. Her views are discussed by many (Fitzpatrick and Whall, 1983; Marriner, 1986; Nicoll, 1986; Meleis, 1985) but Parse (1987) names her as the creator of a new paradigm in the discipline of nursing, the simultaneity paradigm. Rogers defines her own theory contribution as:

> The development of a paradigm for nursing, called the science of unitary human beings. Philosophical and theoretical investigations were directed toward elucidation and further understanding of the nature and direction of unitary human development (Rogers, Curriculum Vitae, 1988).

There has been much written by and about Rogers (see Marriner, 1986, summary). There are audiotapes and videotapes documenting her thoughts, such as the tapes by Sigma Theta Tau, National League for Nursing, Helene Fuld Institutional Award, Meetings Internationale, and Media for Nursing, Inc. These tapes are valued artifacts for future nurse historians.

Hektor, L. M. (1989). Martha E. Rogers: A life history. *Nursing Science Quarterly, 2,* 63–73.

The predominant theme of most of the written articles about Rogers are [sic] on her framework. Many of these writings will provide secondary sources for her biography, including reports of interviews with Rogers (Safier, 1977; Sarter, 1988). One is left with elucidations of the science of unitary human beings, Rogers' views on nursing, on education, and on the state of nursing science. But the tapes and written material provide only part of the picture. Although there are some glimpses of her humor, her originality, her vitality (especially on videotape), there is much more to Rogers than these tapes and writings capture.

The purpose of this life history is to document events in Rogers' personal and professional life that, in turn, shed light on the context and process of the development of the science of unitary human beings. How did this unique woman develop personally and professionally to become a major force in an evolving profession? How did she emerge as the vanguard leader of a new vision of nursing? What can be learned from the life of Rogers that will foster the development of future nurse scientists?

A life history framework was chosen to structure the inquiry. Langness (1965) described the life history approach as "an extensive record of a person's life as it is reported either by the person, or by others, or both" (p. 4). Overall, he states, life histories are descriptive and concerned with biography as a cultural document. This life history will illustrate the ways in which Rogers received, recreated, and transmitted the culture of 20th century nursing.

Rogers has continued for over five decades to be involved professionally and actively committed to change and growth within the discipline of nursing. Her cooperation in this venture provided the opportunity for her to validate documentation of events in her life that she perceived to have influenced the development of her theory.

All quotations in this article were made by Rogers during 3 days of personal interviews conducted on June 27, 28, and 29, 1988, in New York City and verified in a later contact. Interviews were conducted at the same time with two long-time personal and professional associates of Rogers, Joan Hoexter and Gean Mathwig. These sources provided comparative data, as did the interview with Rogers' niece, Katherine Lundy. Throughout this article, quotations from personal interviews with Rogers are referenced by date; quotations from personal interviews with the other sources include the respondent's name and date.

The data have been organized chronologically into four sections for presentation: Part I (1914–1937), Childhood and Early Education; Part II (1938–1953), Years of Work and Study; Part III (1954–1975), The New York University Years; Part IV (1976–1988), Beyond NYU and the Future. Each section begins with a general introduction and summary of the era. This is followed by supportive dialogue and a detailed description of the happenings during the specific years.

PART I

Childhood and Early Education (1914–1937)

The early years of Rogers' life can be characterized by close family life, harmony, fun, and love of knowledge. Rogers developed, early on, a dedication to helping people that continued throughout her life . . . "most of all I wanted to help people, I wanted to *do something.* I didn't want just to talk about it" (June 27, 1988).

Although Rogers' parents had resided in Knoxville, TN, they spent some time in Dallas, TX, which is where Rogers was born. During the first year of her life the family returned to Knoxville. Although Rogers was the firstborn, she never felt she was the oldest child:

> My mother had two sisters and three brothers. Her youngest sister was 18 years younger. One brother was much younger too, and these two were like an older sister and brother to me. I never had a strong feeling of being the firstborn and always had the constraints of an older brother and sister. I was the oldest maternal grandchild. There was always a family to keep you cut down to size (June 27, 1988).

Rogers was barely 3 years old when her father took her to a local airport to see the "local tub," her term for airplane. "I was *sold,*" she said.

> Airplanes were always something special to me. One was in town and my father took me; he lifted me in and we just sat in it. It was a big old thing with benches inside. It was for transporting equipment and there are not many of those airplanes around anymore! My grandmother, now, she was daring! She wanted to take a commercial flight and once she took a plane from Knoxville to Chicago, just because she wanted to ride in an airplane (June 27, 1988).

When asked to describe her childhood, Rogers' early memories of Knoxville included recollections of her father's sprawling old home on Yale Avenue, summer cottages in the mountains, clubhouses, and other aspects of an ordered, peaceful town and genteel lifestyle.

> My paternal grandmother's home was large, with a great big porch. My parents and maternal grandparents had cottages in the Appalachian mountains that were later taken over by the Great Smokey [sic] Mountain National Park. Up until high school, these were summer cottages. There was a clubhouse too and I loved to watch the adults dance. I remember swimming in the river, diving from my father's back and sledding near our home in Knoxville.
>
> There was always family; laughter, an awful lot of fun. We were always in one or another's homes. The women would sew, cook, talk. The men would work (June 27, 1988).

She recounts her early formal education and the first identification of her exceptional intelligence:

> I remember first going to Kindergarten; it was terribly exciting. I discovered I talked too much. I remember the teacher telling me to move away from the table and I was embarrassed. At that time, psychologists were developing intelligence tests,

such as the Simon Binet, and were looking for test subjects. Mother took me and my younger sister to be tested. We were said to be very bright. We were each permitted to skip a grade and the teachers weren't very happy about it. I was entering the fourth grade and they were taking up long division and the teacher kept quizzing me. But I answered all the questions. Math was always one of my favorite subjects.

Rogers' thirst for knowledge began at an early age. She spoke about her love of books and reading that was fostered by her concerned and loving parents:

I had such a large, extended family that I never really wanted for companionship. I liked to go off by myself with a book. By fourth grade, I had read every book in the school library. I used to go to the public library before I was 6. Even before I could read, I was well acquainted with the public library. They had a story hour for preschoolers that I loved. Once I started reading I could take out eight books at a time—I went through the shelves, one after another. When I was in high school, my father was concerned that I was "skimming," not really reading. So my father sat down to discuss the books I was reading with me and found I wasn't skimming!

There were always loads of books in our home and in my grandparents' homes. Books in the attic, in trunks, all kinds of books spilled all over—*Men of Mars,* Buck Rogers; the Greek alphabet I knew by age 10. By sixth grade, I had read all 20 volumes of *The Child's Book of Knowledge* and was into the *Encyclopedia Britannica.* Also, sets of Dickens and Mark Twain (June 27, 1988).

In her description of her high school days, Rogers sketched a picture of a young woman involved in a variety of activities, such as membership in the Junior League and the Methodist church. She learned public speaking, "I was always getting up and speaking," and participated in the Senior class play. Rogers recalls she liked everything about high school. By her senior year, she had completed all the high school math courses and enrolled in a college level algebra course, which she remembered as "great fun." She was, she noted, the only woman in the class. Rogers, as yet not having a clear career commitment, entered the University of Tennessee in Knoxville in 1931 and remained there for 2 years, until 1933:

The University of Tennessee was right there in town; you could go right from Kindergarten to college in Knoxville. The population wasn't as mobile then. I attended the University of Tennessee for 2 years but I didn't know what I wanted to do. I wanted to help people and considered law and medicine. I took the science-med course. It was more substantial than straight pre-med and included more science and math. I took psychology, French, zoology, genetics, embryology and many other courses. My father was worn out buying me fertile eggs to slice up for embryos! An old farmer would always bring eggs that were fertile.

Most of all, I wanted to help people. I wanted to *do something.* I didn't want to talk about it. Social work I didn't know about. It was really serendipitous that I got into nursing. I knew nothing about nursing when I decided to become a nurse. My parents thought that liberal arts education and home economics were good fields for women then. That was what my two sisters studied. "Hen-medics" (women physicians) were discouraged. Nursing was not a very desirable field (June 27, 1988).

Rogers entered nursing school at Knoxville General Hospital in September 1933. She recalls there were only 25 nursing students admitted:

Helen, one of the gals I was friends with, decided to go into nursing at the local hospital. You were listed as you showed up. The list showed, #24, Martha Rogers; #25

Helen! The discipline was Army, pre-Nightingale. You had to stand up for everyone; it really wasn't for me. I left, went home, spent a miserable week. I remember riding the bus one day to the end of the line, looking at all the tired people—working class people, you know, so I went back (to nursing school).

Knoxville General hospital, where I went to nursing school, was a city hospital. It was a medical school prior to being a school of nursing. It was an old frame building with a brick building that was added in the early 1930's for Black patients and a Negro School of Nursing. We had classes together but they had to sit in the back of the room and couldn't talk (June 27, 1988).

Rogers' determination was very apparent during these times.

I discovered there was *no* library in the nursing school when I began my studies there. So I talked to the housemother and we started one. I don't remember if the hospital bought any books for us, but the students and others brought some books in from their homes.

I wanted to see an autopsy to get a feel for what they were like. There was a university student who worked as an orderly who discouraged me from attending, and the more he said it was awful, the more determined I was to go. And I did.

Nurses' "training" was full of surprises and challenges for Rogers, exposing her to a different life-style, language, and social values.

I did enjoy working with people and patients. It was a city hospital serving a very different class of people, with wards of 20 or 22 beds. Across the street was another place for private, obstetrical, and pediatric cases. I didn't really know nursing then; I had no idea about it.

Some of the ward patients had been on the wrong side of the law. I remember one male patient had a tombstone fall on his foot and crushed it when he was hiding loot from a robbery. He said he had to "piss." I had never heard that word! I gave him an emesis basin! I learned a new "language"—I'm not talking about scientific terms but more useful ones! (June 27, 1988).

After completing nurses' "training," Rogers went away to college, partly to please her parents and partly because of her own need for continued intellectual stimulation and growth:

My parents weren't happy that I didn't have a degree and said I needed more education. They thought I was very opinionated. George Peabody College in Nashville, TN, was a good school, a nice place, and that pleased my parents. I didn't realize until I was there that they had Public Health Nursing and that caught my eye. We had very little exposure to that in Knoxville (June 27, 1988).

She received her Bachelor of Science degree in Public Health Nursing in 1937. She was then ready for the larger world, beyond Tennessee. Was it ready for her?

PART II

Years of Work and Study (1938–1953)

These years of work and study began with Rogers' first professional position as a public health nurse in rural Michigan. She spent 2 years in this role before returning to Teacher's College for further study. In 1945, she earned her master's degree from Teacher's College, Columbia University. She was a public health nurse in Hartford, CT, advancing from staff nurse to acting Director of Education. Subsequently, she established the first Visiting Nurse Service in Phoenix, AZ, and became its Executive Director.

Despite the fact that Rogers said she "loved everything about it—everything about those years [in Arizona]," her thirst for knowledge persisted. Therefore, she left Arizona in 1951 and returned to school at the Johns Hopkins University, Baltimore, MD. She said she "had to go back to school." These years were characterized by a high degree of professional involvement, growth, adventure, and movement. Her love of knowledge was a persistent theme and her horizons expanded on all levels.

Rogers described her first position as a public health nurse:

> That was in central Michigan. It was a good job opening, a rural public health position that was recommended by the Director at Peabody. I wanted to travel, see the world, so Michigan was okay with me. What I remember is *snow,* snow shovels, and ashes.
>
> I didn't know how to drive but I knew I had to get a car. Before going to Michigan, I took six driving lessons. When I got to Michigan, the first thing I did was to take a taxi to the automobile factory and buy a car. I drove back into Detroit, down an avenue which was a wide four lane boulevard. The cops stopped me as I was driving the wrong way! They told me to turn around and I did. It was the first time I was driving alone, after all. Anyway, I drove myself from there to the new job; a trip that should have taken 2 hours took 6 (June 28, 1988).

When asked to describe what a typical day was like when she was a public health nurse in Michigan, Rogers gave the following account:

> What I did was straight public health which involved a lot of case finding. Public health nurses planned programs, worked on committees and were "community activists." For example, the Women's Auxiliary of the American Legion met to discuss venereal disease and I was asked to be the speaker. It must have been a good speech because everyone came up to talk to me afterwards and ask questions and arrange for testing.
>
> My days were almost entirely home visits. On any given day I might check out reported cases of communicable diseases or follow up on those or visit mothers with new babies. The last smallpox epidemic in Michigan occurred while I was there and at first, it was thought to be chickenpox. It took someone in Detroit to identify it. Then vaccinations began in earnest. What I liked was seeing people where they were in their homes, and the promotion of health. People in hospitals, after all, are our mistakes.

It is noteworthy that Rogers' first practice role was as a public health nurse, an independent role that seemed to influence her later ideas about nursing. Her theoretical grounding in health and prevention are recurrent themes. These were exciting times in public health nursing, community involvement was stressed, and there was an interdisciplinary approach with nursing as a full and equal member of the health care team. Rogers spent 2 years in rural Michigan, then went to Teacher's College, Columbia University, New York City, to continue her education:

> I liked going to school; I knew I didn't know enough. I sold my car—that was enough to pay tuition with a little left over. Ever since I was a child I wanted to go to Columbia to study. It was highly respected in the community where I grew up; it had the reputation of being a top university (June 28, 1988).

When asked how her parents reacted to this plan, she responded:

> It was taken for granted I wasn't going to be like anyone else. And my father had died one month before . . . he was ill with cancer—but he didn't quit easy. He insisted I go ahead with my plans to return to school (June 28, 1988).

However, at that time, a young Southern woman living alone in New York City was viewed as being in danger, and a room in New York was prearranged by some of Rogers' parents' friends. Soon, however, she relocated to the dorm.

After attending Teacher's College full-time for two semesters, Rogers took a staff position at the Visiting Nurse Association of Hartford, CT. From 1940 to 1945, she attended Teacher's College full-time during the summers and worked in Hartford during the remainder of the year. (Rogers later initiated a similar program plan for graduate students at New York University during her tenure, thus providing for students to complete degree requirements through summer study.) She advanced to the positions of Assistant Supervisor, Assistant Education Director, and acting Director of Education at the Visiting Nurse Association of Hartford, Connecticut.

> In Connecticut, we served the entire community, both upper and lower classes. This was during World War II and there were shifts in the population and the cultural groups in the area. People migrated from Canada to work in war industries; some had limited education and difficulties relocating. There was a settlement house in the neighborhood.
>
> I was assigned a district with 66 different nationalities! I translated pamphlets on health. It was delightful. Professionally, there was a continuation of my ideas about nursing. I thought nursing was a knowledgeable endeavor, and that nurses should be baccalaureate prepared or more. We exercised freedom and autonomy. We were responsible for our own acts. We were never accountable to other disciplines; that accountability would have jeopardized our autonomous position. We had nursing supervision and consultation that was provided by knowledgeable nurses. We had nurses who did nutritional and maternal child consultation.
>
> Communicable diseases had always been a major priority of public health. Tuberculosis was a problem then that was far more acute than AIDS (acquired immunodeficiency syndrome) is now. Nursing has always had major responsibility in regard to communicable diseases in the community and in communicable disease hospitals. Diphtheria was common, and in the hospitals, in an emergency, any nurse might be called upon to perform a tracheotomy (June 28, 1988).

After completing her master's degree, Rogers left her position in Hartford and, true to form, searched for new horizons:

After graduation, my plans were somewhat unclear, and I went home for awhile. I prepared letters and a vita [sic], wrote to Bureaus of Public Health Nursing. There were jobs available and I received many answers. I considered the educational division in Hartford as I had liked it so much there, but I decided on a position in Phoenix. An old, wealthy Arizona family wanted to start a Visiting Nurse's Service and had traveled all over the East looking for a nurse to get it organized. I was hired as the Executive Director to implement their dream (June 28, 1988).

When asked to recall her first days in Phoenix, Rogers talked about the differences in climate and moving out west:

When I left Knoxville it was cold, raining cats and dogs. It was right before Thanksgiving and I wore a wool suit, coat, and gloves. It was a wild flight to Tucson. The plane was old, one of the "slow pokes" (DC-3s), and it was stormy. When we landed in Tucson there was sunshine. My aunt and uncle met me in their lightest summer clothes. I went on to Phoenix and got a room at the Y and several months later got an apartment.

Transportation was always a major issue for public health nurses. At that time, the war was just ending; there were no cars. In Phoenix, there was no public transportation and roads were not paved. Rogers recalled her innovative solution to this problem:

Until someone on the Board found me a Chevrolet coupe, I had an old Model A I used. I remembered these cars from my childhood. We were happy to have any car we could get; the shortage of automobiles made it hard to hire nurses. They needed transportation.

I was able to get my hands on some motor scooters, then I could hire the nurses I needed. I hired a classmate of Gladys Sorenson, now Dean at the University of Arizona, and she was the first nurse to ride a motor scooter.

I called the newspaper to cover the ride . . . "Come this morning," I told them, "or not at all. It won't be news anymore." They sent a photographer and her ride made the front page. Actually I was petrified for her safety. In Phoenix, when it rained, there were rivers of mud, and I followed her on her motor scooter in my Chevrolet that first week. She didn't know it, but I was really worried for her safety.

We designed our own uniforms—navy blue suits. We bought the material and had them tailored. I couldn't see any point in wearing the old fashioned uniforms with aprons.

Rogers recalled the office, which was expanding rapidly, was housed in the Social Service Center. Setting up the services and getting the nurses was an exciting time. Rogers bought office furniture and one of the doctors donated a huge mahogany desk with glass over the top that she described as "beautiful." She also started a staff library. The Executive Director role was varied and multifaceted, allowing Rogers to use her many talents:

I was always calling the newspaper. We were in it at least once a week; I was always doing things to get us publicity. We had a drama group and used our artistic talents. We had a 30 minute play series on the radio. We wrote sketches and I played the nurse's part. I wrote articles for the newspaper and for labor unions. We were active in the community and in nursing organizations.

During these active, busy years, Rogers' ideas about nursing continued to emerge:

The concept of nursing that developed in hospital schools was to follow orders. I believe I was the first nurse in Arizona to have a master's degree. They didn't know what to do with a nurse with a master's degree. "Nurses don't do that sort of thing," I heard all the time. I said, "Yes, they do." I loved everything about those years (June 28, 1988).

Rogers left Arizona to go back to school in 1951, again feeling the need for more education. At that time, there were few Universities offering graduate programs in public health and Rogers selected the Johns Hopkins University in Baltimore. She stated:

I had to go back to school. I didn't know enough. I had too many questions. I earned the MPH and the doctor of science degree, a program that had the same requirements as the Doctor of Philosophy. We took statistics, and courses offered by the different branches of biology. They had the top statisticians there and research facilities.

Students at Hopkins came from a variety of disciplines. For example, there were sanitary engineers, a handful of other health professionals, medical doctors and dentists. The students' ages varied; the basic science students were young; others of us were already full-fledged professionals.

The School of Public Health had a limited number of students enrolled. Everyone knew everyone else really well. Everyone ate in the cafeteria and we had so much fun nobody cared what food they served, or we sat at the local bistro drinking cokes and having all kinds of interdisciplinary discussions. That's an important thing. There is so much more involved in becoming educated than sitting in a classroom. One of the problems of being in school part time is the lack of that kind of interaction and exchange of ideas (June 28, 1988).

When asked if she had begun conceptualizing the science of unitary human beings when she was at Hopkins, Rogers replied:

I started when I was born—collecting more and more facts. New knowledge began to come out—there was the dawn of the Space Age. As for the framework, which comes first, the chicken or the egg? Knowledge doesn't come out of the woodwork. There are new and old world views, ancient history and the Indian philosophies. Things fell into place and ideas grew. Now we're moving into recognizing that there are other ways of thinking. There are no closed doors in science (June 28, 1988).

In looking back, Rogers was unable to single out any educational experience that was more important than any other:

No. They all contributed to many things. None was more important than any other (June 28, 1988).

PART III

New York University (1954–1975)

When Rogers was appointed Head of the Division of Nursing at New York University in 1954, a vital and mutually beneficial association began. These years were characterized by comraderie, humor, debate, and a high level of intellectual growth and development. The science of nursing was developing and the rich garden of knowledge long cultivated by Rogers began to bear new and, what seemed at the time, exotic fruit. Rogers described her introduction to New York University as follows:

> Vera Fry, Head of the Division of Nursing at New York University before me, came for 2 weeks to orient me after I accepted the position. There was a big reception at one of the hotels (June 29, 1988).

Joan Hoexter, RN; PhD, who attended this reception, commented that Rogers wore a beautiful wool dress and a pheasant cloche. Hoexter recalled that all of the faculty who were in place when Rogers became Director of the Division of Nursing left New York University (NYU) except herself. Hoexter states she was "persuaded" to stay.

> I didn't know how anyone could do what she had to do. But she was enthusiastic. She always saw autonomy in practice. She wasn't saying nursing was a learned profession in those days, but she had a great deal of respect for nursing and felt it did not receive enough respect (Hoexter, June 28, 1988).

After Baltimore, Rogers had really wanted to go back out west. However, she recalled that the nursing school directors in that geographic area said that she was "overeducated for a nurse faculty position." She was encouraged to take the position at New York University by Ruth Freeman and so she moved to New York. Rogers described her first sublet apartment in New York City in 1954:

> Now that place had character! It was a large, old apartment building on Wooster Street. There were three floors and a subfloor. There was a dance studio on the top floor. I lived there until January when the city tore down those buildings to make way for middle class housing. The buildings were strangely decorated; the Village [Greenwich] in those days was still "Villagey" in the old sense, Bohemian and charming.
>
> It was a drafty old place. The thermostat for the whole building was in my place and the woman who sublet the apartment to me put a little cage over the thermostat and set it so the tenants couldn't change it. We put ice cubes on the top of it; this would trip the thermostat for several hours and we could warm up.
>
> I had a fireplace and the wind whistled down it. Joan Hoexter and I gathered wood off the streets. I had a woodsman hatchet and we used to hack the wood. It was lots of fun.
>
> The large living room had iron steps up to the roof with lots of plants and things set on them. There were deep windows and a terrace. The woman who sublet the apartment to me was into numerology and had cut all the legs off the furniture. The kitchen was so small you could barely turn around in it! I had a big Thanksgiving

open house that year that lasted all day. I had a deli cook a big turkey—and made a big fire in the fire place. That's the way things were then—open (June 29, 1988).

In recalling her first years at NYU, Rogers expressed her concern about the lack of nursing content in the curriculum:

When I first came to NYU, there was not enough substantive nursing knowledge to know. There is no need to go to college to learn technical skills. We needed nurses with doctorates who knew about research. The only doctoral degrees in nursing at that time were offered by Teacher's College and at New York University by the Schools of Education (June 29, 1988).

When Rogers was asked if doctoral students were initially enrolled in the Division of Nursing, she responded:

Of course, at NYU there was a seminar course for [nurse] doctoral students. When I came I met with the doctoral students. There were about eight students at the time and most of them did graduate eventually.

I made some unilateral changes, adding statistics and later on, physics for students at all levels. That was hard for them and I tutored students in statistics for several years. If you look over the list of [NYU] dissertation titles, you'll see a change from functional topics to [research in] nursing. This was an attempt to focus on people rather than function. Students were free, when they had viable ideas, to pursue them (June 29, 1988).

Rogers was asked if the science of unitary beings was in her head during this time. She responded:

Not specifically, but the idea of a science of nursing *was* there even then. *Educational Revolution in Nursing* was published in 1961, but it was in my head for awhile before that. It was really a naive little book, but it scared a lot of people. *Reveille in Nursing* (1964) came next. It addressed higher education. I had the purple book [*An Introduction to the Theoretical Basis of Nursing Science*] in my head by then.

I first introduced my idea of nursing science to the doctoral students and at that point it was nothing more than a series of statements written by me. We had intellectual excitement. Nobody knew what they were doing. The dissertation seminar had previously been offered by other disciplines and my idea was that the dissertation seminar for nursing students ought to be taught by the Division of Nursing faculty. I taught these seminars as much as I could. This was quite revolutionary for the time (June 29, 1988).

Gean Mathwig, RN; PhD, Professor and Director of the theoretical bases of nursing science at New York University came to NYU in 1963. Martha, she recalled, was marvelous as a seminar leader. "She would change sides to get an argument going!" She described Rogers' impact on the Division of Nursing's scholarly environment as follows:

She supported people in terms of different kinds of thinking. She had avant-garde ideas. She was always creative and independent, and supported that in others (Mathwig, June 27, 1988).

When asked about the academic climate at NYU during those early years, Rogers commented:

There was enthusiasm, students and faculty worked together and everyone got in on the act. We didn't worry about rules or traditions. We were all committed to what we were doing (June 29, 1988).

Joan Hoexter recalls the excitement of those years:

> We would sit in the cafeteria and talk. We were a small faculty at the beginning and everyone taught in all three [program] levels. Most of us were single people so there was much talking about the program outside of work. We all lived near NYU. We ate, slept, and talked together morning, noon and night (Hoexter, June 28, 1988).

Gean Mathwig recollects:

> We worked hard. It was exciting and I enjoyed it. Martha was brilliant, avant garde. We laughed a lot; there was humor, fun, things you don't get in a lot of work situations. The students were as excited as the faculty (Mathwig, June 27, 1988).

If there was a word to sum up Rogers, Gean Mathwig said, it was "worker." Joan Hoexter concurred. She also remembered the "excitement, seeing things going on all around, terribly hard work." However, Rogers' ideas were not always acceptable to everyone:

> Sometimes we wished she would be a little more concerned with the day-to-day issues of the program. Her curriculum approaches didn't always seem sound to us. They seemed [to be] from another world, even then (Hoexter, June 28, 1988).

According to Hoexter, Rogers needed "someone to mind the store," a task that often fell to Hoexter. "I wasn't a *risk taker,*" she said. "Martha *was.* And she was *single minded* in terms of her goals for nursing." She continued:

> People were devoted to her—it's because she can turn off the theory and become a person and have fun. She had this relationship with students, too. She has the ability to attract people and keep people. She had two distinct sides—she works hard and she plays hard (Hoexter, June 28, 1988).

Rogers related the following incident that illustrates her ability to combine these two sides of hard work and hard play:

> When I arrived in New York, I had just graduated from Hopkins and after putting the down payment on my apartment, I was broke. So was Joan. But we wanted to go to the American Public Health Association Convention held in Buffalo, New York, that year. Joan's mother lent us the money to go since neither of us had it! The train we took back from Buffalo must have been a pre-World War I train. It didn't even have normal windows, it had circles. We got stuck on that train. There was a big storm in the western part of New York state. Trees had fallen across the tracks and the train was forced to stop. We ran out of food, although I remember we had plenty to drink. We all shared everything (June 29, 1988).

Hoexter described this same incident as follows:

> Martha arrived in September and in October she and I wanted to attend the American Public Health Association meeting in Buffalo. We barely had the money to get there and didn't have a room. "It'll be O.K.," Martha said, and it was. She knew the Tampax people. They had a suite and we stayed with them.
>
> Then there was one of those historic Buffalo storms. We were stuck and nothing was moving—no trains, no planes, no buses. Finally we got an old, old train out of Buffalo, the Lackawanna line, I think it was. A state room on that train was all we could get. Martha slept in the upper berth. We got up when we thought it was time to be in New York City, but we were stalled and did not know where! There were trees across the track and the train had stopped while we were asleep! I remember all this

as fun. Martha wasn't upset about it at all. "Oh, we'll manage," she said, and we did. There was no food on the train, just some crackers and a few bottles of scotch, but we all had a great time (Hoexter, June 28, 1988).

In addition to her openness and comraderie with the faculty, Hoexter also recalled Rogers' devotion to her family. This bond, discussed earlier, strongly influenced and supported many important decisions in Rogers' early years and was a continuing life theme:

She had tremendously close family ties. She took part of every summer to be with her mother. She would take her mother and a car load of kids, nieces, and nephews, and they would be off to somewhere, like California. One year they went to Hawaii. She was somewhat of an anachronism—self contained, yet a deep sense of family (Hoexter, June 28, 1988).

Rogers' niece, Katherine Lundy, also a nurse, remembered her youth with Rogers with affection. Her visit home every Christmas was a special occasion:

We have pictures of her crawling around on the floor with little kids riding on her back. It was always exciting. I thought her name was "Mrs. Goodrich" and when my parents asked me why, I said "because she is good and because she is rich" (London, [sic] June 29, 1988).

Rogers' family and peers commented on her single-mindedness and determination. Katherine recalled:

When she put her mind to something, *that was it.* She is very single minded towards a goal. Her advice: "set precedents." (London, [sic] June 29, 1988).

Hoexter described Rogers' goal orientation as follows:

You couldn't have worked with anyone more *committed.* Most of the faculty were there because they were committed to Martha. She was a *charismatic* person. She often neglected everything—personal life and department, as she dwelled with ideas. The "drones" kept it going. She was always off in outer space, not concerned over anything day to day. But she always took criticism well. We'd tell her "you have to buy a new dress . . . you have to go to a beauty parlor," and she would. We finally got her into that habit (Hoexter, June 29, 1988).

When asked to comment on her role as an administrator and the day-to-day details of running the department and her personal lifestyle, Rogers responded:

Well, I had a good amount of experience as an administrator. I was used to independent work from my public health experiences and had an educational leadership position in Connecticut and then was Director in Phoenix. I like the idea of working with people. Survival says you learn some things or else.

Delores [sic] Krieger once told me, "You are a lousy administrator! You don't do it like the book says!" I said, "I hope not." The rule of thumb doesn't always work. There were some studies done by psychologists who developed tests to predict who would make a good administrator after they got out of school. Then they decided to try out the test on people who already were successful chief executives of Fortune 500 companies and the like and they all failed (June 29, 1988).

During all these years of work and play, Rogers was moving toward the publication of *An Introduction to the Theoretical Basis of Nursing* (1970). She said:

It just got written. It had to be written. There had to be a book to teach nursing as a science, something for the students to learn in *nursing* or there was no point in having students.

I really started writing it in the mid-60's. I was using some of the chapters in my classes with the undergraduate students and the doctoral students. It was being worked on all the time. I started with an outline I had. The thing was to get it down, to sit down with pencil and paper and write it. Then when I looked at it, I'd ask myself—now, is that really stupid or what? I'd use a little Euclidean logic. I'd write things and throw them away. I'd write out a paragraph or two about something I would think of, jot down ideas and then give them names.

My ideas came from a lifetime of reading, teaching, teachers, students, other faculty. There was no one particular thing that I recall that said "this was it!" I had been living with those ideas for awhile, moving into a new world view. Now, of course, I'm far beyond it. The outlines were there, the framework was laid, and it's a good one, I think. Ideas are changing so fast, there is always more new knowledge that keeps coming, but I see it as elaborations on that basic framework (June 29, 1988).

When reminiscing about the publication of *An Introduction to the Theoretical Basis of Nursing,* Rogers said it was a relief to have it done and recalled her work with the publisher:

F. A. Davis, the publisher, was like family. They hired an artist to do the picture that is on the inside cover. He read the manuscript first and then came to New York City, where we spent time together exploring ideas and getting to know one another.

The small oval picture of the nurse in the left hand corner of the book originally wasn't there! The artist had thrown in an operating table with a group of physicians around it! I suppose the public at that time viewed surgery as esoteric and exciting and that kind of thing just dug in false stereotypes. I was truly angry.

So F. A. Davis found that small oval picture of the nurse and superimposed it over the artists' work. In the original drawing for the book, the edges of the picture of the nurse are curling up now, since it was just pasted on. It's funny in retrospect; the F. A. Davis people always laughed over that whole thing (June 29, 1988).

When Rogers was asked to recall the reactions of people to the book, she said:

Well, there were those who said, "She's crazier than a bedbug!" It was all so new and different. I was trying to get across an idea of life, change, and undirectionality. There were a lot of people who did much misinterpreting and a lot who said she doesn't know what she's talking about. I was told the doctoral students even said, "Oh, she's crazy, but she's nice enough so we don't mind!"

One summer I went to the University of Washington and gave a 3-week seminar. We met all morning, every day. There were 40–50 students. They were very nice, came every day to the seminar and listened but they were convinced I'd lost my buttons! That was all right. I gave speeches all around, not just in New York City where there was some awareness of my basic ideas (June 29, 1988).

When Rogers was asked if she felt criticized, she said she didn't expect anything and did what she thought was important. Her reactions illustrate her independent spirit, commitment to nursing science, and forward thinking:

The criticism wouldn't have made any difference, it didn't really matter to me what people thought of it. I didn't write it to make people happy. Actually, it's been a success far beyond my fondest expectations.

Of course, 10 years later some of the language I originally used became more common. Similar words are now being used in newspapers and magazines, but not when the book was published (June 29, 1988).

When asked to comment on the impact of her 1970 publication, Rogers recalled:

We really began to move in the 70's. There was a lot of thought going into research. The doctoral students were beginning to use the Rogerian framework. The undergrads were really going great guns with it. They were using it by the time the book came out, because they had been "raised" on it. Gean Mathwig was really developing nursing practice on this basis. The undergraduates did not have trouble with it. Then there was not anything that they had to un-learn (June 29, 1988).

Gean Mathwig recalled the impact of Rogers' framework on nursing practice and education:

I tried it in practice and I knew it worked. We had to support students in the beginning. No one had ever conceived of anything other than the medical model (Mathwig, June 27, 29).

Rogers recalled this radical change from nursing using the medical model to using the Rogerian framework was not totally well received by the wider New York University community of scholars, especially the physicians:

The medical school was always anxious to be rid of me, which I took as a compliment. I was tenured then and backed by administration. I would leave when I was ready to leave, not before. Some times I wonder how I got away with it.

When asked to summarize the outstanding memories of those years, Rogers responded:

If there was anything that distinguished the division [nursing], it was the intellectual excitement, the intellectual stimulation, the sharing of ideas by everyone. These were halcyon days in nursing. We had lots of advantages. We had money from Title II and NIMH money. There was more access [to graduate education] for nurses. We made the plans the best we knew how to, the very best they could be, as wild and crazy as we wanted; then we worried about implementing them.

In some ways, we were a way station. People came and moved on. And the first goal was never money. It was learning. We had a commitment that took precedence. It was something different (June 29, 1988).

PART IV

Beyond NYU and the Future (1976–Present)

It is difficult to say that Dr. Rogers has "left" NYU because in truth she has not. Her office is still there; her portrait smiles out on the Division; she is a palpable presence, always. One never knows when one will see her, usually attired in some shade of lavender or purple, walking sprightly through Washington Square Park.

The pace of Rogers' life has not slackened. If anything, her intellectual prowess is more pronounced. Her vision continues to expand. "Beyond the

Horizon'' was the title of her contribution to *The Nursing Profession: A Time to Speak* (Chaska, 1983). In that chapter, she stated, ''the impossible is possible'' (p. 796).

Rogers stepped down as Head of the Division of Nursing in 1975. It was then that her portrait was commissioned. She recalls how the artist examined hundreds of photographs of her. ''It was painted from knowing me as a person.'' Her retirement dinner was a special and gala event held at the Smithsonian Institute in Washington, DC, attended by faculty and alumni. Her retirement gift was uniquely hers, a specially constructed globe.

When asked to elaborate on the years since she stepped down as division head, Rogers noted:

It was a wise decision. It had to do with family matters. I could devote my time to teaching, travelling, presenting my ideas. I didn't legally retire until 1979 and I kept teaching part time until then. Even now I come back and do an occasional lecture now and then. I still have my office here at NYU.

This past year my brother was ill so I spent a lot of time in Arizona with him. But I do continue travelling, speaking, going overseas, lecturing, and presenting workshops. Have ticket, will travel! Sometimes it feels like there is no let up. Articles, all kinds of things. Actually, I often disagree with nurses but we stay good friends anyway! (June 29, 1988).

Safier (1977, pp. 327–328) in her interviews with Rogers, pursued the issues of others' opinions of Rogers' views. Rogers' frank responses confirmed her clear-sightedness and gave evidence of her humor and scope. The following is from Safier's interview with Rogers in 1977:

Rogers: Well, you know, I think that people either think I'm great or they think I should have died a long time ago. Ten or fifteen years ago, when I would give a speech, the first thing I would do would be check how far the windows were from the ground because, really you know, some people got pretty upset. After a while, I suspect, when people asked me to speak it was partly because at least I wouldn't put people to sleep. They had a better idea of what to expect so they didn't have to get angry, because after I spoke I went away. Today it is different. Many more nurses are comfortable with my ideas.

Safier: What do you mean, they were angry with you? What were the ideas you have that upset them?

Rogers: It has varied from time to time. Certainly differentiation of careers and my attacks on antieducationism in nursing have been particularly sore points. Attacks on current euphemisms and the idea of a nurse is a nurse is a nurse, and so on, have been part of it. These, I think, are the things that have been most upsetting to large numbers. When it comes to nursing science, arguments are becoming less frequent. Certainly people are more and more interested in what we are doing in nursing science as far as synergistic man is concerned, and, as far as I know, there haven't been any big fights over it. I think more because it really isn't that well known or that well understood . . .

Continued strides have been made since then in the evolution of nursing science. Gean Mathwig spoke of her great respect for Martha and noted the changes in the nursing profession's view of Rogers that have occurred over time:

She had the courage of her convictions. She hung in there; she stuck with it. The profession owes Martha a vote of thanks. The professional organizations recognize that now (Mathwig, June 27, 1988).

There have been eight honorary doctorates awarded Rogers since 1978 and other honors and awards too numerous to list. This issue of *Nursing Science Quarterly* celebrates Rogers' 75th birthday and the advent of nursing science as well as the documentation of its development.

Although Rogers envisions the future of nursing within the context of rapid change, increasing diversity and new horizons, she reaffirmed that the purpose of nursing has not changed, that of assisting people to achieve maximum well-being. While dreaming of dramatic changes in what is practiced and how nurses work with human beings and their worlds to achieve their goals, Rogers also sees certain themes as recurring in nursing and her own life:

> Public health—that's a theme through my life. That's really what nursing is all about. Hospitals are incidental. Our concern is with people. Hospitals are only one of the places one practices nursing. Our concern is with human beings.

Rogers reiterated her deep and abiding commitment to education, knowledge, and literature. For many years she arose at 5 a.m. to read. Her goal: a book a day. "I was always interested in education," she said. "When I was a little girl I thought I would teach English literature" (Rogers, June 28, 1988).

Another recurrent theme that is reflected is Rogers' ability to "disagree" while remaining friends, her openness, and her belief in women and their abilities:

> Although I'm in favor of the feminist movement, I think there ought to be PEOPLE LIBERATION—everybody, everyone suffers . . . there is *people abuse,* although there is certainly discrimination in this society.
>
> Women aren't stupid. They need to learn to use the resources of the University. At NYU, when I added the statistics requirements, the students had fits. It was rougher on them than I was aware of at the time. Pre-nursing at that time really only required fourth grade arithmetic. You really need a better base in mathematics for statistics. Girls weren't supposed to have enough sense to take math and physics. The requirements for all students were 4 credits in physics, sociology, psychology, and biology. All graduate students needed these. It really went back to gender.

In concluding, envisioning the future and travel in space, Rogers closed with the words, "I'll meet you there!"

Conclusions

Memories are selective. To remember something is not just to repeat it, but as one investigator stated, "to reconstruct, even sometimes to create, to express oneself" (Langness & Frank, 1985, p. 9). It is impossible to recall everything that occurs in the course of a life and, furthermore, pointless. A life is more than the sum of events, of happenings, that occur over the course of time. Undoubtedly, there is a unity of some kind that binds together an individual's life. One is recognized not just by name or the shape of one's physical features, but also by one's character. Over time, individuals reveal somewhat predictable patterns and themes in their lives. This is how one recognizes and appreciates others and oneself.

A variety of themes emerge in the story Rogers tells about herself and in the theoretical and innovative work she has produced over time. These are some of the ways one can come to know her. A new glimpse of Rogers' persona can be realized from these documented life events. Some emerging personal attributes of the theorist described in this work that become apparent are: independence; vision; single mindedness; outspokenness; commitment; hard work; family orientation; and accessibility. Some emergent themes identified in Rogers' personal attributes that can also be found in her nursing science perspective are: autonomy; nursing as a learned profession; concern with health; a view of man as more than and different from the sum of the parts; optimism; and future orientation.

How is it that these themes and unique personal attributes interact with environment and significant others in that environment to enhance the abstraction that is conceived of as culture? Life histories focus on how the culture shapes and molds the individual. In this case, of greater importance is how an individual, specifically Martha E. Rogers, has co-created, received, recreated, and transmitted the culture of 20th century nursing.

In *Saint Genet: Actor and Martyr* Sartre (1963) attempts to reveal what he calls the "fundamental project" of the poet, novelist, and playwright Jean Genet. By "fundamental project" Sartre refers to a nexus of meaning and values, an organizing principle that informs a person's choices. Whether totally by design or, in a word she frequently used, as serendipitous occurrences, Martha E. Rogers' fundamental project could be viewed as change in the discipline of nursing.

It is fitting to conclude with Rogers' statement in "Beyond the Horizon," a chapter she wrote for Norma Chaska's text, *The Nursing Profession: A Time to Speak* (1983):

> The speed of change quickens. The horizon nears. Nursing in the 21st century has a new image. Problems of the 20th century are no longer relevant. New concerns and new visions engage the nurses of tomorrow. Independence of thought and action, creative ideas, human compassion, and enthusiasm for the unknown abound. Diversity is a valued norm. Human health and welfare have new dimensions. Florence Nightingale said it rightly: "No system can endure that does not march." (p. 800).

References

Chaska, N. L. (Ed.). (1983). *The nursing profession: A time to speak.* New York: McGraw-Hill.
Fitzpatrick, J. J., & Whall, A. L. (1983). *Conceptual models of nursing: Analysis and application.* Bowie, MD: Brady.
Langness, L. L. (1965). *Life history in anthropological science.* New York: Holt, Rinehart, Winston.
Langness, L. L., & Frank, G. (1985). *Lives: An anthropological approach to biography.* Novato, CA: Chandler & Sharp.
Malinski, V. M. (Ed.). (1986). *Explorations on Martha Rogers' science of unitary human beings.* Norwalk, CT: Appleton-Century-Crofts.
Marriner, A. (1986). *Nursing theorists and their work.* St. Louis: Mosby.
Meleis, A. (1985). *Theoretical nursing: Development and progress.* Philadelphia: Lippincott.
Nicoll, L. H. (Ed). (1986). *Perspectives in nursing theory.* Boston: Little Brown.
Parse, R. R. (1987). *Nursing science: Major paradigms, themes and critiques.* Philadelphia: Saunders.
Rogers, M. E. (1961). *Educational revolution in nursing.* New York: Macmillan.
Rogers, M. E. (1964). *Reveille in nursing.* Philadelphia: Davis.
Rogers, M. E. (1970). *An introduction to the theoretical basis of nursing science.* Philadelphia: Davis.
Rogers, M. E. (1988). Curriculum vitae.
Safier, G. (1977). *Contemporary American leaders: An oral history.* New York: McGraw-Hill.
Sarter, B. (1988). *The stream of becoming: A study of Martha Rogers' theory.* New York: National League for Nursing.
Sartre, J. P. (1963). *Saint Genet: Actor and martyr.* New York: Basic Books. (Original work published 1952)

CHAPTER 3

Rogers' Early Views: An Ever-Expanding Vision of Nursing

Violet M. Malinski

Prior to the publication in 1970 of *An Introduction to the Theoretical Basis of Nursing,* Rogers had already published two other deceptively slim books. Slender in size but bursting with ideas, these books set the stage for what was to come.

Educational Revolution in Nursing

In the first, *Educational Revolution in Nursing,* published in 1961 by Macmillan, Rogers issued a clarion call for professional education in nursing. She urged that all nurses, regardless of educational preparation, be recognized for their contributions to the welfare of humankind. Simultaneously, however, she called for honestly acknowledging the differences in preparation. Rogers identified the lack of such differentiation as one of the most significant problems facing contemporary nursing. "Experience cannot be equated with knowledge nor can one's practice reflect more than the knowledge one brings to a situation" (Rogers, 1961, p. 5).

Thus "intuitive nursing" was the knowledge realm of the volunteer. The professional nurse, however:

> will possess the knowledge and skills necessary to work in many settings: home, school, industry, hospital, convalescent home, and others. She will be knowledgeably oriented to promoting health, preventing disease, making nursing diagnoses, and determining and implementing measures for the cure and rehabilitation of the ill and disabled. She will work effectively in a peer relationship with other disciplines and will seek the guidance and judgement of qualified persons in her own field. She will be self-directing and will assume appropriate responsibility for guiding the work of technical and vocational practitioners (Rogers, 1961, p. 11).

Such a nurse could only be produced by locating educational programs in university settings that provided a broad base in the liberal arts; the biological, physical, and social sciences; and *theoretical content in nursing.*

In a beginning delineation of this theoretical content, Rogers moved through a philosophical discussion of "Man and the Universe," offering three postulates that contained the seeds of continuous movement, participation in change, and multiple potentials, early ideas that resonated forward and were fleshed out in later writings.

Rogers identified nursing's purpose as helping people attain maximum health and well-being within the theoretical context of the life process. Therefore, she urged nurse-educators to "focus on human beings and the life process" as the basis "for helping man achieve maximum well-being within each individual's potential" (Rogers, 1961, p. 34). Rogers outlined the 5-year baccalaureate program she saw as essential for providing the base for professional nursing, separate and distinct from 2-year programs whose purpose was to prepare technical nurses rather than serve as the lower division of professional education.

The final chapter, "The Road Ahead," presents ideas that are still relevant today. Nurses must be competent in their own field before they can be effective members of an interdisciplinary team. Self-confidence promotes a sense of worth and respect for others, replacing defensiveness and derogation of differences. Recruitors must differentiate among the levels of nursing. Staffing patterns and pay scales need to reflect such differentiation. Finally, "*nurses* [italics added] determine the roles and responsibilities of nurses" (Rogers, 1961, p. 55) in a world where humankind "is no longer bound to planet Earth" (Rogers, 1961, p. 51).

Reveille in Nursing

In her second book, *Reveille in Nursing,* published by F. A. Davis Company in 1964, Rogers expanded on the ideas introduced earlier. She reiterated the call for differentiation according to educational preparation, noting that "professional and technical nurses are no more interchangeable than are medical doctors with medical technicians or engineers with engineering technicians" (Rogers, 1964b, p. 78). Furthermore, Rogers predicted, as more and more tasks become automated, the necessary ratio of technical to professional nurses will decline. As nursing science develops, it will illuminate the life process. Theoretical knowledge must be synthesized from basic research in nursing. The question will shift from "What does the baccalaureate degree graduate *do* that is different?" to "What does the professionally educated nurse *know* that makes her practice different?" (Rogers, 1964b, p. 80).

In this volume Rogers also emphasized the need for nurse-educators to become scholars in nursing, discussing their responsibilities as faculty in institutions of higher learning. She specified the focus of doctoral preparation in nursing: nursing science. She explained the rationale for her support of the Ph.D. as the appropriate credential rather than the professional doctorate (D.N.S. or D.N.Sc.) and for study in nursing science rather than in another discipline. Her concern for people shines through in her call for "knowledgeable compassion'' to replace ''emotional naivete'' and for ''imaginative concern'' that is underwritten by ''substantial scientific knowledge'' (Rogers, 1964b, p. 77).

Nursing Science

In the early 1960s Rogers was also busy with another publication. From 1963 to 1965 she edited a unique journal that was far ahead of its time: *Nursing Science.* The first issue appeared in April 1963; the last in December 1965. Ruth V. Matheney, R.N., Ed.D., served as assistant editor. The editorial board originally consisted of Lulu Wolf Hassenplug, R.N., M.P.H., Elizabeth L. Kemble, R.N., Ed.D., Sister Charles Marie (Frank), R.N., M.S.N.E., C.C.V.I., and Marion Murphy, R.N., Ph.D., and was later joined by Martha Pitel, R.N., Ph.D. This pioneering journal, published bimonthly by F. A. Davis Company, included content on theory development, the emerging science of nursing, nursing research, the process and content of professional education at both undergraduate and graduate levels, and professional practice. Regular features included editorials by Rogers (and the responses they generated in ''Backtalk,'' letters from readers); ''Courage of Their Convictions,'' spotlighting current nursing leaders; ''Demand Reading''; and ''In Capsule,'' highlighting interdisciplinary advances in knowledge.

In her editorials Rogers wrote trenchant commentaries on such topics as:

1. Nursing research of the day: ''Trivial and mediocre studies multiply. Pedestrian investigators whose primary assets are enthusiasm and a 'research attitude' produce absurdities'' (Rogers, 1965b, p. 289). ''Nursing is in grave need of both basic and applied research. But only a miniscule [sic] amount of basic research in nursing has appeared. Consequently, applied research in nursing generally lacks the substance of fundamental concepts'' (Rogers, 1965b, p. 290).
2. Baccalaureate degree education for nurses: ''A value system derogating higher education permeates much of traditional nursing. . . . It takes little investigation to realize that in nursing a baccalaureate degree is not necessarily synonymous with a baccalaureate education'' (Rogers, 1965a, p. 202–203). ''Of growing seriousness is nursing's failure to guarantee society a nurse's safety to practice at a professional level. National State Board Examinations are geared to the hospital school level of preparation'' (Rogers, 1965a, p. 203).
3. Continuous change and the implications for nurses: ''Nursing's unemployables of the next decade are being trained today because nurses have had neither the courage nor the vision to face reality and to take the drastic steps essential to create the indispensable changes that must be made. Vested interests distort the truth and perpetuate misconceptions'' (Rogers, 1964c, p. 463).
4. Accountability: ''Standards of excellence are a means by which nursing fulfills its commitment to the humanity it purports to serve. . . . Professionally, technically, and vocationally educated nurses have a right and a responsibility to seek excellence within the scope of each one's preparation and ability. Society has a right to expect that the most knowledgeable and able in nursing be liable for determining sound standards

for all who nurse" (Rogers, 1964a, p. 72). "Nurses dawdle while society suffers. . . . Concerted action is long overdue" (Rogers, 1964a, p. 73).

A feisty woman, Rogers carried such themes forward throughout her professional career, forever challenging her colleagues to expand their visions of nursing and nurses. She has often said of these early years that when she spoke, she made sure she was on the ground floor with a window nearby in case she had to jump.

The reader of the early 1960s received even more to ponder in the pages of *Nursing Science* through articles such as Dolores Krieger's (1963) "About the Life Process" and Ruth B. Freeman's (1963) "The Nurse as a Writer." Myra Levine (1964) wrote of the need for professional education and development of a body of knowledge in nursing to replace the legacy of the apprenticeship system, where nurses wrote procedures first, then sought the scientific principles to justify them. Imogene King (1964) discussed problems in the development of nursing theory, particularly the area of concept development. Other authors focused on topics such as the role of ecology in nursing science and the mutuality of well-being for human and environment.

Research included Runnerstrom's (1963) "Food Iron Intake and Hemoglobin Levels in Pregnancy," Downs' (1964) "Maternal Stress in Primigravidas as a Factor in the Production of Neonatal Pathology," and Rothberg's (1965) "Dependence, Anxiety, and Surgical Recovery." Practice-related features explored "The Effects of Decreased Barometric Pressure in the Flying Environment" (Foley, 1963), "Oxygen Therapy and Hypoxia" (Streich, 1964), "Maturational Crisis and the Unwed Adolescent Mother" (Clark, 1964), "An Approach to the Nursing Diagnosis of Behavior in a Pediatric Specialty Clinic" (Ohman & Walano, 1964), "A Child's Humor" (Pearson, 1965), and care of the dying (Adamek, 1965; Quint, 1964).

"Demand Reading" urged nurses to broaden their horizons and become familiar with wide-ranging works, such as Carl G. Hempel's *Fundamentals of Concept Formation in Empirical Science,* Mario Bunge's *Intuition and Science,* Oscar Lewis' *Five Families,* Corinne Brown's *Understanding Other Cultures,* Rene Dubos' *The Torch of Life,* G. N. M. Tyrell's *Apparitions,* Lewin's *Field Theory in Social Science,* Selye's *The Stress of Life,* Einstein's *Relativity: The Special and General Theory,* and de Beauvoir's *The Second Sex.*

Educators explored international perspectives on nursing education and service (Fahey, 1965; McKay, 1964), the structure and content of graduate education (Levine, 1965), the purpose of the graduate clinical experience (Putnam, 1964), and specialization (Peplau, 1965). Highlighting the need for clear differentiation among the different programs in nursing, the editorial board prepared and published a recruitment pamphlet in the June-July 1963 issue of *Nursing Science* that could be ordered as a reprint through F. A. Davis Company (see Appendix B). Three different educational paths, preparing three different types of nurses, were identified and described: professional registered nurse programs offered in colleges and universities; technical registered nurse programs, including associate degree and hospital or noncollegiate programs; and practical nurse programs. While respecting the value of each type, the editorial board tried carefully to distinguish the differences among them to permit potential students to make a knowledgeable choice in terms of their own career goals and aspirations.

Planting the Seeds

Over the past years Rogers has been remarkably consistent in her ideas while continually searching for the language to best reflect them. Her emphasis on nursing as both noun and verb, scientific knowledge plus action, is encapsulated in the early use of terms such as "knowledgeable compassion," "knowledgeable intervention," and nursing as a "learned profession." She has consistently maintained that nurses' major concern is people, wherever they are; that nursing theory must illuminate the life process; and that nurses must creatively and imaginatively design ways to facilitate well-being.

Thus she clearly signaled her beliefs that nursing encompasses far more than caring for people who are ill and that the hospital is only one among many potential settings for practice. Rather than "health" Rogers tended to use "well-being," with no reference to signs and symptoms of illness. She identified the nurse's role as one of helping to maximize well-being throughout the life process, noting that the life process is one of becoming and, as such, is an open process.

Early language included words like "equilibrium" and "adaptation," but Rogers soon found them inappropriate, reflecting a closed, mechanistic framework rather than an open one. Similarly, "diagnosis," "intervention," and "prediction" soon disappeared from her writings. Phrases like "infinite future" and "multiple potentials" clearly identified her emerging science as predicated on openness. Energy, evolutionary unfolding and movement, expansion, human interaction with the universe, and man's capacity for change appeared in Rogers' early works and evolved with the continuing refinement of the nursing science.

Rogers identified the environment of the person as the universe. Therefore, it is not surprising that the words "interplanetary" and "intergalactic" appear in her early writings, forecasting her ongoing fascination with nursing in space. In later years she has written and lectured extensively on the space age and the role of nurses in space exploration, as will be seen in later chapters.

Rogers' early work provided the impetus for her controversial positions and seminal achievements in every facet of nursing. She has never confined her efforts to one arena but has embraced them all, with notable contributions to nursing education, research, science, and practice, as well as nursing's professional and political agenda. Through her awareness of infinite potentials, she has shared an ever-expanding vision of nursing that knows no boundaries.

References

Adamek, M. E. (1965). Some observations on death and a family. *Nursing Science, 3,* 258–267.

Clark, A. L. (1964). Maturational crisis and the unwed adolescent mother. *Nursing Science, 2,* 112–124.

Downs, F. S. (1964). Maternal stress in primigravidas as a factor in the production of neonatal pathology. *Nursing Science, 2,* 348–367.

Fahey, E. (1965). Elements of comparative nursing education. *Nursing Science, 3,* 145–161.

Foley, M. F. (1963). The effects of decreased barometric pressure in the flying environment. *Nursing Science, 1,* 170–186.

Freeman, R. B. (1963). The nurse as a writer. *Nursing Science, 1,* 156–162.

King, I. (1964). Nursing theory: Problems and prospect. *Nursing Science, 2,* 394–403.

Krieger, D. (1963). About the life process. *Nursing Science, 1,* 105–115.

Let's recruit! *Nursing Science, 1,* 77–84.
Levine, M. E. (1964). "Not to startle, though the way were steep. . . ." *Nursing Science, 2,* 58–67.
Levine, M. E. (1965). The professional nurse and graduate education. *Nursing Science, 3,* 206–214.
McKay, R. (1964). A comparative approach to the development of nursing education. *Nursing Science, 2,* 125–137.
Ohman, E. N., & Walano, D. (1964). An approach to the nursing diagnosis of behavior in a pediatric specialty clinic. *Nursing Science, 2,* 152–158.
Pearson, G. A. (1965). A child's humor. *Nursing Science, 3,* 94–108.
Peplau, H. (1965). Specialization in professional nursing. *Nursing Science, 3,* 268–287.
Putnam, P. A. (1964). A reappraisal of the graduate field laboratory. *Nursing Science, 2,* 464–470.
Quint, J. C. (1964). Nursing services and the care of dying patients: Some speculations. *Nursing Science, 2,* 432–443.
Rogers, M. E. (1961). *Educational revolution in nursing.* New York: Macmillan.
Rogers, M. E. (1964a). Editorial: Professional standards: Whose responsibility? *Nursing Science, 2,* 71–73.
Rogers, M. E. (1964b). *Reveille in nursing.* Philadelphia: Davis.
Rogers, M. E. (1964c). Editorial. *Nursing Science, 2,* 462–463.
Rogers, M. E. (1965a). Editorial. *Nursing Science, 3,* 202–205.
Rogers, M. E. (1965b). Editorial. *Nursing Science, 3,* 288–294.
Rothberg, J. (1965). Dependence, anxiety, and surgical recovery. *Nursing Science, 3,* 243–256.
Runnerstrom, L. (1963). Food iron intake and hemoglobin levels in pregnancy. *Nursing Science, 1,* 187–197.
Streich, U. (1964). Oxygen therapy and hypoxia. *Nursing Science, 2,* 48–57.

SECTION TWO

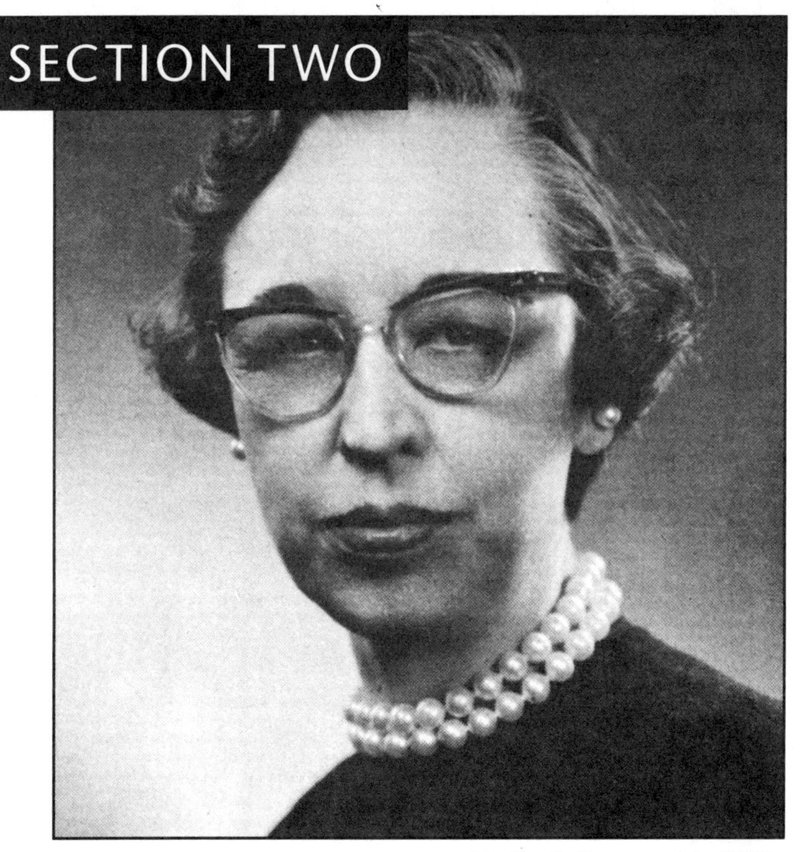

Martha E. Rogers, early 1950s.

Education and Research

Section Editors

Elizabeth Ann Manhart Barrett

Violet M. Malinski

CHAPTER 4

Revolution and Reveille in Nursing Education and Research

Elizabeth Ann Manhart Barrett and
Violet M. Malinski

Martha E. Rogers, as the head of one of the largest and foremost educational programs for nursing, served as an innovative thinker and articulate spokesperson for professional education for nurses. "Rogers called for an educational revolution in nursing and, indeed, for the past 30 years has been an educational revolutionary" (Barrett, 1990a, p. 303).

From the beginning her commitment to nursing, as a learned profession and an academic discipline, was characterized by a unique and abstract body of knowledge about nursing's phenomenon of concern—people and their world (Rogers, 1986). The knowledge of the discipline has continued to emerge over time. This knowledge, variously termed nursing science or the science of nursing, is from Rogers' purview what she has now called the Science of Unitary Human Beings.

From the beginning Rogers believed that "professionally educated nurses are independent practitioners prepared to knowledgeably provide health services to individuals, families, groups, and communities. They are accountable for their own acts and liable to the public they serve. They are peer participants in collaborative judgments made with professional personnel in other fields" (Rogers, 1985a, p. 382).

A major commitment in Rogers' career was toward actualizing these ideas through nursing science–based education. To this day she continues to teach students of all ages both formally and informally as well as nationally and internationally.

Martha Rogers arrived at New York University (NYU) in 1954, the day after she was awarded the doctor of science degree from Johns Hopkins University. She had accepted the position of chairperson of the Department of Nurse Education in the School of Education. At that time she was the only nurse on the faculty with an earned doctorate (M. E. Rogers, personal communication, July 10, 1992).

Rogers immediately began laying groundwork for what was to become a revolution in nursing education. She began by working toward her goal of achieving excellence in educational programs preparing nurses. She believed that if nursing education was to take place in institutions of higher learning, then the requirements for nurses must be comparable with and as rigorous as those in other disciplines. This was not the prevailing situation at that time.

Prior to Rogers' arrival, New York State had approved the School of Education to award both Ed.D. and Ph.D. degrees. The dozen or so doctoral students who were enrolled had elected the Ed.D. route, primarily because there was no foreign language requirement (M. E. Rogers, personal communication, July 10, 1992). Early on, the dean of education selected Rogers for a committee charged with differentiating the Ed.D. and the Ph.D. degrees. Subsequently, Rogers convened an all-day nursing faculty meeting for the purpose of deciding which doctoral degree would be offered for nurses. The group concluded that since the NYU faculty was moving toward knowledgeable nursing, the Ph.D., which offered a major in nursing and required a dissertation, would be more appropriate than the Ed.D., which provided a major in education and required a research project. Additionally, students in nursing were currently taking most of the course work required for the Ph.D. Rogers emphasized that it was not a case of better or worse, but rather at NYU the most appropriate degree for their mission was the Ph.D. (M. E. Rogers, personal communication, July 10, 1992).

Laying groundwork for changing the master's and especially the baccalaureate programs was much more difficult. This required an educational revolution that has echoed through most of nursing. Rogers became a key revolutionary both in developing the platform of needed changes and as a leader in communicating her position on these changes while implementing them in the nursing programs at NYU.

As a supporting rationale Rogers cited the work of Brown in 1948 in the landmark report *Nursing for the Future,* where she delineated professional, technical, and vocational paths in nursing. About the same time the Ginsberg report recommended "that institutions of higher learning recognize their responsibility for establishing programs providing for the professional and technical education of nurses. Furthermore, Montag in 1951 initiated junior college preparation of technical registered nurses (Rogers, 1963b, p. 400–401).

Rogers instituted curriculum changes at NYU that initiated science-based nursing beginning with the baccalaureate degree as the foundation of professional practice. During these early years Rogers became increasingly active in professional nursing organizations. As one of many examples of networking, in 1957 and 1958 she collaborated with Esther Lucile Brown of Boston University School of Nursing and R. Louise McManus, Division of Nursing Education, Teacher's College, Columbia University, as well as other members of the National Deans Committee. Led by Brown, their purpose was to develop a position paper on (1) the role of university schools of nursing in the improvement of patient care and health teaching; (2) faculty growth and development; (3) interdisciplinary courses on both the undergraduate and graduate levels; and (4) interpretation of nursing and nursing education (Brown, 1958). Reading letters in Rogers' correspondence file that were exchanged by these leaders was like visiting nursing's professional education roots and personally experiencing a part of that history. A profound sense of mutual respect and collegiality was apparent among these women.

As early as 1959 Rogers was using the term "nursing science" and discussing appropriate content for baccalaureate degree programs as preparation for professional practice, master's degree programs as preparation for specialist practice, and doctoral degree programs as preparation for research, college teaching, or administrative positions in education or service (Rogers, 1959). Rogers was moving full steam ahead into perhaps the most important decade in the annuls of nursing education.

Educational Revolution

The 1960s were the time in Rogers' career when massive changes would occur in nursing, and she was often an important catalyst in evoking them. When she published *Educational Revolution in Nursing* (Rogers, 1961), the ideas were different; the seeds of nursing science were beginning to germinate. Montag later recalled, "For so long nursing had been thought of as simply a branch of medicine, and not a very significant one at that, that to have someone claim there is a body of nursing knowledge and then proceed to present it to nurses in writing is a real breakthrough. She has placed emphasis on science, the science of nursing" (Montag, 1979, p. 3). The revolution had begun.

Three papers from 1962 and 1963 (Rogers, 1962a, 1962b, 1963c) presented in this volume likewise reveal Rogers' seminal thinking regarding knowledgeable nursing. Her message was loud and clear. Apprenticeship training could not be equated with education obtained in college and experience was not a substitute for education. She emphatically proposed that the notion of nursing as a vocation be replaced with the conviction that nursing is a learned profession.

Another seminal idea emerged. "The traditional identification of nursing as 'doing' is being replaced by an understanding of nursing as a body of knowledge, unique in its aggregate of knowledge, and when applied representing the practice of nursing" (Rogers, 1962b, p. 3). She quoted Gardner to warn that "an educational system grudgingly and tardily patched to meet the needs of the moment will be perpetually out of date" (cited in Rogers 1962b, p. 5). She knew then what she still maintains today: nursing's uniqueness flows from its knowledge base, not from activities of practicing nurses (Rogers, 1962b, 1990). Furthermore, she proposed that "undergraduate students will not be pushing back the frontiers of knowledge. Rather, they will be gaining a toe-hold in the doorway that can lead to new frontiers" (Rogers, 1962b, p. 6). To best pursue these new frontiers, they would need to go on to master's and doctoral education in nursing science.

During the early 1960s the three careers in nursing (professional, technical, and vocational) were more clearly articulated. Furthermore, Rogers noted that the professional did not build on the technical (Rogers, 1962a, 1963c). The National League for Nursing developed a resolution endorsing the three careers in nursing ("Resolved," 1962). Rogers was president of the New York State League for Nursing during the period and her curriculum vitae at that time revealed numerous presentations of speeches, papers, and other professional activities. Rogers eloquently urged her nursing colleagues to stand up and be counted as they moved the preparation of registered nurses into the mainstream of higher education. She warned that "bold, forthright action on the part of courageous, responsible leaders in nursing is desperately needed to meet the challenges of a changing world" (Rogers, 1963a). Indeed, as role model, Rogers was a woman of courage and commitment.

In 1964 Rogers published *Reveille in Nursing,* which first presented comprehensive background knowledge of higher education. Second, she further described what would be required for the evolving world of nursing to become a peer discipline in the world of higher education. Readers were encouraged to explore the references that could "act as a lantern to the curious traveler" (Rogers, 1964b, p. vi). Opening up new vistas for students through exposure to references crossing numerous diverse disciplines was to become a hallmark of Rogers as educator. *Reveille* also presented further evolved roots of the Science of Unitary Human Beings.

As early as 1963 Rogers (1963b) proposed that the legal definition of nursing had been outgrown. She simultaneously worked diligently to establish a "valid" baccalaureate curriculum at NYU. She objected vehemently to allocation of college credit for hospital training, as was the case for diploma graduates seeking baccalaureate degrees at that time.

> The allocation of advanced standing credits for nursing courses taken in a noncollegiate program . . . cannot be equated with nursing courses which demand substantial prerequisites for their comprehension. There can be no justification for the continuation of general nursing programs. They should have ceased a long time ago. And I say this knowing that I am chairman of a department in which such a program exists. We must not permit this to continue. A baccalaureate program should be set up on the same basis as other baccalaureate programs in higher education are set up. Advanced standing should be granted on the same basis that advanced standing is granted in other areas of the institution of higher education (Rogers, 1962a, p. 6).

In 1964 the above changes were instituted and a "valid" 5-year baccalaureate program based on the science of nursing was instituted (Rogers, 1970a). No longer was college credit given for hospital training (M. E. Rogers, personal communication, July 10, 1992). Rogers believed that "failure to differentiate careers in nursing denies all nurses opportunity to realize their full potentialities" (Rogers, 1964a, p. 73). And always, she advocated a respect for these differences. Also administrative changes took place. Rogers' title changed to Head of the Division of Nursing in the School of Education, Health, Nursing, and the Arts Professions.

Meanwhile, Rogers continued to develop the nursing science knowledge base at NYU. In 1963 (Rogers, 1963c) and 1964 (Rogers, 1964b) the emergent formulations and language still reflected the traditional causal old worldview. Initially, she spoke of an "adaptive" life process (Rogers, 1962b). Her definitions of nursing science and nursing practice continuously evolved. A major change occurs from the 1963 view of "man as a unified biophysical-psychosocial organism" (Rogers, 1963c, p. 3) to the 1964 view of "MAN as an indivisible phenomenon" (Rogers, 1964b, p. 37). Furthermore "the life process is a becoming" (Rogers, 1964b, p. 38).

Key 1964 definitions printed in *Reveille in Nursing* (Rogers, 1964b) are presented below. Italics have been added by the authors to indicate words that Rogers later deleted or changed.

Nursing Science: A body of scientific knowledge characterized by descriptive, explanatory and *predictive* principles about the life process in *MAN*. These principles rest on a view of *MAN* as an indivisible phenomenon in constant *interaction* with all *parts* of the environment. *This body of knowledge develops through synthesis and resynthesis of selected knowledges from the humanities, the natural and social sciences* and any other sources of knowledge for new concepts and new understandings (the *unifying* principles and hypothetical generalizations of nursing science) about *MAN* and his environment. Its system of *concepts* is acquired by reasoning.

Nursing Practice: The process by which the body of scientific knowledge (nursing science) is used for the purpose of assisting human beings to move *in the direction of maximum* well-being. This process is subsumed under two major categories, namely;

1. *Evaluative and diagnostic*—the process of *determining* the position of an individual, family, or group on the *continuum of minimum to maximum* well-being. This process utilizes knowledge and understanding of descriptive and exploratory principles, observation, and intellectual skill.
2. *Interventive*—the process of *determining* and initiating discriminative action based on *predictive principles.*

These are continuous and concurrent processes characterized by ongoing modification, alteration, revision and change (Rogers, 1964b, pp. 37–38).

Sometime during the second half of the 1960s Rogers made the quantum leap from viewing nursing science as based on an old worldview to conceptualizing nursing science as based on a new worldview. She does not recall any particular time but describes the changes as continuously evolving. "Nursing science had continuous input from doctoral students" (M. E. Rogers, personal communication, July 10, 1992). From 1965 until *An Introduction to the Theoretical Basis of Nursing* was published in 1970 (Rogers, 1970b), drafts of the book in typed form were used with students. For several years Rogers established a seminar with doctoral students who had nearly completed course work or were A.B.D. (had completed all but the dissertation). Every 2 weeks a group of 18 to 24 students met in Rogers' apartment in Greenwich Village to explore the evolving postulates and principles of the science. She noted that these groups had a kind of unity few groups ever achieve. She recalls these sessions as "loaded with ideas and dreams" or, as a former student recently remarked, "those days had a touch of magic." "Some of the students were also faculty, but it didn't matter. Everyone was an equal. Students were the ones that made it real" (M. E. Rogers, personal communication, July 10, 1992).

Further Evolution of Baccalaureate, Master's, and Doctoral Education at New York University

Rogers maintained that undergraduate, master's, and doctoral programs comprised a sequence of ever more complex learnings. Like professional education in other fields, the transmission of theory was the distinguishing characteristic. She emphasized that the science of nursing was not a summation of facts and principles drawn from other sources. Nursing was an emergent, new product; it was what she called a Science of Man (Rogers, 1971). This title was later changed to the Science of Unitary Human Beings.

Thus for Rogers, "Nursing's educational system had to include both undergraduate and graduate education in the science of nursing or neither will exist. . . . This body of knowledge consists of abstract principles arrived at by scientific research and logical analysis, not technical skills and the fruits of practical experience'' (Rogers, 1968, p. 11).

With the emergence of the science of nursing and the advent of ''valid'' baccalaureate education, graduate education built on the foundation of general and professional education. The baccalaureate curriculum incorporated the following three areas of learning:

> . . . 1) broad general knowledge in the arts and sciences (a characteristic of all college graduates), such as written English and literature, foreign language, mathematics, logic, history, economics, government, art, music, and an introduction to the psychological, sociological, biological, chemical, and physical worlds; 2) advanced general education in courses having relevance for nursing, such as, anatomy and physiology, genetics, embryology, microbiology, organic chemistry, anthropology, social psychology, comparative religion, philosophy, and biostatistics; and 3) the nursing major—in which students learn of nursing's rich heritage of the past and evolve a philosophy of nursing for the future, pursue learning in the science of nursing and develop beginning competence in its utilization, and are introduced to tools and methods of investigation that can enable them to exploit knowledge for the enhancement of practice and the betterment of man (Rogers, 1969b, p. 35).

Such a baccalaureate degree program, as previously mentioned, has been in place at NYU since 1964. The elaboration of the body of nursing knowledge was ongoing under Rogers' direction. Faculty committees, workshops, and seminars had long before embarked on the ''task of trying to identify and develop a body of scientific knowledge specific to nursing'' (Rogers, 1970a, p. 2). Eventually the ''bare bones of potentially productive issues began to accumulate flesh and blood'' (Rogers, 1970a, p. 2).

In 1967 a one-semester graduate course already in the curriculum was revised. It introduced the philosophy, principles, and theories of the emerging science of nursing and its implications for practice. While ''these curriculum revisions had their inception some 15 years earlier,'' Rogers noted that further changes must continue to take place (Rogers, 1970a, p. 3).

Although traditional majors in the master's program at NYU still continued to exist in 1970, Rogers reminded colleagues that ''any idea that the traditional majors are here to stay is a denial of reality'' (Rogers, 1970a, p. 6). She noted that these majors evolved from an earlier time oriented to segmentation of humans. Advanced study at the master's level properly consisted of an extension in scope, depth, and understanding of what was then viewed as the unique phenomenon of nursing; that is, the human development of the whole person (Rogers, 1970a). During the 1970s traditional majors were eliminated and master's education at NYU shifted to a generalist stance.

At the doctoral level scientists and scholars were prepared. In the 1960s doctoral research began to focus on human beings rather than nurses and their functions. The prescientific era in nursing was coming to an end. In 1968 Rogers pointed out that the Division of Nursing at NYU had the largest enrollment of doctoral candidates in nursing in the nation. She maintained that students sought to study at NYU in order to pursue the creative elaboration of nursing science as it was developing there (M. E. Rogers, unpublished material from files, 1968).

Meanwhile Rogers took a position against the federally funded nurse-scientist doctoral programs that were preparing nurses with doctorates in other disciplines such as physiology, psychology, sociology, and anthropology. At NYU the Division of Nurse Education "refused to be beguiled into treading the primrose path to a piece of parchment" (Rogers, 1971, p. 111). She further maintained that clinical doctorates bypassed the essential theoretical basis of nursing (Rogers, 1971).

Deploring what she termed a traditional and persistent anti-intellectualism and antieducationism in nursing, she proposed that these attitudes were responsible for many nurses' reluctance to contend with substantive knowledge in the discipline of nursing. She cried out loud and clear for "continuing efforts to design and implement graduate programs of structure and substance." She pleaded for "new ways of thinking and doing else our students will be penalized and the health of people will suffer" (Rogers, 1970a, p. 8).

She later opposed "Joint Appointments" and the "Unification Model" as examples of antieducationism manifesting through a return to apprenticeship and as denial of something substantive to know in nursing. She termed these types of phenomena as "the doing syndrome." Instead, she cautioned that "without mutual respect for difference in knowledge, skill, and expertise that identify and differentiate educators, practitioners, administrators, and researchers, there can be no growth or goodwill. The public has a right to expect that they will not be sacrificed on the altar of obsolescence" (Rogers, 1980, p. 7).

From the beginning, the educational revolution concerned imparting to nursing students knowledge about human beings and ways to promote their health and well-being. Because Rogers views health as a value judgment and maintains that health is defined by people for themselves, she has preferred the term "well-being" in recent years.

> A nation's first line of defense in building a healthy people lies in maintenance and promotion of health. Any society that concentrates its health dollars and its health services on care of the sick will never be a healthy society. . . . Community health services are needed to transcend "sick services." This is not to suggest that care of the sick is unimportant (Rogers, 1967, p. 5).

Yet, she emphasized that only a few are sick and nursing is concerned with all people. Hence, this belief greatly influenced the nursing educational programs at NYU and other schools of nursing.

Educational Update

Although Rogers' ideas on nursing education were primarily developed in the 1950s and 1960s, their relevance remains timely today. One such example (Rogers, 1985a) is reprinted in this section. "The Nature and Characteristics of Professional Education for Nursing" was published in 1985; however, it was written nearly two decades before and was published in its original form.

Rogers argued that professional education does not exceed the quality of the faculty. According to statistics reported by her, only 6.2 percent of full-time faculty teaching in baccalaureate and higher degree programs held doctoral degrees in 1970. She viewed faculty as a community of scholars with academic freedom and maintained that nurse-educators required earned doctorates if they were to transmit theoretical knowledge in nursing to students.

In 1985, Rogers also addressed the future of nursing education. She focused on entry levels and licensure, advocating what has come to be known as the SAIN (Society for Advancement in Nursing) proposal, reprinted in Chapter 31. Continuing to endorse complete professional autonomy of the baccalaureate graduate and continuing to denounce antieducationism and dependency, she viewed separate examination and licensure for the independent nurse (IN) with a baccalaureate degree in nursing as essential for full professional autonomy and stature. This has yet to be realized; only the future will reveal the success or failure of such a proposal. Perhaps if such autonomous practice can be demonstrated by a sufficient number of nurses, then legislative changes to update current practice of baccalaureate and higher degree nurses may be more readily forthcoming. Readers are referred to the SAIN proposal for licensure of the independent nurse that appears in this volume.

Rogers' egalitarian philosophy has consistently characterized her lifelong interactions with students. She set the tone for collegial interchange through mechanisms such as faculty and students communicating on a first-name basis. But more than that, Rogers conveyed to students a genuine sense of respect and a belief that they were capable of achieving far beyond their current levels. She continuously challenged students to reach beyond their grasp. In her encouragement of students she did not make it easy for them but she conveyed they could accomplish the task at hand.

Rogers has always extended herself to students. She was, and continues to be, available and accessible regardless of where students are studying. Appreciatively, a student wrote to Rogers in the 1960s, "May you continue to bring dignity to the hearts of nursing generations" (M. E. Rogers, unpublished materials from files, 1968). In the 1990s a student wrote, "If you get to the next dimension before I do, please reserve a seat for me along side of you on a moonbeam" (M. E. Rogers, unpublished materials from files, 1991).

Research

In her 1970 book Rogers provided examples of significant research questions derived from nursing science. For her, curiosity and compassion spearheaded the need to know that "mankind" may benefit.

> The "whys" of human behavior and human endeavor, immersed within a universe of mystery and magnificence, must be sought diligently and with imagination. Only as the "whys" become understood can there be "hows" knowledgeably designed to achieve nursing's goals (Rogers, 1970b, p. 111).

The way of perceiving person and environment offered by this nursing science suggested exploration of such ideas as (1) the topology of the human field; (2) motion—its nature and speed—and imposed motion and developmental patterns; (3) the relationship between environmental sound patterns and developmental processes, between sound patterns and individual rhythms; (4) field correlates of thought transmissions; and (5) perceptions of time passing (flying, dragging, standing still, timelessness). These and other ideas became the focus of early doctoral research beginning in the 1960s at NYU and continuing in various forms across the country in the 1990s.

Consistently Rogers' focus has been use of the research process to develop the knowledge, the science of nursing, from which the application or art of nursing will flow. She has said over and over that one cannot apply what one does not possess. It is up to nurses to develop the nursing knowledge that will inform nursing practice.

Rogers mentored doctoral students conducting basic research through dissertations required for the Ph.D. degree at NYU for 25 years. Since her official retirement in 1979, she has continued to informally mentor many master's, doctoral, and postdoctoral students, and faculty conducting research in various colleges and universities.

While she maintained that nursing needs both basic and applied research, the paramount need for basic research in the science of nursing was a continuous theme as this type of research is essential in the creation and testing of new knowledge. She insisted that doctoral preparation was required to abstractly conceptualize and conduct basic or applied research as principal investigators.

Basic research in the Science of Unitary Human Beings at NYU evolved in tandem with the evolution of the science itself. Ference (1986) described in detail this progression and traced the field manifestations of humans and their environments that were the focus of study. Initially, while assumptions of the Science of Unitary Human Beings were stated, the conceptual framework of the studies reflected many sciences other than nursing. In 1977 Rawnsley, a doctoral candidate at Boston University, was considered the first researcher to frame her research solely within the Science of Unitary Human Beings. Since then numerous studies, both quantitative and qualitative, continue such theory-testing and theory-generating research. These studies add to the ever-changing, open-ended Science of Unitary Human Beings.

Rogers clarified differences between knowledge and use of knowledge as they respectively concerned basic and applied research. She emphasized that the application of knowledge grew out of previous knowledge rooted in basic research. She warned against a fascination with methodology and urged researchers to focus on necessary theoretical substance. She further warned against testing theories from other disciplines, maintaining that such knowledge contributed only to the other field, not to nursing. Yet, she noted that "when knowledges from other fields are useful to nursing they can be used just as nursing knowledges may have equal significance for other fields" (Rogers, 1969a, p. 35). However, trying to sum up knowledges from other fields, she warned, would never constitute new knowledge of nursing, nor did the study of nurses and their activities constitute nursing research. Research in the science of nursing was viewed as the foundation for providing knowledgeable nursing services (Rogers, 1969a).

Rogers (1967) cited the abuse of informed consent through experimental research as a national dilemma in 1967. Advocacy and adherence to client's informed choices has been a consistent theme in Rogers' philosophy of education, practice, and research.

While acknowledging that the term "clinical research" was probably an effort to differentiate applied research concerned with human beings from study of nurses, she increasingly has urged complete discontinuation of the term "clinical" because it derives from the medical model and refers to direct observation of the "patient" in clinical settings. Rogers proposes that this research be termed applied research since "clinical means investigation of a disease in the living subject by observation as distinguished from controlled study . . . something done at the bedside" (Rogers, 1987, p. 122).

Rogers recently noted the growing body of research concerned with the Science of Unitary Human Beings (Barrett, 1990b; Malinski, 1986; Sarter, 1988). Multiple quantitative and qualitative methodologies are endorsed by her as appropriate (Rogers, 1992). Some tools specific to this science have been developed, and she reminds researchers that others also are needed as well as new methods. Rogers' new way of thinking based on a new world view presents a future for nursing research that is as essential as it is infinite (Rogers, 1987, 1992).

Summary and Conclusions

In summary, Rogers articulated the need for baccalaureate education as the base on which to build graduate and doctoral programs in nursing. Located "squarely within the framework of higher education," education of professionals in nursing "demands a fusion of liberal arts; biological, physical, and social sciences; and theoretical content in nursing" (Rogers, 1961, p. vii). Proclaiming nursing to be a learned profession and an academic discipline, Rogers not only actualized her ideas through establishing nursing science–based programs at NYU but also created the Science of Unitary Human Beings. While recognizing the contributions of technical and professional nurses, Rogers advocated that the differences between the two groups be acknowledged in licensure and practice. She insisted that the traditional definition of "nursing" as a verb concerned with doing be replaced with the definition of "nursing" as a noun identified by a body of nursing knowledge that served as the basis for nursing practice.

Equally important was Rogers' contention that doctoral education was the appropriate and necessary base from which to conduct basic and applied nursing research. She guided many nurses in the conduct of research concerning unitary human beings and their unitary environments. She noted the growing body of knowledge emerging from this research. Although she endorsed quantitative and qualitative methods as well as the development of new methods, she proclaimed the necessity of focusing on theoretical substance.

The accomplishments of Martha E. Rogers as they relate to nursing education and nursing research are truly astounding! Future generations will do well to heed her wisdom. "Education is for the future; yesterday's methods will not suffice for tomorrow's needs" (Rogers, 1961, p. 33). Many claiming the title "nurse" will thank her for recognizing that education and research in the Science of Unitary Human Beings enrich nursing's capacity to fulfill its societal mandate.

References

Barrett, E. A. M. (1990a). The continuing revolution of Rogers' science-based nursing education. In E. A. M. Barrett (Ed.), *Visions of Rogers' science-based nursing* (pp. 303–317). New York: National League for Nursing.

Barrett, E. A. M. (Ed.). (1990b). *Visions of Rogers' science-based nursing.* New York: National League for Nursing.

Brown, E. L. (1958). *The role of university schools of nursing in the improvement of patient care and health guidance.* Unpublished manuscript.

Ference, H. M. (1986). Foundation of a nursing science and its evolution: A perspective. In V. M. Malinski (Ed.), *Explorations on Martha Rogers' science of unitary human beings* (pp. 35–44). Norwalk, CT: Appleton-Century-Crofts.

Malinski, V. (Ed.). (1986). *Explorations on Martha Rogers' science of unitary human beings.* Norwalk, CT: Appleton-Century-Crofts.

Montag, M. (1979, May). *Martha E. Rogers' day.* Paper presented at the retirement party for Martha E. Rogers, Division of Nursing Alumni, New York University, New York.

Resolved. (1962, March). *New York State League Lines for Nursing,* pp. 1, 3.

Rogers, M. E. (1959, May). Nursing science. *New York State League Lines for Nursing,* pp. 2, 5.

Rogers, M. E. (1961). *Educational revolution in nursing.* New York: Macmillan.

Rogers, M. E. (1962a, March). *Untitled.* Paper presented at the Council of Member Agencies, Department of Baccalaureate and Higher Degree Programs, National League for Nursing, Williamsburg, VA.

Rogers, M. E. (1962b, June). *Nursing charts her course.* Paper presented at the Annual Lectureship, School of Nursing Medical College of Georgia, Athens, GA.

Rogers, M. E. (1963a). Editorial. *Nursing Science, 1,* 222–223.

Rogers, M. E. (1963b). Editorial. *Nursing Science, 1,* 399–405.

Rogers, M. E. (1963c, November). *Educating the nurse for the future.* Paper presented at the Annual Meeting of Directors and Supervisors of Public Health Nursing in New York State, Albany, NY.

Rogers, M. E. (1964a). Editorial. *Nursing Science, 2,* 71–73.

Rogers, M. E. (1964b). *Reveille in nursing.* Philadelphia: Davis.

Rogers, M. E. (1967, February). *Nursing science: Research and researchers.* Paper presented at the Annual Conference on Research and Nursing, Division of Nursing Education, Teachers College, Columbia University, New York, NY.

Rogers, M. E. (1968, October). *Doctoral education for nurses.* Paper presented at the Sigma Theta Tau Program Meeting, Rutgers University, College of Nursing, New Brunswick, NJ.

Rogers, M. E. (1969a). *Nursing research: Relevant to practice?* Unpublished manuscript.

Rogers, M. E. (1969b). Preparation of the baccalaureate degree graduate. *New Jersey Nurse, 25*(5), 32–37.

Rogers, M. E. (1970a). *Graduate education in nursing at New York University.* Revised unpublished manuscript.

Rogers, M. E. (1970b). *An introduction to the theoretical basis of nursing.* Philadelphia: Davis.

Rogers, M. E. (1971). *Future directions of doctoral education for nurses.* (DHEW Publication No. NIH 72-82). Bethesda, MD: U.S. Government Printing Office.

Rogers, M. E. (1980, October). Obsolescence revisited: The doing syndrome. *SAIN Newsletter,* pp. 6–7.

Rogers, M. E. (1985a). The nature and characteristics of professional education for nursing. *Journal of Professional Nursing, 1,* 381–383.

Rogers, M. E. (1985b). Nursing education: Preparing for the future. In *Patterns in education: The unfolding of nursing* (pp. 11–14). New York: National League for Nursing.

Rogers, M. E. (1986). Science of unitary human beings. In V. Malinski (Ed.), *Explorations on Martha Rogers' science of unitary human beings* (pp. 3–8). Norwalk, CT: Appleton-Century-Crofts.

Rogers, M. E. (1987). Nursing research in the future. In *Changing patterns in nursing education* (pp. 121–123). New York: National League for Nursing.

Rogers, M. E. (1990). Nursing: Science of unitary, irreducible human beings: Update 1990. In E. A. M. Barrett (Ed.), *Visions of Rogers' science-based nursing* (pp. 5–11). New York: National League for Nursing.

Rogers, M. E. (1992). Nursing science and the space age. *Nursing Science Quarterly, 5,* 27–34.

Sarter, B. (1988). *The stream of becoming: A study of Martha Rogers' theory.* New York: National League for Nursing.

CHAPTER 5

Untitled

Martha E. Rogers

It is a privilege to be here and to have this opportunity to speak before you. Williamsburg is an ideal spot in which to seek the perspective that comes from uniting the past and present as we direct ourselves to knowledgeable and wise planning for tomorrow.

In planning the comments I wish to make this morning, it seemed useful to bring with me some supplementary material, which has been distributed. The references were selected for the contribution they might make in stimulating new ideas, raising our sights, and directing our thinking toward a rapidly changing future. They have been drawn from logic, philosophy, economics, the basic sciences, automation, and the exploration of outer space. Most of these are available in paperback: an added advantage.

You also have before you a mimeographed statement entitled, "Selecting Your Career in Nursing." The Department of Nurse Education at New York University receives frequent requests from young people seeking information concerning nursing as a career. Many of these letters contain quite specific questions. Others of them are more general, such as the one from a third grader who wrote, "I am in the third grade. I want to be a nurse. Tell me all about it." The volume of such letters made it increasingly difficult to answer them as it was felt they should be answered. Consequently, the questions that were asked were used as a basis for developing mimeographed material that might be sent in response to requests for information. I might point out that one of the reasons this material was developed is because we believe that young people seeking a career in nursing should have accurate and forthright information on which to make their decision. Unfortunately, there is little in the literature that provides specific answers to many of these questions.

The third piece of material which was distributed includes the report of a New York State League for Nursing workshop held in January 1962 for state league board members, local league presidents, and state committee chair-

---

Rogers, M. E. (1962, March). *Untitled.* Paper presented at Council of Member Agencies, Department of Baccalaureate and Higher Degree Programs, National League for Nursing, Williamsburg, VA.

men. The seven goals developed in this workshop should be of interest to the group at this meeting. The first resolution should be of particular interest to this group and is closely related to some of the points I wish to make in a few minutes. Specifically, it was unanimously agreed that generally accepted definitions of professional, technical, and vocational occupations be used rather than defining the levels in nursing according to existing educational programs.

Dr. Savage has laid a very excellent foundation for this meeting and has raised a number of critical questions which we should examine carefully. Any discussion of critical areas such as is planned for this afternoon and the next two days has to be carried out within a framework of definitions, assumptions, and predictions of the future. Some predictions for the future in the light of current trends would seem to be a significant point of departure. Many of the events taking place today are disturbing. These events are having a direct impact on nursing, and nurses are faced with making some critical decisions directly related to these changes. In trying to predict what may happen in the next ten to twenty-five years, one cannot help treading on the threshold of fantasy. The world of reality and the world of science fiction are increasingly close together.

Some major changes already taking place, and reported with increasing frequency in newspapers and on radio and television, presage identifiable changes that must be made in nursing. One of the most significant is the move toward more and more automation. Automation is here to stay. It is already having a marked economic impact on our society. Unemployment is becoming a major problem in many of our larger industrial cities, and it can be expected to grow markedly unless forward-looking steps are taken.

Yesterday, the *New York Times* carried a statement that read as follows: "Automation Seen in United States Farming. . . . The revolution in agriculture which already has drained away more than half the farm's population while producing huge surpluses of many crops still has a long way to go."[1] President Kennedy has requested a public works program—a project also related to the impact of automation. With automation we can expect to have an increase in production and concomitantly a decrease in man-hours of labor. The proposed twenty-hour week which has appeared in the newspapers is not so strange as one might think.

This is not the first time that man has faced a shortening of work hours coupled with increased production. The first industrial revolution represented the bringing in of machines, cutting down of man-hours of work, and an increased amount of leisure time. It seems likely that the future will see this on a much larger scale. It is already taking place and can be expected to increase. The effect of automation can be expected to be felt first by blue-collar workers, the group perhaps least able to use added free time effectively.

Automation in industry, agriculture, and education will be accompanied by automation in health services. The increase in automation will demand more and better educated, more knowledgeable and wiser people. This group is already in very short supply in all fields. It can be expected to get worse unless we move rapidly to lessen this shortage. Man is being asked to make

[1]*New York Times,* March 25, 1962.

decisions for which there are no precedents. Though the past can give us many clues and information on which to build, some of the events we are now facing and will face require new and undreamed of answers.

I would like to quote from Donald Michael in the pamphlet *Cybernation: The Silent Conquest.* "Cybernation presages changes in the social system so vast and so different from those with which we have traditionally wrestled that it will challenge to their roots our current perceptions about the viability of our way of life."[2] Our value systems, our cultural patterns, and our political ideologies can be expected to undergo radical change.

A second major event taking place that will have a growing impact on how we plan for the future in nursing relates to the exploration of outer space. Such exploration has been ongoing for some time, with manned space travel a more recent accomplishment. The scientific discoveries that make these explorations of outer space possible coupled with the knowledge gained from such exploration is contributing along with other factors in forcing us to revise our concepts of man and the life process. We must look at man and his relationships with other parts of the universe within a new context. Old explanations are no longer valid. The mysticism of the Vitalists and the Cartesian mind-body dichotomy are giving way to a concept of man as an integral part of the universe, and of the life process as an adaptive process. One of the things that space exploration is doing is giving us a new vision of man's smallness—a concept that is frightening to many. It is interesting to note that in the last year man seems to be handling this fear in part by humor. The joking literature includes more and more delightful stories and cartoons. Humor is a wonderful thing. Perhaps one of the things we need to do is laugh at ourselves more often. New beliefs, behaviors, and goals far different from those we now hold must be developed. If we do not develop them, man may move toward increasing frustration and fear. Man must have meaningful purpose in his striving if he is to move forward.

Another major factor to be considered is the role of government. One of the things that occurs in an increasingly complex world is a concomitant increase in complexity of organization. As organization increases, benefits occurring under simpler patterns give way to new benefits appropriate to changing organization. Current trends suggest that government may play an ever larger role in education, business, industry, health services, and many other aspects of American life.

Political ideologies are also undergoing change. By virtue of living in a dynamic universe, in which change is inevitable, this can be expected as a reality of life. Another point that cannot be overlooked is man's desire for the products of technology which will further contribute to promoting change. In short, we can expect that the future will be characterized by a greatly expanded demand for learned persons, by an increasingly larger role of government in all aspects of American life, by increased production coupled with markedly fewer man-hours of labor, and by vast expansion of automation in health services. The latter will affect diagnosis and therapy habilitation and rehabilitation in all of the health services. Electronic devices such as the cardiac pacemaker and others are already in use. Many, yet unimagined, can be expected to appear. A quotation from Donald Price has relevance for us as we look ahead.

---

[2]Michael, Donald N., *Cybneration: The Silent Conquest,* Center for the Study of Democratic Institutions, Box 4068, Santa Barbara, California, 1962, pp. 14–15.

"We must learn to think without making use of the patterns or models taken for granted in most of the textbooks." What is the relevance of these predictions for the areas of discussion facing us this week? Change is occurring rapidly. There is great urgency in our need to plan wisely and well, to move quickly to set and implement goals for change, change that will not wait for us to dally over making decisions.

The predictable future supports an overwhelming need for nursing as a learned profession. The concept of nursing as a learned profession is an exceedingly difficult one for nurses to envision as it currently exists. Such a concept does not currently exist except in a very embryonic form.

To achieve such a concept of nursing demands a completely new look, for it is quite different from that which we have held in the past. Nursing was initiated as a vocational occupation and has so developed. Nursing has not yet bridged the gap between vocational training and learned education. Until a concept of nursing as a learned profession exists, little progress can be made toward developing examinations to test a professional level of knowledge and competence. Moreover, those who are to prepare such tests must possess the knowledge and competences characterizing learned professional education and practice.

I do not believe that it is possible to achieve a concept of nursing as a learned profession simply by asking how nursing is different from medicine or from some other group. Such an approach is, of itself, revealing of attitudes and thinking inconsistent with the development of a profession. Recognition of nursing as a learned profession and internalization of such a concept must be followed by a clear differentiation of the occupational careers in nursing.

Individual differences in ability and motivation must be reconciled with man's right to human dignity and the employment of his resources in useful productive labor. One of the tragedies growing out of our unwillingness to make decisions differentiating nursing careers is exemplified in our denying almost all nurses any opportunity to achieve excellence. We talk about poor, good, and best nurses as though the number of diplomas and degrees determined the excellence of practice. It does not.

Rather each one of these levels represents a career in itself and if we are to give people an opportunity to achieve excellence within the framework of their preparation, we must clearly indicate for what it is they are prepared. Furthermore, we must look at preparation according to what it prepares the person for rather than the piece of paper the person holds. At this point in time a particular degree is not a guarantee of level of preparation. Perhaps the following comments will stimulate some thinking.

At the present time there is a wide variety of programs preparing nurses. If we use generally accepted definitions such as those listed in the issue of the *New York State League Lines* which you have in your hands, it becomes apparent that a large number of programs in nursing are at a vocational level. This is true of practical nurse programs, of many diploma programs, and of the nursing portion of some of our baccalaureate programs. Why do I say this? What are the characteristics and purposes of higher education? How can a faculty person with little or no college education be expected to teach at a college level? How can a person who has had no upper division or graduate study in nursing teach nursing at a college level? Many of the textbooks in nursing are of less than college level. There is very little in nursing texts that can be considered of an upper division college level. Obviously, textbooks comprehended by students in a noncollegiate program who possess neither the general education nor the substantial basic science background on which to build are not appropriate texts for a school purporting to offer upper division nursing education.

But these are the texts that we tend to use throughout our educational programs. We must face these and other facts. In our desire to achieve recognition and to get under the umbrella of higher education, we have impugned the integrity of higher education and I might add that persons in higher education have also been party to this. In this process we have derogated the value of all programs in nursing. We have a responsibility to do something about this matter.

Learned persons in the future regardless of field must possess a broad foundation of knowledge. In the days ahead, this is going to become increasingly important. Man must possess the knowledge that will enable him to adapt to a new and strange future. We can expect that the next ten to twenty-five years will present events well beyond those which any of us can foresee today. The knowledges which may be expected to enable man to grow, to adapt, to create are found in the liberal arts, the creative arts, the earth sciences and space sciences, the basic sciences (biological, physical, and social), logic and philosophy, history, mathematics, communication, and languages. College graduates of the next decade will probably not be able to understand many of the things going on around them because it is impossible to get into a college education the amount of knowledge necessary to real understanding.

In looking at nursing as a profession, beyond the broad foundation, we must move to further depth in selected areas of knowledge consistent with the social ends for which nursing knowledge is to be used. The foundation of general education and the added depth in selected areas, provides the base without which it is not possible to comprehend nursing theory. To refer back to a comment made by Dr. Savage concerning courses labeled for nurses, all of us are well aware that such courses have rather generally represented courses of less than college level. As we develop an organized body of theoretical knowledge based on the aforesaid foundations, the situation should be very different.

I would like to indicate briefly what I believe nursing theory to be. Moreover, in its methods of development it does not differ from other professional fields. There are numerous theories in existence directed toward explaining man, the life process, and different aspects of the universe. New theories are being developed continuously. The more one knows, the more one is aware of the little one knows. Theories must be constantly tested, revised, developed. A particular theory may well be shared with many disciplines. It is in the particular aggregate of theories that nursing knowledge achieves its uniqueness. Nursing knowledge precedes and is the basis for nursing diagnosis and knowledgeable intervention for predictable outcomes. Accuracy of diagnosis and outcomes will be limited by the nurse's knowledge and the continually changing interaction of man with all parts of the universe.

Through observation, knowledge, and intellectual skill, the learned professional nurse evaluates individual and group level of biophysical, psychosocial functioning on the continuum of minimum to maximum well-being. Such determination will be dependent on preceding theoretical content in nursing.

Theoretical content in nursing is dependent on preceding general and science education. Nursing diagnosis is dynamic, requires continuous revision and varies with time and space. It provides the basis for knowledgeable intervention. Knowledgeable intervention is directed toward helping the individual and group move toward maximum adaptation within the framework of nursing knowledge.

I would like to make a few further comments concerning the areas listed for our discussion. I have already indicated briefly what I believe to be some of the characteristics of the nursing major. The fusion of the liberal arts, the basic sciences, and nursing theory constitutes a unified whole. Each step in developing this whole depends on a previous step. Quite obviously then the allocation of advanced standing credits for nursing courses taken in a noncollegiate program or of a lower division level, regardless of the school year in which taken, cannot be equated with nursing courses which demand substantial prerequisites for their comprehension. There can be no justification for the continuation of general nursing programs. They should have ceased a long time ago. And I say this knowing that I am chairman of a department in which such a program exists. We must not permit this to continue. A baccalaureate program should be set up on the same basis as other baccalaureate programs in higher education are set up. Advanced standing should be granted on the same basis that advanced standing is granted in other areas of the institution of higher education.

The basis on which we have allocated credit for noncollegiate preparation in nursing is highly invalid. It is amazing that nursing has been permitted to do this. At the point upper division nursing theory is taught, it is dependent on prerequisites for its comprehension. The individual who presents nursing courses which did not have these prerequisites will not have had upper division nursing theory. A basic baccalaureate curriculum provides a baseline against which to determine the appropriateness of advanced standing for a given course. It is true that there are many ways in which we learn, and not all of them are in formal education. However, formal education represents the major source of basic facts which we acquire. Our society invests enough money in education for one to feel that perhaps society thinks this is the most efficient and economical way in which to learn.

I am not sure how much we can do about master's curriculums until we develop our baccalaureate curriculum. In general, I would say that a large part of the nursing content in any graduate program in nursing today properly belongs in an undergraduate curriculum. Characteristics of graduates of baccalaureate programs in nursing which prepare for professional practice are rooted in the knowledge graduates possess and in the intellectual skill with which it is used. Many of our baccalaureate programs prepare for vocational and quasi-technical practice in nursing. Our stronger programs, and this is true of some of the general nursing and basic baccalaureate programs, have achieved good technological education. Until we achieve a concept of nursing as a learned profession, I am not sure to what extent we can move towards education for a learned profession. Perhaps in our discussion this week, we may achieve some of this.

I would like to end these comments with a quotation from Alfred North Whitehead, "When ideals sink to the level of practice, stagnation is the result."

CHAPTER 6

Nursing Charts Her Course

Martha E. Rogers

E. H. Carr, eminent historian, in his recent volume entitled *What Is History* writes, "The belief that we have come from somewhere is closely linked with the belief that we are going somewhere."[1] A concept of man as evolving world-stuff and man's mind as the agency by which evolution can reach new levels of achievement is carrying man, with unprecedented speed, toward fulfilling his urge to trod new roads and to seek new understandings. The rapidity of change is forcing man to make decisions for which there are no precedents. Facts we have been taking for granted are moving daily into the realm of scientific fiction. A whole new way of life involving our values, employment, education is emerging in the onslaught of automation. Roots reaching deep into the past are being disturbed, and many human beings are fearful of the opening up of an expanding universe beyond comprehension.

Time magazine (June 1, 1962) reports that psychiatrist Viktor E. Frankl of the University of Vienna has stated that he finds that 81 percent of Americans indicate they have experienced "existential vacuum"—a doubt that life has any meaning.[2] In the midst of multiple scientific advances and technological leapfrogging, it should not seem strange that men stop to question. Out of such questions can emerge new understandings, new strengths, new goals. Man's capacity to transcend the tangible realities can be mobilized to give renewed meaning to the purpose of life and to seek new ways of achieving them. Man's potential for greatness need not be swallowed up in the smallness engendered by our shrinking planet.

Just as Copernicus and Keppler forced men to new views of their place in the universe—threatening in those days—so can man achieve further revision of this relationship and, in so achieving, reach new heights.

But to achieve dynamic stability in the turmoil of change which can be anticipated in the next 5 to 10 or 20 years will demand an exceedingly large quantity of courage, faith, imagination, and knowledge. Experience is no longer a substitute for learning. Nor can learning be achieved by just living.

Rogers, M. E. (1962, June). *Nursing charts her course.* Paper presented at Annual Lectureship, School of Nursing, Medical College of Georgia, Athens, GA.

The nonspecialized adaptive powers of youth must be developed so that rapid and effective responses to an unknown future can be brought into play. The need for interdisciplinary cooperation between the life and physical scientists has led to the new field of bionics. Among the health disciplines, no one discipline possesses the gamut of knowledges necessary to achieve man's health potential.

New knowledge is revising man's concept of himself and his world. Roles and responsibilities of health personnel are undergoing dramatic change. Society's needs and demands for health services in the future will be radically different from those with which we are currently familiar. Moreover, there is increasing cognizance that a society in which health personnel concentrate predominantly on care of the ill can never be a truly healthy society.

The evolutionary forces impinging so heavily and directly on our society are not without their counterforces. Threatened institutions strive forcibly to repress individuals and groups demanding progressive action. Society's welfare becomes secondary for those who seek to maintain the status quo.

As nursing charts her course for the days ahead, there can be no room for navigators of narrow vision and shortsightedness. Society's welfare must rise paramount. Nursing education and practice sufficient unto the past are highly inadequate for the future. The predictable health needs of people demand of nurses a learned profession. A concept of nursing as a learned profession must replace the concept of nursing as a vocation. The traditional identification of nursing as "doing" is being replaced by an understanding of nursing as a body of knowledge, unique in its aggregate of knowledge, and when applied representing the practice of nursing. Elizabeth Kemble, dean of the School of Nursing at the University of North Carolina, has said, "Much has been written and said concerning the spirit, art, and science of nursing. No one will deny the importance of all three in the effective practice of nursing. But the noble spirit alone is not enough. The art of nursing falls short of its goals even with a fine spirit. It is only when nursing practice is based on a theoretically sound foundation that the spirit and art can come into full being."[3] The uniqueness of nursing will not be found in asking what the nurse does that is different from that which workers in other disciplines do. Nor does the difference between professional, technical, and vocational workers in nursing lie in the difference between the activities of each. The uniqueness of nursing rests on a concept of nursing as an organized body of theoretical knowledge. This body of knowledge is rooted in the humanities, and the biological, physical, and social sciences. Through selection, synthesis and resynthesis, and searching into the farther reaches of these areas, there exists an aggregate of theories which goes beyond the foundation and which represents the core of nursing knowledge on which professional practice in nursing depends. The explanatory and predictive principles of nursing make possible nursing diagnosis and knowledgeable intervention directed toward predictable goals. Nursing focuses on human beings. The practice of nursing is directed toward helping man achieve the maximum well-being within each person's potential.

Already nursing is late in moving ahead decisively and forthrightly in designing a future consistent with man's anticipated health needs. Creative, intelligent planning is imperative and the need for action is urgent. Clear, unequivocal interpretation of the careers open to potential students of nursing must replace the meretricious recruitment of students into programs inconsistent with the individual's goals and abilities. Thomas Griffith in *The Waist-High Culture* points out that "of all the wastes in American society, not the cutting down of forests but the stunting of intellectual growth is our most costly squandering of resources."[4] When applied to nursing the continued costly squandering of youthful minds in apprentice training programs in nursing is far too costly in the face of the evident superiority of multipurpose educational institutions for the preparation of (1) vocational nurses in high school programs, (2) technical nurses in associate degree programs, and (3) professional nurses in baccalaureate degree programs.

Plans for the future must reach beyond functions studies and identification of activities. This is not to say that such studies may not serve a useful purpose. But, in the words of Alfred North Whitehead, "when ideals have sunk to the level of practice, stagnation is the result."[5]

Preparation of learned professional practitioners in nursing is essential if nursing is to meet its responsibilities to society. Without such persons, technical nurses, currently prepared in hospital diploma schools, associate degree programs, and the majority of baccalaureate programs, cannot move forward. Concomitantly to the extent that learned professional nursing leadership and direction is absent or unused, society's welfare is jeopardized. Educators must recognize that modifications of the traditional hospital school pattern whether in a hospital school or included as part of a baccalaureate program can only reflect John W. Gardner's comment that "an educational system grudgingly and tardily patched to meet the needs of the moment will be perpetually out of date."[6]

The education of nurses belongs squarely within the framework of multidiscipline educational institutions. The education of the professional practitioner in nursing demands a strong foundation in the humanities and sciences taught at both lower and upper division college levels. The significant relationship of a college of nursing is with the liberal arts college of the educational institution. Students majoring in nursing must possess knowledge in English, history, logic, and philosophy; in foreign language, mathematics, biology, physics, and chemistry; in psychology and sociology, political science, and economics. They must possess knowledge and understanding of the biopsychosocial organism—gained through study in physiology, microbiology, genetics, embryology, biophysics, and biochemistry; in social psychology, anthropology, literature, history, philosophy, economics, and political science.

They must know and understand the theoretical concepts of nursing—incomprehensible without a liberal and nonspecialized foundation. Their professional education focuses on human beings. Undergraduate students will not be pushing back the frontiers of knowledge. Rather they will be gaining a toehold in the doorway that can lead to new frontiers. Graduates of such programs assume responsibility for themselves and others. They seek the guidance of specialists in nursing and work in a peer relationship with other disciplines.

Nursing specialization begins at the graduate level. Articulation and coordination of baccalaureate, master's, and doctoral programs is significant. Theoretical content in nursing is expanded and deepened. Investigatory skills are strengthened and leadership ability grows to fuller stature. At the doctoral level the scientist, the researcher, or the university teacher is prepared to seek new frontiers and to share both knowledge and the challenge of creative ideas with students.

The science of nursing grows as those nurses possessing the knowledge and tools gained in high quality doctoral study in nursing endeavor through conceptual creativity to state explicitly the unifying characteristics and the hypothetical generalizations and theories of this emerging science. Only as such nurses establish connections between different phenomena and identify the predictive principles can there be technological application.[7] "Observation and experiment do not provide the conceptions without which inquiry is aimless and blind."[8] Nurse-scientists must engage in pushing back the frontiers of knowledge. They must have a philosophy of the nature of man and the world in which he lives. They must possess intelligence.

The rebuilding of undergraduate and graduate curriculums in nursing that must take place, if technologists, and professional practitioners, specialists, and scientists are to be prepared, is already making frightening demands on a shortage of qualified faculty members. At the same time one can be confident that nurses today, as in the past, will grasp this challenge enthusiastically and will be unafraid to reach for the stars.

The waters through which nursing must steer her course are filled with many "sacred cows." In 1791 Thomas Paine in his *Rights of Man* makes a statement as relevant in its application today as when it was written. "Titles are like circles drawn by the magician's wand to contract the sphere of man's felicity. He lives immured within the Bastille of a word, and surveys at a distance the envied life of man." Status which is dependent on titles and words is ephemeral. It lacks the substance of reality and leads to loss of self-confidence. "Achievement of prestige will be bulwarked by more than status words and symbols."[9]

Traditional roles, attitudes, and values must give way as nurses seek excellence for all who nurse. In our failure to clearly differentiate careers in nursing according to generally accepted criteria, we deny the majority of nurses opportunity to achieve excellence. In the struggle to achieve for mankind maximum well-being within each individual's potential, all who nurse should have opportunity to find growing satisfaction, renewed vision, and replenished courage.

The wholeness of man and the universe, the unity of knowledge, and the challenge of a promising and exciting future can be extrapolated from a quotation from Pythagoras written 7000 years ago. "There is geometry in the humming of the strings. There is music in the spacing of the spheres."

There is a future in nursing that stretches far beyond the dreams of Florence Nightingale, whose vision prompted her to say, "May we hope that when we are all dead and gone, leaders will arise who will lead far beyond anything we have done."

Tomorrow belongs to all of us. In meeting the challenges of today, we are also preparing for an unknown tomorrow.

References

1. Carr, E. H., *What Is History,* Alfred A. Knopf, N.Y.
2. *Time,* Vol. LXXIX, No. 22, June 1, 1962, p. 48.
3. Kemble, Elizabeth, "Foreword," *Unity of Nursing Care,* University of North Carolina School of Nursing, June 1960.

4. Griffith, Thomas, *The Waist-High Culture,* Harper and Bros., N.Y., 1959.
5. Whitehead, Alfred N. as quoted in McGlothin, William J., "The Place of Nursing Among the Professions," *Nursing Outlook,* Vol. 9, No. 4, April 1961, p. 216.
6. *Pursuit of Excellence:* (Education and the Future of America), Panel Report V of the Special Studies Project, The Rockefeller Brothers Fund, Published by Doubleday & Co., Inc., Garden City, N.Y., 1958, p. 33.
7. Hempel, Carl G., *Fundamentals of Concept Formation in Empirical Science,* The University of Chicago Press, Chicago, Illinois, 1952.
8. Nagel, Ernest, "The Philosopher Looks at Science," *Medicine and the Other Disciplines,* International Universities Press, N.Y., 1960, p. 24.
9. Rogers, Martha E., *Educational Revolution in Nursing,* Macmillan, N.Y., 1961, p. 60.

CHAPTER 7

Editorial

Martha E. Rogers

Bold, forthright action on the part of courageous, responsible leaders in nursing is desperately needed to meet the challenges of a changing world. Halfway measures will neither suffice nor succeed. Evasion of responsibility for determining and implementing definitive steps in the education and practice of nurses consistent with present and predictable health needs of people negates nursing's fundamental humanitarian aims. Arguments over terminology serve only to confuse the uninformed and to deny the reality of contemporary and emerging events.

A diminishing naivete in evaluating health services characterizes growing numbers of the population. Society is increasing its demands for responsible leadership among the health disciplines. The trend toward preparation of educated men and women for the complex task of building a healthy society is as unmistakable in nursing as is the trend toward an increasingly well-educated public.

The preparation of Registered Nurses is moving inexorably into the main stream of higher education. Academic aims have been broadened. Social concern is taking on new dimensions. Apprentice training is being replaced by technical education in associate degree programs. Professional education in nursing is emerging in baccalaureate and higher degree programs.

As hospital schools move back into the pages of history, as one era of significant service gives way to another of even greater promise, it is true there will be many a backward, nostalgic look. Pressures of the moment may loom as giant shadows for the myopic. But nursing, like the rest of the world, is in transition.

Rapidly changing times demand the mobilization of strong visionary, and resourceful leaders. Knowledge and wisdom must join hands with courage and conviction. Integrity of spirit and strength of purpose are essential ingredients.

Planning for transition in nursing is urgent. Nursing is obligated to provide the leadership that binds the past and future and that transcends the present "that the nursing needs of the people will be met" now and in the

Rogers, M. E. (1963). Editorial. *Nursing Science, 1,* 222–223. Reprinted with permission.

days ahead. Self-direction is imperative. Nursing carries full responsibility for determining and implementing sound, forward-looking measures basic to providing the educational programs and nursing practice that will safeguard the public welfare. This responsibility can neither be delegated nor abnegated.

Equivocation, delay, dependency endanger the future. Concerted, forthright planning and action are overdue. Society will not long tolerate an erratic course nor will the changing times permit it. Strong, courageous leadership in nursing must move forward vigorously and definitively. The time is now.

CHAPTER 8

Educating the Nurse for the Future

Martha E. Rogers

Educating the nurse for the future is of itself a misnomer. Of the numerous events taking place in nursing perhaps most obvious is the fact that there is no such person as "the nurse." Dramatic revisions in the education, roles, and responsibilities of health personnel in general are already in the making. A variety of nursing personnel has emerged in response to social and health needs and the demands of people. Vocational, technical, and professional practitioners, nurse specialists, and nurse scientists are engaged in a multiplicity of activities.

Because nursing is no more static than any other aspect of society, we are engaged in a period of sweeping transitions in nursing. As a result, older securities have been shaken and new tensions aroused. The impact of geometrically advancing knowledge in the natural and social sciences, technological know-how, and changing social values are [sic] making demands on nurses of a hitherto unheard-of nature. *Nursing has outgrown its legal definitions.* The advent on the health scene of professionally educated nurses is quite new. The historical accident that placed the preparation of nurses under hospital control is in process of rectification. Trends and recommendations in the nation's educational system bring into bold relief the obsolescence of traditional patterns of education in nursing. The nurses we prepare today will be the nursing leaders 20 years from now.

Transition in nursing education and practice is proceeding apace even though forthright statements of facts; clearly defined goals; and organized, forward-looking, courageous leadership in nursing may be weak. The "fallacy of gradualism—the notion that every change must be approached by slow degrees . . . ,"[1] abrogation of responsibility, and failure to exercise self-determination too often promote chaos and perpetuate subservience to an outmoded

Rogers, M. E. (1963, November). *Educating the nurse for the future.* Paper presented at the Annual Meeting of Directors and Supervisors of Public Health Nursing of New York State, Albany, NY.

system. But Sister Charles Marie of Catholic University has pointed out that "whether we will it or not the professionally incompetent (the incompetent in general) will be left behind for social forces greater than ourselves or our profession are sweeping out-moded systems and their agents from their strongholds."[2]

Responsibility for nursing quality and quantity, its dimensions and its bounds, rests with nurses. Decision making for the education and practice of nurses is our full responsibility. Either nurses move forward now, forthrightly and decisively, to make forward-looking decisions based on broad knowledge and facts or others will make them for us. Identifiable vested interests are endeavoring to do just this and, on occasion, are supported by shortsighted persons in and out of organized nursing. Human welfare cannot be further jeopardized through our apathy or neglect or through narrow vision and dedication to expediency. Nor should we forget that all persons are not equally able to make all decisions. The total quality of nursing practice will be no greater than the knowledgeable leadership that must be provided by professionally educated staff nurses, nurse-specialists, and nurse-scientists. Concomitantly, the excellence of nursing services is equally dependent on the effective interaction of professional, technical, and vocational nurses striving toward a common goal and working effectively with society and other health disciplines in a concerted effort to achieve maximum health for all people.

The New York State Office of Public Health Nursing has brought together here leaders in public health nursing services and in nursing education from across New York State so that perspectives for the future in nursing—significant for public health in the future—may be explored jointly and with central concern for the public welfare. Though nursing services and nursing education differ in the specific purposes and responsibilities of each, they share equally in the ultimate goal of better health for society and are equally responsible for nursing's commitment to human welfare. Nurses have tended to hold education suspect although this is in process of change. Fortunately it is to the educated portion of the population regardless of field to whom society looks for leadership.

Every major step forward creates inconvenience and dislocations. Therefore, it does not seem amiss to include in this paper a short story taken from Louis Nizer's *My Life in Court.* It goes as follows: ". . . a farmer, before sunrise on a cold and misty morning, saw a huge beast on a distant hill. He seized his rifle and walked cautiously toward the ogre to head off an attack on his family. When he got nearer, he was relieved to find that the beast was only a small bear. He approached more confidently and when he was within a few hundred yards, the distorting haze had lifted sufficiently so that he could recognize the figure as only that of a man. Lowering his rifle, he walked toward the stranger and discovered he was his brother."[3]

The kaleidoscope of nursing is being brought into focus. The complexity of knowledge and skill required to safeguard the recipients of nursing services today and tomorrow makes mandatory the identification of a nucleus of professionally educated nurses distinct from those whose preparation is technical or vocational in nature. And as Howard S. Becker writes, "Professions, as commonly conceived, are occupations which possess a monopoly of some esoteric and difficult body of knowledge . . . The body of knowledge over which the profession holds a monopoly consists not of technical skills and the fruits of practical experience but, rather of abstract principles arrived at by scientific research and logical analysis."[4] McConnell, Anderson, and Hunter, discussing "The University and Professional Education," state, "The University is justified in asking that the professional school emphasize the theoretical foundations of professional practice and that a fundamental body of scholarly knowledge should be the core of professional education and that the acquisition of skills and techniques should be a secondary, if necessary concern."[5] W. J. McGlothlin in his book *Patterns of Professional Education* writes, "the movement of professional education is in the direction of knowledge and away from skills."[6] Marshall Robinson, dean of the graduate School of Business, University of Pittsburgh, writes, "Educational efficiency suggests that we should push a larger portion of the student's education about the artistic elements (the art of practice) of each field onto those who hire our graduates . . . so far, the schools who have done it have not suffered. They have delivered a brighter product, one that is able to learn and integrate what is learned. They have delivered a student who moves into his career knowing that he has serious knowledge gaps and is eager to fill them."[7]

Moreover, experience is not a substitute for knowledge. A syndicated newspaper column appearing in the nation's newspaper this past August (1963) points out rather forcibly some handicaps of experience in current times.

Is experience the best teacher? Not always. Richard Barbour, guidance director of the San Diego (California) public schools, recently was visited by two young engineers who, some years before, he had helped in making their vocational choices. At the time of their visit they were trying to modernize a well-established but rundown factory. When asked the most significant lesson their work had taught them, they said the most important thing they had learned was "not to rely too much on past experience in solving new problems."

During the ensuing discussion the young men pointed out that they had found it vital to think in new categories rather than in old ones. "You have to explore the unfamiliar and the unknown," they agreed. "Things change so fast, experience can be a handicap."

It took guidance-director Barbour some time to realize the full import of this statement. He had heard the same idea expressed by scientists engaged in advanced, far-out research, but the two young engineers were talking about down-to-earth production problems. He realized that even in factories, things are changing so fast that experience may be a handicap, and the same is true in selecting a career.

"The only thing we can be sure of," Mr. Barbour later wrote in *Together* (September 1962), "is that our offspring will have to be flexible. They will have to scrap old skills and information, acquire new training, and cope with constant and far-reaching changes." It is futile to educate for nonexistent jobs.

Nursing, as a learned profession, assuming its responsibilities to society within the broad fabric of emerging social, economic, scientific, and educational events, takes on new dimensions. Definitions are revised and clarified. Nursing science and nursing practice emerge as clearly different conditions of nursing.

Nursing science is a body of scientific knowledge characterized by descriptive, explanatory, and predictive principles about the life process in man.

These principles rest on a view of man as a unified biophysical, psychosocial organism in constant interaction with all parts of the environment. This body of knowledge develops through synthesis and resynthesis of selected knowledges from the humanities and natural and social sciences for new concepts and new understandings. Formulation of the unifying principles and hypothetical generalizations of nursing is under way and baccalaureate and graduate curriculums are being rebuilt to provide professional education.

Nursing practice is the process by which this body of knowledge, nursing science, is used for the purpose of assisting human beings to achieve maximum health within the potential of each person. It is the process by which the body of scientific knowledge (nursing science) is used for the purpose of assisting human beings to move in the direction of maximum well-being. This process is subsumed under two major categories, namely: (1) *Evaluative and diagnostic*—the process of determining the position of an individual, family, or group on the continuum of minimum to maximum well-being. This process utilizes knowledge and understanding of descriptive and explanatory principles concerning man and his environment, observation, and intellectual skill. (2) *Interventive*—the process of determining and initiating discriminative action based on predictive principles. These are continuous and concurrent processes characterized by ongoing modification, alteration, revision, and change. The central concern is with human beings in multiple settings—not with things.

Education for professional practice is offered only in colleges and universities. These programs prepare for the broad scope of nursing practice and require substantial knowledge in the liberal arts; biological, physical, and social sciences; and upper division nursing theory with its related laboratory study. Students in nursing are integral parts of the total student body throughout their educational program. Courses in nursing are taught by qualified college faculty in nursing and are dependent on prerequisites in general education and the basic sciences for their comprehension. Nursing courses represent only a portion of the courses taught at a senior college level. Laboratory study in nursing represents regularly scheduled courses. Many community resources such as hospitals, public health agencies, and schools provide the settings for laboratory study.

Graduates are prepared to assume professional responsibility for promotion of health and prevention of disease, and for nursing diagnosis, therapy, and rehabilitation. They are prepared to work directly with human beings. They assume increasing responsibility for themselves and for appropriate guidance of registered nurse graduates of associate degree and hospital school programs, practical nurses, and auxiliary personnel. They work in a peer relationship with professional personnel in other disciplines. These programs provide the foundation for nurses who wish to go on for master's and doctoral study in nursing. Master's programs begin the process of specialization. They build on a broad undergraduate base. Doctoral study moves further into the complexities of nursing science. Here are prepared the university teachers, the researchers, and scientists.

The educational program is directed toward developing enduring values, *not* just for immediate utility; it teaches the broad principles that can be unified to meet novel situations and that will provide the basis for continued learning. The school of nursing's *one* significant tie is with the school of liberal arts and sciences within the institution of higher learning of which the school of nursing is an integral part. Instruction in the humanities is the responsibility of persons knowledgeable and competent in these areas. Persons teaching in the biological, physical, and social sciences are biologists, physicists, chemists, psychologists, sociologists, and other specialists within these broad fields. Nursing science and its related laboratory study are taught by nurse faculty members expert in their own field and possessing the usual preparation expected by colleges and universities for college and university teaching.

Within the nursing profession, as within other professional groups, a large number of nurses are those who must have an equally 'excellent' educational program but whose scope of knowledge and responsibility is consistent with a level of preparation and practice different from and less demanding than professional education and practice. The registered nurse has made and is continuing to make a tremendously significant contribution to human health and welfare. The ongoing need for technically educated nursing personnel should be as obvious as the need for professionally educated nurses, though the proportionate numbers are likely to decrease markedly with automation, programming, etc. of nursing tasks. Technical education is of junior college level and includes a leavening of the liberal arts and sciences. The uniquely significant role of educational institutions in providing the liberal foundation and the specialized training needed in today's world, coupled with the demonstrable superiority of associate degree programs over hospital-controlled programs in the preparation of registered nurses, further supports innumerable recommendations of more than half a century: specifically, the education of nurses belongs squarely within the framework of educational institutions. Evidence of a geometrically advancing increase in enrollments in junior and community college programs in nursing and a concomitant percentage decrease in hospital schools is documented. For example, in September of 1962, admissions to schools of nursing in California were distributed with approximately one third to hospital schools, one third to associate degree programs, and one third to baccalaureate degree programs. It has been predicted that in less than 4 years all education of nurses in California will be located in educational institutions. Nor is this trend peculiar to California. Florida is reported to be moving rapidly. As of this fall, approximately 20 associate degree programs are ongoing in New York State and the recent Report of the New York State Governor's Commission on Education for the Health Professions recommends that these programs "should be given every encouragement, because they, too, meet the major criterion that education for the health professions should be provided in an educational rather than a service environment."[8] Let me clarify: education for the health profession does *not* mean that all persons will be professionally educated.

The relatively recent advent of practical nurse programs with their heavy government subsidies raises some critical questions concerning the variety of nursing personnel needed for the future. The Ginsberg[9] report of 1948 recommended two levels of nurse preparation, the professional and the technical, and proposed the absorption of practical nurse students into the technical level of preparation for those so competent and in-service training for an aide group. Subsequent studies have tended to support this in spite of increasing numbers of practical nurses. Practical nurses themselves point to the inadequacies of their preparation for the job to be done and are continuing to propose lengthened programs.

Will continued federal aid to practical nurse programs improve or further dilute the quality of nursing service? Might quality be strengthened by less diffusion of our energies? Biology teaches us that the more narrowly specialized the organism, the more subject it is to extinction. Is there an ecological niche for each of these groups that can profitably provide the sustenance that will make for quality in nursing services? What about the impact of technology and automation? Might we not better look to identification of the numbers of kinds of nursing personnel according to the needs of the society we purport to serve rather than to vested interest groups among nurses and among groups outside of nursing?

As a result of recently expanded federal support, specifically the National Manpower Training and Development Act, for widespread training and retraining of large segments of the population, which has included training programs for practical nurses, New York State has, as of this September, an additional 23 schools of practical nursing. At the same time that massive numbers of minimally skilled nursing personnel are being loosed upon an unwitting public to join hands with technically prepared registered nurse graduates of our associate degree and hospital schools in caring for New York State's ill and handicapped, professionally educated leadership, knowledgeable and competent to make the judgments and provide the direction that can safeguard human welfare, are [sic] notably absent or unused. This is a frightening situation. And we cannot deny that we have contributed to its development through our own failure to foresee the nursing needs of people within the context of changing times, to clearly differentiate vocational, technical, and professional levels of preparation and practice, and to take forthright action in pushing ahead. Will our concern for people be great enough to overcome our adherence to tradition?

How much do we really want nursing quality? Achievement of nursing quality demands that we must not only clarify the roles and responsibilities of the different kinds of nursing personnel but we must move honestly into clear, definitive, sound recruitment programs. It is morally reprehensible to recruit into hospital programs young people whose abilities, interests, and goals are consistent with baccalaureate education in nursing. Educators have long recognized the importance of helping young people select educational programs consistent with each person's intellectual potential and motivation. Although much needs to be done to improve the educational guidance of young people, nursing has made limited use of the knowledge already available.

Hospital and associate degree programs are not the first part of baccalaureate degree programs. Professional and technical education represent two different careers in nursing. The intellectual demands for each are different and the responsibilities for which each group is prepared are also different. Young people must be told about the different careers in nursing and be given an opportunity to select the career appropriate for each person. Too often potential students of nursing are denied a choice through our failure to provide accurate information or through our dissemination of misinformation. Nor can baccalaureate programs or their products be compared with associate degree and hospital school programs and products. They are measured against different criteria, goals, purposes. They are not comparable. Not better than but different from.

The level and quality of nursing practice is dependent on the education which precedes it. "Living and seeing may give some acquaintance with things but never an understanding of things."[10] All who nurse must have opportunity to achieve excellence within the scope of each person's preparation and ability. All who nurse are entitled to the satisfaction that comes with a job well done.

Might honest recruitment lead to increased admissions to schools of nursing in place of the now shrinking percentage of high school graduates seeking a career in this field? Will the fine recommendations for recruitment of college-bound youth into true professional schools of nursing in colleges and universities flower or will they founder because we were "too little and too late"? Neither society nor nursing can afford Lewis Mumford's criticism that "our own leaders are now living in a one-dimensional world of the immediate present, unable to remember the lessons of the past or to anticipate the probability of the future."[11]

Many centuries ago the Roman poet Horace wrote, "There are no footprints pointing backward." Change in nursing or in anything else does not wait upon formal declarations for its existence. Actions taken in august bodies may confirm, refute, or propose postponement of what is already reality. But change will not be denied.

Differentiation of careers in nursing will not be found in studies of functions. Nor will the surgeon general's consultant group recommendation for another study of "nursing education today" result in more than time-consuming, dollar-reducing repetition. Rather, we had better heed Alfred North Whitehead's warning that "when ideals sink to the level of practice, stagnation is the result."[12]

We have been asking the wrong questions in our efforts to differentiate levels of nurses and to differentiate nursing from other disciplines. The difference does not lie in what each does but in which each knows. The kind and amount of knowledge and its utilization for human betterment clearly differentiate groups within nursing and between nursing and other disciplines. Professional, technical, and vocational education have well-established criteria. Our problem lies not with what constitutes generally understood terminology but with ourselves. Perhaps a further quotation from Whitehead is not out of place. "Where attainable knowledge could have changed the issue, ignorance has the guilt of vice."[13]

Not only must the careers in nursing be stated forthrightly and honestly but the levels of instruction which must be provided for the respective kinds of nurses must represent levels of education well beyond those which, traditionally, have been provided. A few months ago *Harper's* magazine (April 1963) reported an exciting experiment in teaching average three-year-olds how to read. And they loved it. Second-graders are studying Euclidean geometry, and adolescent space enthusiasts are taking for granted Einstein's world of curves. Those who are responsible for instruction of students must seek learning and relearning for themselves. Programmed instruction and teaching machines, an amazing variety of visual aids, creative teaching, and research findings must become parts of the learning environment of both students and teachers. Nor is the learning and relearning limited to teachers. The age we live in is making demands on all nurses for continued learning. Moreover, continued learning helps to bridge the gap between the past and the unknown future.

Modern nursing's search for quality is as old as modern nursing. Visionary leaders in nursing have struggled long and hard, with courage and imagination to foretell the future and to create the changes that would further define and strengthen quality nursing. And nursing's search must surely have met with some measure of success else the phenomenal growth in kinds and numbers of nurses sought round this planet to serve man's welfare would not be so large. The ideals of human service that have motivated nurses for more than a century are no less great today than they have ever been. The urge to move forward, to forgo obsolescence in past achievements, that human welfare may be better served, is strong.

Contemporary nursing constitutes a major social force. It is continually molding and being molded by the culture in which it exists. Man's capacity for initiating change is also the capacity of nurses for envisioning the future and determining sound direction in the great task of building a healthy society.

A quotation from Charles F. Kettering sounds a pertinent note on which to close. "The past is gone and static. Nothing we can do will change it. The future is before us and dynamic. Everything we do will affect it."

References

1. Mumford, Lewis, *In The Name of Sanity,* Harcourt, Brace & Co., NY, 1954. p. 95.
2. Sister Charles Marie Frank, "Freedom to Achieve," *New York State Nurse, XXXIV,* Jan. 1962. pp. 3–6.
3. Nizer, Louis, *My Life In Court,* Doubleday & Co., Inc., Garden City, NY, 1961. p. 443.
4. Becker, Howard S., "The Nature of a Profession," *Education for the Professions,* The Sixty-first Yearbook of the National Society for the Study of Education, Part II, University of Chicago Press, Chicago, Ill., 1962. p. 35.
5. McConnell, Anderson, and Hunter, "The University and Professional Education," *Education for the Professions,* The Sixty-first Yearbook of the National Society for the Study of Education, Part II, University of Chicago Press, Chicago, Ill., 1962. p. 259.
6. McGlothlin, W. J., *Patterns of Professional Education,* G. P. Putnam's Sons, Inc., NY, 1960. p. 174.
7. Robinson, Marshall A., "Applied Sciences—Deep and Shallow." Unpublished paper presented at NLN Council of Baccalaureate and Higher Degree Programs, Phoenix, Arizona, November 14, 1962.
8. New York State Committee on Medical Education, *Education for the Health Professions,* Albany, NY, 1963. p. 31.
9. Ginsberg, Eli (edit.), *A Program for the Nursing Profession,* The Macmillan Co., NY, 1948.
10. Bunge, Mario, *Intuition and Science,* Prentice-Hall, Inc., Englewood Cliffs, NJ, 1962. p. 23.
11. Mumford, Lewis, *In The Name of Sanity,* Harcourt, Brace & Co., NY, 1954. p. 4.
12. Whitehead, A. N., as quoted in McGlothlin, W. J., "The Place of Nursing Among the Professions," *Nursing Outlook,* Vol. 9, No. 4, April 1961. p. 216.
13. Whitehead, A. N., as quoted in *The University and World Affairs,* The Ford Foundation, NY, 1960. p. 13.

CHAPTER 9

Editorial

Martha E. Rogers

Deeply ingrained attitudes yield slowly, even to overwhelming evidence.
—Eli Ginsberg

Decision to study the "present system of nursing education" as recommended by the Surgeon General's Consultant Group in Nursing has been announced jointly by the boards of directors of the American Nurses Association and the National League for Nursing. In the face of overwhelming evidence, nursing "leaders" propose to sponsor a time-consuming, dollar-reducing, re-examination of an out-moded system. Whitehead's words are indeed prophetic, "When ideals sink to the level of practice, stagnation is the result."[14] In 1959 Margaret Bridgman pointed out that "it is unquestionably true that the preparation of nurses would not have lagged so far behind the demand if educational developments had kept pace with those in other fields."[2]

In 1948 Esther Lucile Brown prefaced her report on Nursing for the Future with these words, "For a quarter of a century leaders of nursing education have striven with almost unparalleled zeal but with distressingly small results . . . to create a sound and socially motivated form of nursing. Long ago they became convinced that a system of apprenticeship . . . was no longer adequate to prepare nurses . . .

Josephine Goldmark's distinguished report, *Nursing and Nursing Education in the United States,* published in 1923 under the auspices of the Committee for the Study of Nursing Education, concerned itself with the problem of the reorientation of professional practice to meet new health and social goals, and made specific recommendations for education of such reorientation. Three years later the Committee on the Grading of Nursing Schools began its prodigious task, to which nearly ten years and a quarter of a million dollars were devoted . . ."[3]

Esther L. Brown's report on *Nursing for the Future* was itself a thorough and painstaking investigation sponsored by the National Nursing Council. Concerning this study, "First, and most important, was the decision to view nursing service and nursing education in terms of what is best for society—

Rogers, M. E. (1963). Editorial. *Nursing Science, 1,* 399–405. Reprinted with permission.

not what is best for the profession of nursing as a possibly 'vested interest.' "[3] Professional, technical, and vocational education were differentiated. The need for a professionally educated group of nurses was stressed. She further wrote: "Almost without a dissenting voice those who are conversant with the trend of professional education in the United States agree that preparation of the professional nurse belongs squarely within the institution of higher learning. So convinced are they that they consider this conclusion above argument."[3] and ". . . we recommend that the term 'professional,' when applied to nursing education, be restricted to schools . . . that are able to furnish professional education as that term has come to be understood by educators."[3]

Agnes Gelinas noted "The Brown Report points out that the present inadequacies in nursing service are due primarily to an outmoded educational system."[5]

At the same time that Esther L. Brown was pursuing her investigation, the Committee on the Function of Nursing chaired by Eli Ginsberg and sponsored by the Division of Nursing Education, Teacher's College, Columbia University undertook to examine "a selected group of problems centering around the current and prospective shortages of nursing personnel."[6] This committee recommended two categories of nursing personnel and stated "By professional nurses, we mean collegiate-trained nurses who hold a baccalaureate degree."[6]

The Department of Higher Education of the National Education Association in 1951 adopted the following resolution:

> Whereas, health needs of the civilian population and military personnel are making increasing demands for the services of professionally and technically prepared nurses, and,
>
> Whereas, education for nursing is now predominantly outside higher education, with emphasis on apprenticeship training,
>
> Be it resolved: That institutions of higher learning recognize their responsibility for establishing programs providing for the professional and technical education of nurses.[4]

In 1951 Mildred Montag initiated her epoch-making, and no longer experimental, demonstration of junior college education for technical Registered Nurse practice. Demonstrably, Registered Nurses can be prepared in associate degree programs as well as or better than in hospital schools and in a shorter time. "Focusing on helping students gain desired objectives, the [associate degree] nursing faculty reduces repetitive practice to a minimum,"[11] whereas in hospital schools "emphasis is placed on learning through practical use of knowledge." Graduates of associate degree programs are prepared to carry the same responsibilities as are graduates of hospital schools. They are qualified for examination for licensure as registered nurses and interestingly enough their mean score performance on the national licensing examinations is somewhat higher than the mean scores for hospital school graduates. The successful development of associate degree programs in nursing provided for a realistic appraisal of patterns of nurse education according to generally understood criteria in use by educators. Nor does any informed person confuse associate degree education with valid baccalaureate education.

In 1947 the President's Commission on Higher Education had stated that "a full four years of college is not necessary . . . for education on the technician level . . . Training for these jobs is the kind the community colleges should provide."[13] This point was further confirmed and strengthened a decade later in the Second Report of the President's Commission on *Education beyond the High School.*

The recent Report of the New York State Governor's Commission on *Education for the Health Professions* recommends that associate degree programs in nursing "be given every encouragement, because, they, too, meet the major criterion that education for the health professions should be provided in an educational rather than a service environment."[9]

A compilation of studies sponsored by the American Nurses Association and the American Nurses Foundation during the years 1950 to 1957 was published in 1958 under the title, *Twenty Thousand Nurses Tell Their Story.* Hughes, Hughes, and Deutscher, authors of this volume, wrote "Now profession has become, in the English language, the word to designate an occupation of the highest possible prestige and status. . . . Some occupational groups, putting the chicken before the egg, assume that by calling themselves professions, they automatically will be accorded high prestige."[8] They further state that the population on which they are reporting "chose nursing from a pool of 'womanly' vocations which require some special skill and education but not a great deal of either."[8]

In 1957 the Committee on the Future of the National League for Nursing studied changing needs in nursing service and nursing education with direct consideration of social and health trends in the foreseeable future. The results of this study were published in a booklet titled Nurses for a Growing Nation. Based on the kinds of activities in which registered nurses were currently engaged the committee recommended proportionate numbers for three broad levels of practice and the educational preparation necessary to safely carry the responsibilities within a given level. Graduates of hospital schools and associate degree programs constituted one level, and it was recommended that these persons constitute approximately 67 per cent of the total. A second level, requiring baccalaureate education, was needed in about 20 per cent of the positions, and approximately 13 per cent were needed who would possess graduate education.

Differentiation of levels of nurse preparation and practice is implicit in the organizational structure of the National League for Nursing. Note the names of the following departments: (1) Department of Baccalaureate and Higher Degree Programs, (2) Department of Diploma and Associate Degree Programs, and (3) Department of Practical Nurse Education.

The American Nurses Association in its "Goal Three" has given formal recognition to the fact that professional education in nursing is of at least baccalaureate degree level.

It is interesting to note that William Bishop, speaking before the N.L.N. Convention in 1959, commented on the misinterpretations of Florence Nightingale's teachings, rampant among many nurses, and stated that, "It is really an extraordinary thing that there should be this subservience to an outmoded system . . . It is indeed remarkable that one of the most forward-looking women who ever lived should [be misinterpreted and thus used to] exercise an inhibitory effect upon progress and experiment."[1]

Nursing has outgrown its legal definitions. The complexity of knowledge and skill required to safeguard recipients of nursing services today and tomorrow makes mandatory the identification of a nucleus of professionally educated nurses distinct from those whose preparation in nursing is technical and vocational. That baccalaureate education is different in kind and amount from associate degree and hospital school programs is beyond argument. A year ago the National League for Nursing initiated the development of baccalaureate level achievement tests in nursing. But at the present time, in no place is society guaranteed a minimum safe level of professional practice in nursing, and at least one state education department has made this point explicit. That baccalaureate degree graduates perform significantly better on national Registered Nurse licensing examinations than do hospital school and associate degree graduates has no more relevance than that college freshmen perform significantly better than tenth grade students on a tenth grade English test.

It is therefore incomprehensible that *Nursing Outlook* in October 1963 would carry a statement concerning nurse licensure prepared by the staff of the N.L.N. test services in which it is implied that baccalaureate programs differ from hospital schools only in "breadth of liberal education" and "higher flights of professional education," and that one examination for diploma and baccalaureate degree graduates is ample "Because that's what the boards of nursing want and designate."[10] Perhaps we all might ponder Whitehead's statement that "Where attainable knowledge could have changed the issue, ignorance has the guilt of vice."[15]

"We seem fatuously unwilling to learn from our own mistakes."[15] And to paraphrase Sister Charles Marie, "It is time the Rip Van Winkles in nursing woke up."[12] Change does not wait upon pronouncements by august bodies. Are there those who would substitute planned chaos for planned transition? What is the price to society of nursing's failure to act with foresight and knowledge upon massive evidence crying for long overdue implementation in the name of human welfare? Will the fine recommendations for recruitment of college-bound youth into true professional schools of nursing in colleges and universities flower or will they founder because we were "too little and too late"?

What motivations underlie this recommendation of the Surgeon General's Consultant Group? What hidden agenda might have been brought to bear in the action taken by the boards of directors of the A.N.A. and N.L.N. to implement this recommendation? Who is competent to determine standards of education and practice in nursing? Has Lavinia Dock and Isabel Stewart's warning against "influences that sap [nurses'] independence and integrity" been for naught?

I believe there are more instances of the abridgment of the freedom of the people by gradual and silent encroachments of those in power than by violent and sudden usurpation.

—James Madison
June 16, 1788

References

1. Bishop, William: Florence Nightingale and Her Message for Today. Paper presented at N.L.N. Biennial Convention, Philadelphia, May 14, 1959.
2. Bridgman, Margaret: Development and Purpose of Collegiate Programs in the Evolving System of Education for Nursing. The Yearbook of Modern Nursing—1959. G. P. Putnam's Sons, New York, 1959, p. 239.
3. Brown, Esther Lucile: Nursing for the Future. Russell Sage Foundation, New York, 1948, pp. 17, 77, 138. College and University Bulletin. 3:2 (Apr.) 1951.

4. Gelinas, Agnes: Our Basic Educational Programs. Amer. Jour. Nursing 49:47 (Jan.) 1949.
5. Herrick, C. Judson: The Evolution of Human Nature. Harper and Row, New York, 1961, p. 194.
6. Ginsberg, Eli (Ed.): A Program for the Nursing Profession. Macmillan Co., New York, 1949, pp. IX, 9.
7. Hughes, E. C., Hughes, H. M., and Deutscher, I.: Twenty Thousand Nurses Tell Their Story. J. B. Lippincott Co., Philadelphia, 1958, pp. 3, 50, 235.
8. New York State Committee on Medical Education: Education for the Health Professions. Albany, NY, 1963, p. 31.
9. NLN Testing Services Staff: Let's Examine. Nursing Outlook 11:749 (Oct.) 1963.
10. Nursing Education Programs Today. National League for Nursing, New York, 1962, pp. 11, 12.
11. Nursing Education Programs Today. National League for Nursing, New York, 1962, pp. 11, 12.
12. Sister Charles Marie: Nursing Needs More Freedom. Amer. Jour. Nursing 62:53–55 (July) 1962.
13. The President's Commission on Higher Education: Higher Education for American Democracy. Harper and Brothers, New York, 1947, vol. I, p. 69.
14. Whitehead, A. N., as quoted in McGlothlin, W. J.: The Place of Nursing among the Professions. Nursing Outlook 9:216 (Apr.) 1961.
15. Whitehead, A. N., as quoted in The University and World Affairs. Ford Foundation, New York, 1960, p. 13.

CHAPTER 10

Editorial

Professional Standards: Whose Responsibility?

Martha E. Rogers

When an organization under the suppressing force of extreme equalitarianism reaches a sufficiently dead level of mediocrity, it may be ready prey to the vitality of men who are prepared to step in with personal force and initiative.

—John W. Gardner

It is beyond argument that a profession is responsible for setting its own standards. Yet within these oft repeated words lies a Pandora's box of unresolved controversy, confusion, and contumacious refusal to face the reality that if there are to be professional standards they will be set by learned professional personnel. Fervently embracing mediocrity, the sciolists in nursing adamantly refuse to examine today's reality and tomorrow's promise. Advocates of extreme equalitarianism cast a pervasive smog designed to blind even the most astute and while demanding freedom for themselves would deny it to others. Hostility and indifference to learning implies a contemptuous concern for human dignity and social welfare.

The time is past for endless squabbling over matters of little import. Social welfare demands that compromise on fundamental issues cease. The focus of nursing is clear for those who care to look. The historical accident that placed the preparation of nurses under hospital control is in process of rectification. Junior and community college associate degree programs have more than demonstrated their superiority over hospital schools in the preparation of Registered Nurses for technical practice. The complexity of knowledge and skill required to safeguard the recipients of nursing services has made mandatory the identification of a nucleus of professionally educated nurses distinct from those whose preparation is technical or vocational in nature. Baccalaureate and graduate curriculums are being rebuilt to provide true professional edu-

Rogers, M. E. (1964). Editorial. *Nursing Science, 2,* 71–73. Reprinted with permission.

cation in nursing. Standards of excellence incontrovertibly differentiate professional, technical, and vocational careers in nursing. How long will the suppressing force of extreme equalitarianism be permitted to deny excellence to nurses and to society?

Standards are overt signs by which nursing recognizes society's stake in nursing education and nursing services. Standards of excellence are a means by which nursing fulfills its commitment to the humanity it purports to serve. Standards point to an attainable goal—not an accomplished fact. Professionally, technically, and vocationally educated nurses have a right and a responsibility to seek excellence within the scope of each one's preparation and ability. Society has a right to expect that the most knowledgeable and able in nursing be liable for determining sound standards for all who nurse.

Succinctly stated is John W. Gardner's question, "How can we provide opportunities and rewards for individuals of every degree of ability so that individuals at every level will realize their full potentialities, perform at their best and harbor no resentment toward any other level?* Nursing has outgrown its legal definitions. Insipidities and absurdities no longer suffice to veil the direct relevance to nursing of Gardner's question. Nor does facing this question relieve responsibility for determined action. Failure to differentiate careers in nursing denies all nurses opportunity to realize their full potentialities. Resentment is magnified and vested interest groups in and out of nursing have fallow ground for plowing under socially significant goals.

Nurses dawdle while society suffers. Professional standards set by carefully selected, professionally educated personnel in nursing are critically urgent. Excellence will not be achieved by invalid distortions and denial of differences. Concerted action is long overdue.

Setting professional standards is the responsibility of the profession. But glib words are not enough. Their meaning must be plumbed and their implications made explicit. Human welfare must take precedence over expediency. Human dignity must be recognized. How much do nurses want quality nursing?

WHOSE RESPONSIBILITY?

---

*Gardner, John W.: Excellence. Harper & Row, Publishers, New York, 1961. p. 115.

Many nurses are afflicted with a peculiar condition which might be diagnosed as "symbol syndrome." This condition tends to be characterized by massive psychobiological reactions to certain words, such as: professional, technical, vocational, apprentice, levels, degrees, et cetera. Or there may be a wide range spectrum response to such variables as omission of caps, starch shortages, and others. In its particularly severe stages, the sensory modalities may undergo complete rejection of all new stimuli.

CHAPTER 11

Editorial

Martha E. Rogers

. . . among all the benefits that could be conferred upon mankind I find none so great as the discovery of new arts, endowments, and commodities for the bettering of man's life. For I saw that among the crude people in primitive homes that authors of inventions and discoveries were consecrated and numbered among the Gods. . . . But above all, if a man could succeed, not in striking out some new invention, however useful, but in kindling a light in nature—a light which should in its ray rising touch and illuminate all the border regions that confine upon the circle of our present knowledge; and so spreading further and further should presently disclose and bring into sight all that is most hidden and secret in the world, that man would be the benefactor indeed of the human race.

—Roger Bacon

Few more critical problems face nursing today than the paucity in numbers and the nature of the preparation of scientists and researchers in nursing. Without such persons education and practice in nursing must fail to advance and nursing will cease to fulfill its commitment to human welfare.

"Research" is a glowing word in our society. Third graders look up words in the dictionary and call it research. Clerks tabulate long lists of figures and call it research. Nurses collect multiple specimens of urine and call it research. The public views the technological wonders that speed man's journey, relieve his boredom, foster his comfort, add years to his life, and that are beginning to replace his old organs with new . . . and is unbelievably willing to support all manner of proposals providing they are clothed in the magic term "research."

The most mundane and mediocre of accomplishments parade under this prestigious sounding term. Enthusiasm and a research attitude are mistaken for substantial knowledge and creative conceptualization. Nurses, unequipped with scholarly knowledge and tools, attempt to wring professional recognition out of multiplying numbers of trivial investigations.

While one may expect that all professionally educated nurses (meaning no less than a valid baccalaureate degree education with an upper division major in nursing) will initiate and exploit knowledge for the enhancement of

Rogers, M. E. (1964). Editorial. *Nursing Science, 2,* 379–380. Reprinted with permission.

nursing practice, such persons possess neither the knowledge nor the tools necessary for true research. Master's degree programs extend nursing knowledge and the tools of study. These graduates are properly expected to be able to identify and resolve more complex problems and to exploit knowledge with greater sophistication than will baccalaureate degree graduates. Independent scholarly research and peer participation in interdisciplinary and interprofessional investigations justifying the appellation "research" require doctoral degree preparation that moves the student further into the complexities of nursing science and supplies essential methodology and tools not previously included.

Ignorance of the meaning of true research, a long standing task-oriented tradition, too frequent derogation of scholarly learning, and an almost pathological dependency on other groups are self-defeating. Would-be scientists and researchers in nursing whose doctoral study prepares them to be psychologists or sociologists, physicists or physiologists, or statisticians are severely handicapped by the narrowness and inadequacy of their preparation for productive research in nursing—the study of the life process in MAN. Research in nursing and the development of nursing science languishes in spite of fine intentions.

Nurses who lack broad knowledge, superior conceptual capacity, and the ability to far transcend Poincaré's "heap of stones" will not evolve the unifying principles and hypothetical generalizations which constitute the core of professional education in nursing. Nor can society afford Jacques Barzun's "cults of science, research, and creativity" so well illustrated by nursing: in the application of dollars to maintain mediocrity, in enthusing praise of superficiality, and in support of impoverished and shallow ideas.

We must cease advising the unqualified and unable that all nurses should do research. We must cease looking to other disciplines for pat answers in nursing. Researchers in other disciplines may study nurses ad infinitum to test theories in their own fields but they do not possess the knowledges necessary to develop and test theories in nursing. Only nurses, highly qualified and competent, creative and intelligent, can create the conceptual base, develop the ideas and theories, and implement scholarly research in nursing. Only as nurses are competent in research in their own field can they be peer participants in developing creative ideas which integrate the knowledges of a variety of fields.

True researchers in nursing will contribute far beyond their numbers and without their contributions leaping obsolescence will increasingly endanger the lives of those we purport to serve. Excuses and dilatory tactics are dangerous substitutes for responsible, decisive action.

CHAPTER 12

Editorial

Martha E. Rogers

Recent legislative action has provided monies to perpetuate increasingly dangerous obsolescence through funneling dollars from Washington into demonstrably inadequate patterns of education in nursing. Society, potential students of nursing, and nurses are critically penalized while those who try to hold back the hands of time fight a battle already lost.

We are living in a new era: one as critically different from the industrial age as the industrial age was from the agricultural era that preceded it. But whereas the agricultural revolution lasted more than 8,000 years, the industrial revolution was a short 200 years. Today's socioeconomic order—the age of cybernation—is a matter of a decade.

Machine techniques and skills are already in advance of man's educational achievements. The nationwide thrust of the community college movement, the philosophy underlying the National Manpower Training and Development Act, and the National Science Foundation's support of multiple projects designed to raise the quality and level of education from kindergarten through college and university are but a few of the many forces already at work to provide education consistent with today's world.

And the moment of truth is coming for nurses—far sooner than most people realize. Only educational institutions possess the resources that can prepare for the future. Every effort must be made to develop these resources to their maximum and to use them honestly in the education of nurses. Perpetuation of hospital schools beyond the most urgent need to span today's rapid transition is more than a disservice. It is tragic disregard for the society we purport to serve. It is selfish unconcern for the students we recruit. And the efforts of some hospital schools to disguise their outdatedness through the subterfuge of using a community college association to signify something it doesn't is also unfortunate.

Nursing's unemployables of the next decade are being trained today because nurses have had neither the courage nor the vision to face reality and to

Rogers, M. E. (1964). Editorial. *Nursing Science, 2,* 462–463. Reprinted with permission.

take the drastic steps essential to create the indispensable changes that must be made. Vested interests distort the truth and perpetuate misconceptions.

Legislators and the public are dependent on knowledgeable, forward-looking leadership in nursing for sound direction. Nursing's failure to present a united front that takes cognizance of changing times and is more concerned with the public good than with the status quo is only too well known.

Society cannot afford a sentimental view of nursing education and practice. Else the horror stories will increase and the unemployables will multiply. The American Hospital Association's role in negating sound legislation for nursing through short-sighted action and misinformation is deplorable. That nurses would sacrifice the social good for "peace at such a price" cannot continue. Nurses are no less committed to the ideal of human service today than they have ever been. But commitment must be made explicit in concerted action.

Sound legislation at that uses the taxpayer's money wisely and honestly demands intelligent, aggressive action by nurses and by the citizenry. Where will we be when the 89th Congress meets next year?

CHAPTER 13

For Public Safety: Higher Education's Responsibility for Professional Education in Nursing

Martha E. Rogers

That there is critical need for professionally educated nurses to coordinate with learned professional personnel in other fields should need no belaboring. Documentation and recommendations for its accomplishment abound. Public safety demands it and humanitarian values support it. Institutions of higher learning are indispensable to its achievement.

Time has kaleidoscoped with sweeping advances in science and technology. The status quo is ephemeral and quickly lost so rapid are the innovations that crowd our doorsteps. Preparation of professionally educated nurses for the world of tomorrow—already upon us—demands a vision of the future: a vision that extends and strengthens nursing's long commitment to human service and that will not be dissipated by loyalty to petrified opinion.

Experience is no longer a substitute for learning—if it ever was. Compassion for the human predicament dictates knowledgeable performance by those who would provide and guide professional practice in any field. This is no less true for nursing than for any other learned discipline.

The nation's colleges and universities carry a signal responsibility for providing the learned men and women to whom a contemporary society looks for leadership (albeit sometimes fearfully). Changing values are reflected in growing amounts of tax monies in support of higher education. Expanding college enrollments, by no means altogether attributable to social pressures and em-

Rogers, M. E. (1969). For public safety: Higher education's responsibility for professional education in nursing. *Hartwick Review, 5,* pp. 21–26. Reprinted with permission.

ployment demands, are further evidence of man's insatiable curiosity for the knowable and the unknown. Youth is demanding relevance in its struggle to be heard.

Rapid expansion of educational opportunities at all levels testifies to massive, on-going efforts to conserve and enhance the nation's intellectual potential and to insure future productivity of youth. Second graders are studying measurement, prediction, and inference. Junior high school students are happily gathering hypotheses for their science projects. The community college movement reflects technological advances that require fourteen (14) years of education for a person to compete with a machine. Demands abound for adult education opportunities. In every instance stress is placed on emphasizing general education and on de-emphasizing specific job skills. For as Alfred North Whitehead noted more than thirty-five (35) years ago "a properly trained worker can pick up specific job skills in no time."

Full colleges and universities are faced with further clarifying their philosophy and purposes. Conservation, transmission, and advancement of knowledge are taking on new dimensions germane to the future. Undergraduate and graduate schools of the arts and sciences, core of the higher learning, are undergoing critical scrutiny. Professional schools, except as they are relevant to the future, will be eliminated. Innovation is the order of the day though many have yet to grasp its full implications. Rearranging tradition cannot be mistaken for creative educational development.

Long cherished assumptions about man and his world are fast becoming antiquated. The higher learning, whether in the arts and sciences or in professional schools, must be directed toward preparing youth for a world not yet imagined. Broad knowledge, fundamental principles, capacity to perceive and use knowledge in novel ways—these things must characterize those who graduate from our colleges and universities. Equally relevant is McGlothlin's point that "history makes clear that professional schools began to improve as the use of practitioner teachers diminished."[1]

Faced with growing public demand and the high cost of higher education, tax supported institutions are increasing their enrollments. Competition for qualified faculty is acute. Private institutions are facing a dollar crisis only partly relieved by allocation of tax monies, predominantly in support of research.

Not only is financing of higher education of grave concern but professional schools are notably even more costly than general education. Yet it is the professional schools that must provide the nation's lawyers and theologians, dentists and medical doctors, engineers, clinical psychologists, professional nurses, and professional personnel in a range of fields. An institution's commitment to professional education is of itself a commitment to social welfare as demanding as its commitment to other areas of the higher learning. This is not to propose that all colleges and universities need provide professional education. Rather it is to make clear that colleges and universities have a direct responsibility for providing professional schools adequate in number and quality to meet the needs of society.

The critical responsibility carried by colleges and universities for the preparation of professionally educated nurses is manifest. In fulfilling this responsibility colleges and universities must maintain their integrity as institutions of higher learning and concomitantly guarantee the integrity of the professional schools of nursing. Professional education in nursing is as substantial as professional education in law, engineering, medicine, dentistry and other such fields. The educational unit in nursing must be coordinate with other schools and colleges within a university. The faculty in nursing, consistent with the overall philosophy and purposes of the institution of higher learning in which the nursing unit is located, must hold professional autonomy in determining the nature of the professional curriculums, the theoretical content and clinical learnings to be transmitted in the nursing major, the purposes for which this knowledge is to be used, the selection of its students, and the determination of standards by which the excellence of the educational programs will be measured. This is equally true of both undergraduate and graduate programs in nursing. Anything less than full professional responsibility by qualified nurse faculty denies academic freedom and perpetuates fraud upon the unwary and unknowing, who, seeking professional education in nursing, find themselves caught in an amorphous ambiguity of power struggles, conflicting purposes, and impoverished learning.

Colleges and universities must demand excellence and encourage imaginative innovation. They are responsible to the students they recruit for guaranteeing that a baccalaureate education is a concomitant of the baccalaureate degree which the graduates will be granted (and similarly for graduate education and graduate degrees in nursing).

True professional education in nursing is of relatively recent vintage though verbal and written protestations that nursing is a profession abound. The term "profession" has been used so loosely, so long, by nurses that its ambiguity is a major problem. At the same time discussion of the role of institutions of higher learning in professional education in nursing presupposes a common understanding of the terminology used.

Nursing is a learned profession. This does not mean that all nurses either are or should be professional workers. It does mean that by definition, nursing as a learned profession has a range of distinguishing characteristics in common with other learned professions.

The inseparability of professional education and the higher learning is noted widely in the literature. Such education is an integral part of full colleges and universities. Howard S. Becker in discussing "The Nature of a Profession" has written, "Professions, as commonly conceived, are occupations which possess a monopoly of some esoteric and difficult body of knowledge. The body of knowledge over which the profession holds a monopoly consists not of technical skills and the fruits of practical experience but, rather, of abstract principles arrived at by scientific research and logical analysis."[2]

Hall and Thompson have noted that "In medicine, law, or engineering practitioners possess skills not held by laymen, but possession of scarce skills is not enough to distinguish professions from other occupations. The master plumber, or printer, the watchmaker, and the airline pilot possess skills not generally held by laymen, but they are seldom regarded as professions. What distinguishes the obvious professions from other skilled occupations is that the skills of the professional are derived from abstract knowledge of cause-and-effect relationships, or theory."[3]

The distinguishing characteristics of professional education in nursing is the transmission of nursing's body of abstract principles arrived at by scientific research and logical analysis—not a body of technical skills. This is not to deny the importance of technical skill but rather to make clear that it is nursing's theoretical knowledge that identifies nursing as a profession. It is the utilization of this knowledge in service to people that determines the nature of nursing services. It is this body of knowledge that encompasses nursing's descriptive, explanatory, and predictive principles which guide its practitioners and make possible professional practice: a fulfillment of nursing's scientific humanitarianism.

The preparation of professional practitioners in nursing is speeding up—in large part a reflection of leap-frogging scientific and technological advances and changing values. So rapid is the speed of change that George S. Counts has commented that "as our feet tread the earth of a new world our heads continue to dwell in the past."[4]

The world of reality is forcing educational change. Already it has been proposed that with the installation of automated equipment in hospitals nurses will have as much as 40% more time to spend with patients. (One might also note the 50% time saving that would increase patient care hours if nurses ceased engaging in non-nursing activities.) Microsensors are monitoring temperature, pulse, respiration, and blood-pressure. Soon wireless monitoring devices will be on the market. Pacemakers may be controlled from a central station and stand-by systems worn like wristwatches. Pills containing micro-TV cameras can be expected to transmit pictures of the digestive tract. Space hospitals are nearing the launching pad. It has been proposed that, as well as caring for space travellers and serving as space quarantine centers, such hospitals might well provide therapeutic environments for conditions such as those involving cardiac pathology and emotional disturbances. The capacity of orbiting hospitals to provide varying levels of gravity will add further dimensions to the armamentarium of intervention and health promotion.

Central computers are linking together community health and welfare agencies as personnel feed data into a common storage system. Planning and implementation of health and welfare services take on vastly new dimensions when a telephone system makes possible retrieval of significant data in moments.

Changing values about man's responsibility to man are being translated into law. The public is demanding social and health services of a nature and quality clearly beyond that currently available. Meanwhile automation threatens man's privacy. The immorality of human experimentation without informed consent of the individual has become a national issue. Power struggles are reminiscent of Ardrey's *Territorial Imperatives.*

But machines and technology are not a substitute for people. Rather their impact is in the change they generate in the kinds of jobs that must be done; in the differences in the nature and amounts of knowledge needed to do the jobs, not just tomorrow but today: a task that must be dealt with by higher education and by nursing as well as by others.

A profession exists for social ends. Its direct responsibility is to the people it purports to serve. This takes precedence over all other relationships. The nursing profession exists to serve society. It does not exist to serve the ends of another profession. Nursing, as a learned profession, has no dependent functions. It, like all other professions, has many collaborative functions—indispensable to providing society with a higher order of service than any one profession can offer. Nor does one profession delegate anything to another profession. Each profession is responsible for determining its own boundaries within the context of social need.

Nursing is concerned with people—all people—of whom only a segment is ill. A nation's first line of defense in building a healthy people lies in maintenance and promotion of health. Any society that concentrates its health dollars and its health services on care of the sick will never be a healthy society. There is critical need for a concept of community "health services" to transcend the all too common concept of "sick services." This is not to suggest that care of sick is unimportant. Rather the sick reflect our failures in promoting and maintaining health. The sick do need nursing services and in reality consume the largest number of nursing hours.

No one group holds the key to human health and welfare. Dramatic revisions in the education, roles, and responsibilities of health personnel are in the making. New fields are emerging. There is no such person as "the nurse."

The complexity of knowledge and skill required to safeguard the recipients of nursing services today has made mandatory a concept of nursing as a 'learned profession' and the identification of professionally educated nurses clearly distinct from those whose preparation is technical or vocational in nature. Baccalaureate curriculums are being built and re-built to provide professional education as this is understood in our country. Associate degree nursing programs are rapidly replacing hospital schools. Only educational institutions provide the resources and learning indispensable to the preparation of either professional nurses or nursing technicians in modern society. Planned transition is beginning to replace the planned chaos still propagated by vested interests in nursing, hospitals, and medicine.

The evolution of professional education in nursing is directly related to the identification of nursing's theoretical base. Nursing is concerned with human beings—specifically the life process in man. Nursing's body of scientific knowledge seeks to describe, explain, and predict about this life process. The phenomenon at the center of nursing's purpose is a unified whole; more than and different from the sum of its parts. A description of biological man, or psychological man no more describes MAN than a description of hydrogen describes water. Nor does a summation of these add up to MAN.

If one asked a biologist "What is biology?" and he responded "It is the study of the biological world" this answer might be less complete than one wanted but neither would one expect him to give a complete picture of biological science in a paragraph or even in a year. Moreover, one would no doubt be aware that biological principles of today may not hold true tomorrow. For example, the conventional meanings of concepts like homeostasis, adaptation, and steady-state are demonstrably antiquated.[5] New terms are being introduced such as homeokinesis. The science of nursing is concerned with homeodynamics.

Nursing's science—its system of concepts—is acquired by reasoning. It seeks to push back the frontiers of knowledge and those who seek to push back frontiers must have come close to those frontiers themselves. Nursing science is *not* a summation of facts and principles drawn from the basic sciences and other disciplines. It is a new product. It encompasses nursing's scientific principles that guide nursing practice.

Baccalaureate degree education in nursing is the cornerstone of nursing's educational system. Its one essential tie is with the college of arts and sciences in the institution of higher learning in which the college of nursing is located. The central focus of baccalaureate education in nursing is direct nursing services to people—all people wherever they may be. Baccalaureate degree graduates constitute nursing's hard core of professional practitioners. These graduates must assume increasing responsibility for themselves and for appropriate guidance of registered nurse graduates of associate degree programs and hospital schools, practical nurses and auxiliary workers. Graduates of baccalaureate degree programs are the source of graduate students in nursing; the future clinical specialists, supervisors, teachers, and researchers.

Nursing needs not only professionally educated personnel but it is also in great need of that large body of registered nurses possessing equally excellent preparation for technical practice. Technical education in nursing (just as in other fields) differs from professional education in the amount and scope of knowledge and responsibility appropriate to each. Technical education is of junior college level. The uniquely significant role of educational institutions in providing the liberal foundation and specialized training indispensable in today's world makes explicit the dangerous obsolescence of apprentice-type programs no matter how modified. Nor do the wide range of various relationships developed by many hospital schools with educational institutions do more than provide a stop-gap to bridge transition. Hospital schools do not become college programs whether associate degree or baccalaureate. Hospital schools prepare their graduates for the *same career* in nursing as do associate degree programs. As sound associate degree programs have developed there is extensive evidence that this results in more registered nurses, better prepared to meet the demands of today and tomorrow. Technical education is not the first part of professional education. It is complete in itself. It prepares for a career worthy of honor in itself. Its products are entitled to respect for the knowledge they possess and the services they are equipped to render.

For years nurses have been asking what is the difference between what baccalaureate graduates (professional) do and what hospital and associate degree nursing graduates (technical) do. And when one asks the wrong questions one of course gets the wrong answer. The difference between the two groups lies in what each knows. It is the body of knowledge possessed by each group that differentiates the practice of each group. Nor is this a derogation of hospital school and associate degree graduates. Hospital school and associate degree graduates have every right to be proud of the career they have chosen and to seek excellence in their practice.

For the small percentage of hospital school and associate degree graduates in nursing who decide to change their career goal professional education in nursing is available in full colleges and universities. Such students are not going back. Such students have never had professional education in nursing. Transfer college credit is properly granted these applicants on the same basis as for any other student. Courses taken previously are evaluated for their equivalence in scope, level, and content to the courses for which substitution is requested. Acceptable completion of college work must be testified to by a regular college transcript. Courses taken in a hospital school and taught by a faculty member from a nearby college are generally not the equivalent of college courses and as such are not properly acceptable for transfer college credit. Associate degree nursing programs do include general education courses for which transfer college credit may be granted. The nursing courses taken in hospital schools and associate degree programs are not the equivalent in scope, level, and content to upper division professional nursing courses and are not therefore properly accepted for advanced standing or transfer college credit.

While we can expect that there may always be a few nurses who change their career goals every effort should be made to assist potential students of nursing to select the right career and right program in the beginning. Honest recruitment, clearly explaining the different careers in nursing is urgent. It is morally reprehensible to recruit into associate degree nursing programs and hospital schools those whose abilities and goals are consistent with professional education and practice. The numbers of angry young people who leave nursing disillusioned and disappointed might then be decreased. What intellectual wastelands do we sow when professionally educable young people are recruited into technical programs? Nursing's professional and technical career choices must be presented honestly without the equivocation and misinformation inherent in talk of 'types of programs'—an evasion of reality that might be labelled 'Games Vested Interests Play'. Nursing offers preparation for two careers: professional and technical. Slowness to apply clearly different criteria in evaluating professionally educated practitioners and technically educated practitioners is a further source of confusion. Differentiating licensure is long over-due. Society has a right to be guaranteed a minimum level of professional practice as well as the present licensure for the R.N. level of practice.

The nature and levels of education and practice in nursing must be geared to mushrooming revisions in all areas of American life. All nurses must seek learning and re-learning for themselves consistent with the career in nursing they have chosen and consistent with the level of practice for which they are prepared. Perpetuation of out-dated patterns of preparing nurses beyond the shortest possible time necessary to provide preparation for all nurses in educational institutions could make its own contribution to the nation's unemployables. This is equally true for out-dated programs offered in educational institutions.

The education of nursing's technical and professional practitioners will not exceed the quality of the nurse faculty. The 1967 Edition of the ANA *Facts About Nursing* reports that one-fourth of the nurses teaching in hospital schools do not themselves possess undergraduate college education. By what alchemy, then, can they purport to be teaching anything at a college level. By comparison approximately 70% of nurses teaching in associate degree programs in nursing possess a master's or higher degree. Concomitantly, every one of the United States has a law requiring a college degree for public school teachers.

Preparation for full college and university teaching is at the doctoral level. Bernard Berelson has pointed out that "The Master's degree . . . cannot be retained as the acceptable degree for college teachers." Concomitantly, the 1967 Edition of the ANA *Facts About Nursing* reports that although 88% of baccalaureate degree faculty are reported to hold master's or higher degrees only 6.4% of these have completed a doctoral degree. What fallacies do we perpetuate when we grant baccalaureate degrees in the absence of baccalaureate education? The implications for graduate education are equally serious. Nonetheless there are those who are party to an increase in the numbers of baccalaureate degree and graduate programs in the absence of even minimally qualified faculty and further dangerously dilute the numbers of qualified persons available.

Colleges and universities must carry their own weight of guilt to the extent they contribute to mushrooming numbers of schools and programs and the dilution of numbers of qualified faculty with subsequent second and third rate education that foolishly equates numbers with quality.

Nurse educators are equally guilty. Too frequently excuses and dilatory tactics are used to evade responsibility. Value systems defaming scholarly achievement coupled with substitution of prestigious sounding mediocrity for substantial achievement in creative endeavor have also delayed responsible concern for scholarly learning among nurse educators.

Of further consequence is the failure of many to recognize society's needs and to comprehend nursing as a learned profession. The dead-end aspects for nursing science (and ultimately public safety) of the would-be scholar, scientist, and researcher in nursing whose doctoral study prepares her to be a psychologist or sociologist, a physicist or physiologist, or statistician are more than unfortunate. Such persons are severely handicapped by the irrelevance and inadequacy of their preparation for productive, scholarly work in nursing. Their potential for contribution to the elaboration of nursing's science languishes in spite of fine intentions.

Nursing's practitioners are the products of nursing's educational system. An unwitting public is being victimized by the addition of massive numbers of minimally skilled workers to care for patients at the same time that hospital and associate degree registered nurse graduates are forced by an obsolete system to spend one-half their time in non-nursing activities which could well be done by lesser prepared persons. Concomitantly professionally educated practitioners coming out of valid baccalaureate degree programs in nursing are not only spending much time in non-nursing activities but they are also frequently denied opportunity to practice at the level of their preparation and to provide the knowledgeable judgement indispensable to safe nursing services (and beyond the ken of technical practitioners). Professional and technical nurses are not interchangeable. Hospital school and associate degree graduates are no more comparable to baccalaureate degree graduates than dental hygienists are comparable to dentists.

Employing agencies must take immediate steps to recognize career differences in employment practices. The professionally educated nurse—meaning valid baccalaureate graduate—must have freedom to use her knowledge and skills for human betterment. Her greater responsibility must carry tangible evidence in the granting of appropriate authority and in salary differential.

The emergence of professional education and practice in nursing is an expression of nursing's history, a recognition of changing times, and a vision of the future. Change in nursing is a reality. Bernard Baruch's comment that "every man has a right to his opinions but no man should be wrong about his facts," needs heeding; so too, does Whitehead's comment that, "Where attainable knowledge could have changed the issue, ignorance has the guilt of vice."

Colleges and universities have the same responsibility for professional education in nursing that they have for professional education in any other field. They are liable for the educational programs they offer and for the validity of the degrees they grant. They are responsible for maintaining their integrity as institutions of higher learning and for supporting excellence in the professional education of nurses no less than for any other professional program.

They must guarantee academic freedom to the faculty in nursing and must be forthright in their expectations of professional responsibility. At the same time nurse faculties must recognize that academic responsibility goes hand in hand with academic privilege.

Except as institutions of higher learning meet their responsibility for supporting valid professional education in nursing public safety is jeopardized and community health services impoverished. A society which purports to value health cannot afford nursing judgements which are not based on the substantial learning available only in colleges and universities.

College and university faculties in nursing are charged specifically with providing professional education in nursing commensurate with the degree to be granted. They constitute an integral part of the higher education. They are directly responsible for the development, implementation, and interpretation of a philosophy of professional education in nursing. The professional faculty in nursing must represent a community of scholars. Unless they do they cannot purport to offer professional education in nursing nor to fulfill their responsibility to the institution of higher learning, nor their responsibility to the students they recruit and the public that is ultimately served.

Contemporary nursing is a major social force. It is continually molding and being molded by the culture in which it exists. Man's capacity for initiating change is also the capacity of nurses for envisioning the future and determining sound direction in the great task of building a healthy society.

References

1. McGlothlin, William, *Patterns of Professional Education.* New York: G. P. Putnam's Sons. 1960.
2. Becker, Howard S., "The Nature of a Profession," *Education for the Professions.* The Sixty-first Yearbook of the National Society for the Study of Education, Part II. Chicago, Ill.: The University of Chicago Press. 1962.
3. Hall, R. D., and Thompson, J. D., "What Do You Mean Business Is a Profession?," *Business Horizons.* Vol. 7, No. 1, Spring 1964.
4. Counts, George S., "The Impact of Technological Change," *The Planning of Change.* New York: Holt, Rinehart and Winston. 1962. p. 21.
5. Shaefer, Karl (Editor), *Man's Dependence on the Earthly Atmosphere.* New York: The Macmillan Co. 1962.
6. Rogers, Martha E., *Reveille in Nursing.* Philadelphia: F. A. Davis Publishers. 1964.

CHAPTER 14

Graduate Education in Nursing at New York University

Martha E. Rogers

No system can endure that does not march.
—Florence Nightingale

For nearly 40 years New York University, through the educational unit in nursing in the School of Education, has offered programs of study for nurses leading to undergraduate and graduate degrees. Until the middle 1950s these programs, like all other programs for nurses across the United States, focused predominantly on providing management skills and teaching methods. Nurses were identified according to employing agency (ie, hospital nurse, public health nurse, school nurse, and so on) and courses purporting to be in nursing generally dealt with how to be a supervisor, administrator, counselor, or teacher in hospital, public health agency, school, and so on.

Undergraduate upper division courses in nursing (in contrast to courses dealing with functions of nurses) did not really begin to emerge until after 1950, spurred on by Brown's *Nursing for the Future,* the Ginsberg Report, and Bridgman's *Collegiate Education in Nursing.* Initiation of community college programs in nursing (which are today rapidly replacing hospital schools throughout the nation) brought into sharp focus major fallacies in baccalaureate degree programs, forcing re-examination of the philosophy, purposes, and content of baccalaureate education in nursing. As baccalaureate programs began to incorporate more complex learnings and to increase the scope and depth of their offerings graduate programs for nurses began to take on new characteristics.

In 1957 the National League for Nursing Council of Baccalaureate and Higher Degree Programs published "Guidelines for Master's Degree Programs in Nursing," reflecting changes already then under way in a number of col-

Rogers, M. E. (1970, October). *Graduate education in nursing at New York University.* Unpublished manuscript, New York University, Division of Nursing, New York.

leges and universities and setting in motion many revisions in M.A. programs throughout the United States.

At New York University the faculty in the Division of Nurse Education had already (prior to the guidelines) incorporated majors in nursing as an integral part of the program leading to an M.A. degree. Course sequences in medical-surgical nursing, psychiatric–mental health nursing, parent-child nursing, and public health nursing provided students with advanced knowledge in these speciality areas within the framework of the graduate program. Subsequently a graduate major in cancer nursing was initiated—to be discontinued 3 years later. Two additional nursing majors were added which still continue, namely: rehabilitation nursing and nursing in child psychiatry.

As nursing sought with diligence to make explicit its rightful place within the nation's system of higher education, undergraduate and graduate faculties in nursing were forced to examine the nature and level of instruction that would justify inclusion of nurse education within the framework of colleges and universities. Apprentice training, no matter how modified, could not be equated with college education. Experience could no longer be deemed a substitute for learning. Recognition that the identification and development of a body of substantive nursing knowledge was essential to continuing viability of higher education in nursing emerged and began to grow.

In 1955 the Division of Nurse Education admitted its first associate degree nursing graduate to baccalaureate degree study and concomitantly initiated critical examination of the division's undergraduate and graduate programs. The graduate programs underwent significant revisions. Nursing majors (as indicated earlier) were established. Functional minors were retained and both were encompassed within the broad philosophy and purposes of graduate education developed by the faculty. It is worth noting that students participated in these developments—a practice that has been continuous in the division for many years.

At the same time that these changes were taking place, the division also embarked on the long-range task of trying to identify and develop a body of scientific knowledge specific to nursing. Faculty committees, workshops, and seminars were instituted. Three doctoral candidates, in a joint effort, focused their dissertations on trying to evolve principles of nursing with two outcomes. First, they all secured their doctoral degrees, and second, it was evident that the approach which they used (an approach which interestingly enough was also being suggested by nurses in other places) would not provide the theoretical base nursing sorely needed.

Many blind alleys were explored. Difficulties in thinking in terms of broad principles in contrast to nursing's tradition of dealing with facts and rules of procedure sometimes blocked progress. Nonetheless direction was maintained and the bare bones of potentially productive ideas began to accumulate flesh and blood.

Before 1960 these ideas, though still embryonic, were already being incorporated into the doctoral program. Doctoral research began to focus on human beings rather than on nurses and their functions. Research findings began to appear that could later take on new and enlarged meanings as they would become lodged within an organized conceptual system.

A logical plan for incorporating nursing's emerging body of abstract knowledge into the instructional process was evident. Quite properly this had been initiated first in the doctoral program. The elaboration of a body of abstract knowledge is dependent on scientists and scholars, in whatever the given field, for its accomplishment.

The baccalaureate degree program—the core of nursing's education system—provides the foundation on which graduate study builds. Sound articulation between baccalaureate, master's, and doctoral programs is inherent in the philosophy and purposes of higher education. The development of substantive baccalaureate level education for learned professional practice in nursing as this is understood in our society constituted the next step in transition.

In 1964 a basic baccalaureate curriculum providing a liberal foundation and based on broad scientific principles specific to nursing was established. High school graduates, transfer college students, college graduates seeking preparation for a professional career in nursing, and registered nurse hospital and associate degree graduates whose career goals were now directed toward professional education in nursing were admitted to study. The performance of graduates of this program (though the number is still small) provides a strong evidence of the validity of the nursing science base and its relevance for professional practice in nursing and for social betterment.

In 1967 the third step in incorporating these knowledges into the division's educational programs was put into motion. Through a one-semester course (already in the curriculum but now revised) the philosophy, principles, and theories of nursing science were introduced and implications for nursing practice indicated. An ad hoc committee of the faculty participated actively in designing this course and a number of the faculty participated in various ways in its instruction. Student evaluations of this course were considered carefully in its evolution. The extent to which this foundation (for it was so designed) has been built upon as students have pursued study in their selected areas of concentration in nursing has varied. *The curriculum revisions being discussed now had their inception some 15 years ago.* They constitute a logical outgrowth of continuing and uninterrupted effort and concern that the education of our students at all levels shall encompass the best we know how to offer.

Today's events add a further dimension to the nature of curriculum changes that must take place. Present and predictable realities speak loudly to Robert Hutchin's statement that ". . . the most practical education is the most theoretical one." (*The Learning Society.* New York: Frederick A. Praeger, Publishers. 1968. p. 8). Alvin Toffler in *Future Shock* speaks clearly to a future already here and demanding substantive innovation of a nature scarcely yet imagined.

In the real world, newspapers, articles, books, speeches, legislative hearings, and public demonstrations bear active testimony to the irrelevance, inadequacy, and impoverishment of health services and health resources. Human safety is *daily* jeopardized by professional incompetence and social irresponsibility among vested interests in hospitals, medicine, and nursing. A Chicago court, this year, ruled the registered nurse and the hospital criminally negligent as well as the medical doctor whose specific negligence resulted in the amputation of a child's leg. Why? Because although the nurse and the hospital had notified the medical doctor more than once of the situation neither the registered nurse nor the hospital had taken overt action to prevent the outcomes.

Statistical data provide demonstrable evidence that the United States is by no means the healthiest nation on this planet. Maternal and infant death rates in the United States exceed those of a number of other countries (some of which countries are deemed "underdeveloped"). Persons on waiting lists for admission to psychiatric clinics have as high recovery rates as do those admitted to care. So-called extended care facilities and so-called community health centers are generally limited to narrowly conceived sick services by medical doctors and *do not provide health services* which require the range of professional personnel for their provision.

The public is demanding health services of a nature and amount not yet even imagined. And the public is increasingly intolerant of irrelevant and miniscule modifications of traditional patterns and practices regardless of the health field involved.

The nature of professional education commensurate with massive changes in all aspects of contemporary life is equally subject to criticism. New cosmologies are emerging to explain better the nature of man and his becoming. Many traditional methods of teaching are not only financially untenable but they are notably outmoded. Technological advances provide instructional tools of major import. Third-graders are learning things today that only a decade ago were reserved for college students. New knowledges are rapidly making obsolete many cherished beliefs—scientific and otherwise.

Nursing cannot afford to exemplify Counts' comment that ". . . as our feet tread the earth of a new world our heads continue to dwell in the past." ("The Impact of Technological Change," *The Planning of Change.* New York: Holt, Rinehart, and Winston. 1961. p. 21). Continuing education for all nurses must be stepped up. Educational programs must be designed to prepare students for the world of tomorrow. Unless we in nursing have the courage and imagination to take the necessary steps, nursing will contribute its own share of unemployables to the future. This is not said to frighten anyone but it *is* said to make clear that not only is change inevitable but we must also exercise our capacity for initiating, directing, and implementing change—with vision and with fortitude.

As the nation stands on the threshold of major governmental, political, and economic unrest, the financial problems that have long beset higher education have become critical. State governments have been forced to buy out private colleges and universities and are finding themselves with physical plants they do not have adequate dollars to staff and operate. Some states have built new plants without adequate consideration of or provision for operating expenses—the primary item of which is faculty salaries. The City University of New York system is faced with having to deal with a new open admissions policy at the same time that economics is forcing a decrease in the number of faculty. Tax monies come from the people, and although we may and often do disagree with the ways in which governmental bodies allocate public funds (and rightly so), nonetheless there are realistic limits to public financial liability.

New York University has a sizable dollar deficit and other major universities face even larger deficits. Actual operating costs are approximately double tuition income, and foundations are no longer the ready source they used to be. Endowments are more difficult to secure and only innovative and forward-looking proposals stand a chance of significant funding from such sources.

Budgets must be balanced. Education must be improved. Faculty salaries must be increased commensurate with a competitive market. More students must be served. Man's humanness must be preserved and his capacity for creative development enhanced amidst the inroads of technology. Respect for human differences must find its way into the nation's value system. Achieving this diverse set of objectives demands a clearly new approach to higher and professional education—to what we teach and to how we teach it.

McConnell, Anderson, and Hunter have stated quite specifically that "the university is justified in asking that the professional school emphasize the theoretical foundations of professional practice; that a fundamental body of scholarly knowledge should be the core of professional education and that acquisition of skills and techniques should be a secondary, if necessary, concern." ("The University and Professional Education," *Education for the Professions.* The Sixty-first Yearbook of the National Society for the Study of Education, Part II. Chicago: The University of Chicago Press. 1962. p. 259). Not long ago I had a high ranking officer in the military nurse corps say to me (and to some others who were present) that the intelligent young graduate of a baccalaureate program in nursing who possessed a substantial knowledge base could pick up skills in no time. Her concern was that they have the knowledge base. There is *no* evidence that multiple hours of laboratory experience results in a better professional practitioner. On the contrary there is a great deal of evidence that given a substantial theoretical base the integration of learnings in the clinical setting can take place in far less time than is often supposed. This is *not* a suggestion to do away with all laboratory courses. But that better graduate education can be achieved with greater emphasis on nursing's theoretical base and with fewer laboratory hours than currently exist here finds extensive support in the literature and in the real world.

The high cost of professional education is directly related to the high cost of laboratory courses. Further a disproportionate emphasis on laboratory hours is closely related to the apprentice origins of such education and—true to American pragmatism—tends to deny the value of theory. Polanyi's statement that "Almost every major systematic error which has deluded men for thousands of years relied on practical experience" (*Personal Knowledge.* Chicago: The University of Chicago Press. 1958. p. 183) should be noted.

Equally fallacious is the old idea of a teacher on one end of the log and the student on the other end. Education is considerably more than a dialogue. Multiple methods of transmitting knowledge are available. And just as research is not dependent on rats and laboratory coats for its pursuit, neither are many of these methods dependent on expensive machinery and highly specialized technical personnel for their conduct.

The faculty in the Division of Nurse Education is charged with evolving and implementing the transmission of knowledge to students that human beings may be better served. Curriculum development, evaluation, revision, and innovation are integral responsibilities of all college and university faculty. These are continuous, ongoing activities that never cease. The evolution of graduate education in this division is a continuous process. That what is going on here has meaning for other nurse-educators finds substantiation in the fact that in the past two years consultation has been provided to one or more colleges and universities in more than half of each of these United States, the District of Columbia, and a number of foreign countries.

Faculty must be responsive to the needs of students and to the needs of society and at the same time maintain the integrity of the higher learning and fulfill their responsibilities for the preservation, transmission, and advancement of knowledge. They must possess the vision to see deeply into the future, to plan wisely for change, and to dare to be innovative. These are difficult tasks and require the concerted efforts of many, including students.

Nursing is in the throes of rapid change. In a period of transition, retention of the present areas of major concentration in nursing coupled with an underlying foundation in the theoretical basis of nursing provides a bridge to future change. And be assured, after graduation, no matter where you are or what you may be doing, you will face immediacy in your own responsibility for evolving further change. *No* proposal has been made to discontinue the present graduate majors at this point in time. But any idea that the traditional majors in nursing are here to stay is a denial of reality. Their denouement has already begun in a number of educational institutions, and new areas of concentration in nursing are being initiated.

The functions of nurses with graduate preparation are in an equally great state of flux. For decades nurses have administered and supervised things and rules. Only as baccalaureate and graduate education in *nursing itself* began to emerge was there a move toward administering and supervising nursing. Even today the majority of nurses holding administrative and supervisory positions have no knowledge in nursing beyond that secured in a hospital school and this is true as well for many of those who hold baccalaureate and master's degrees. There are those who propose that advanced education in nursing is unnecessary for the nursing service administrator and supervisor. If this is true, one might equally well ask, "Need this person be a nurse?" In view of the present level and quality of nursing services, to propose that one does not need advanced knowledge in nursing in order to administer and supervise nursing is, it seems to me, explicit denial of our responsibility for even minimal human safety.

With the advent of nurses prepared for advanced clinical practice, most of whom are also prepared for functional responsibilities in teaching or in clinical administration/supervision, a myriad of roles began to evolve. In the service setting the nature of an individual's responsibilities are probably more often a reflection of the situation and the individual's own ingenuity in carving out a place for herself within a generally outmoded system. Those qualified to do so and who take on the formal title of administrator or supervisor are also bringing new dimensions of safety to patient care and evolving new roles. Not infrequently the roles of the advanced practitioner in nursing and the advanced practitioner who holds the title of supervisor or administrator are quite similar. There is a potentially predictable convergence of advanced practitioner and supervisor/administrator roles inherent in the current trends in community-oriented health services and facilities for acute and convalescent care.

What is the purpose of master's degree programs in nursing? For what should graduates of these programs be prepared? What can we predict for the future?

Master's degree programs build upon the undergraduate foundation. As undergraduate programs move more nearly toward providing a baccalaureate education along with the baccalaureate degree and as nursing moves to licensure for professional registered nurse practice as well as the present licensure for technical registered nurse practice, graduate education can expect to have a more consistent base and one that has a growing social and educational significance. Undergraduate education in nursing has undergone considerable strengthening in recent years. However nursing's slowness to evolve an organized conceptual system with all that this means has been a major deterrent to providing true professional education. As nursing's body of abstract knowledge becomes incorporated into undergraduate programs, the characteristics of professional education come into view. Moreover, as undergraduate education improves, much of what has been and is often included in master's programs will be properly included in baccalaureate degree programs. This kind of change is not peculiar to nursing. For example, today's high school graduate may possess more learning than the college graduate of a few years back. Today's college students may be introduced to the same mathematical concepts that second-graders are learning. Children take for granted a world that adults are still struggling to accept.

Flexibility and the capacity to deal with rapid change equably is indispensable. Students must be given broad knowledge and basic principles that can be pulled together in novel ways for unpredictable uses. Except as students, whether undergraduate or graduate, are introduced to a continually expanding organized body of abstract knowledge specific to nursing, there will cease to be either need or justification for higher education in nursing.

Students must be helped to develop a concept of self and a professional commitment commensurate with responsible leadership, initiative, and innovative action. Master's degree candidates must be introduced to investigatory tools and skills beyond those possessed by baccalaureate graduates if they are to recognize and resolve more complex problems and contribute effectively in making the larger judgments requiring greater analytical skill based on advanced knowledge in nursing.

Economic developments, governmental and political trends, technological advances, value shifts, population characteristics, and other factors must be viewed in their interrelatedness and examined according to their impact on the health and welfare of society and their implications for nursing education and practice.

A profession exists for social ends. Nursing knowledge must be translated into practice. The functional knowledges and skills which will enable master's degree graduates to use their knowledge meaningly whether through transmitting it to students or using it in the clinical and community setting in advanced practice and in the administration and supervision of nursing are further adjuncts to master's programs. Doctoral students must be prepared to add to nursing's body of theoretical knowledge and to validate its relevance for the world of reality.

How then does one develop a curriculum that will prepare such persons? What are the areas of knowledge that need to be encompassed? The hard core of graduate education in any field is firmly rooted in the scientific base specific to a given field. Advanced study in a selected area of a given field emerges out of the aforesaid foundation and represents an extension in depth, scope, and understanding beyond the undergraduate level. Cognate courses relevant to the scientific core of a given field enhance understanding and contribute to the overall goals of a program of study.

Graduate education in nursing builds upon undergraduate education in nursing. An organized body of scientific knowledge specific to nursing provides the foundation necessary to identify the validity of the graduate program. Areas of concentration appropriate to graduate education are logical outgrowths of nursing's organized conceptual system. Nursing is concerned with human beings; with man as a synergistic system; a unified whole. Man neither exists as nor can he be perceived by knowledge of his parts, whether these be atoms, molecules, cells, or circulatory systems or physical, biological, psychological, or social attributes. The parts do not identify the human being, nor does a summation of parts add up to a human being. The science of nursing is directed toward describing, explaining, and predicting the nature and direction of man's development. *The science of nursing is the study of human development.* Core courses in the science of nursing and related areas provide the base from which to evolve learnings to be included in areas of concentration. Cognate courses in general education, philosophy, and the basic sciences add further dimensions to study.

The nursing majors as currently identified evolved out of an earlier period oriented to segmentation of man and learning. They are inconsistent with present knowledge and with public demands for health services commensurate with today's world. As the faculty members in the various graduate majors have explored together the nature of the courses they teach, multiple areas of overlap have been identified. Ambiguity in attempts to clarify differences between majors has emerged. Students are requesting opportunity to take courses in nursing in other majors as well as in the major sequence which they have selected. The need for re-examination of what should constitute graduate areas of concentration has become apparent. Transition is inevitable but the nature of transition must be determined carefully and wisely.

The ways in which nursing knowledge is to be used constitute a further area of concern for those who would design curriculums for the future. The nature and delivery of health services are subjects of major public criticism. Efforts on the part of the various health fields to deal with public criticism are generally lacking in social awareness, imagination, and relevance.

Organized medicine is spending large sums of money to deny society knowledgeable nursing services by endeavoring to recruit nurses out of nursing and into medicine; by proposing legislative action to do away with registered nurse licensure; and by a number of other equally reprehensible and socially unconcerned acts.

Nursing has been equally remiss in failing to initiate thoughtfully aggressive and socially responsible leadership in health services. A traditional antieducationism underwrites many nurses' reluctance to grapple with a substantive body of knowledge in nursing. The problems of coping with escalating change are large.

Only those who have the courage and the vision to look into the future and to design and implement educational programs that are oriented to socially significant goals and that encompass substantive scientific knowledge in nursing will persist. Graduate education in nursing appropriate to the past is no longer meaningful to the future.

As the Division of Nurse Education pursues its continuing efforts to design and implement graduate education of stature and substance, there must emerge new ways of thinking and doing else our students will be penalized and the health of people will suffer.

CHAPTER 15

Ph.D. in Nursing

Martha E. Rogers

New York University awarded its first Ph.D. degree to a nurse through the educational unit in nursing nearly 40 years ago. In the first 25 years following this award only a small number of nurses matriculated for doctoral study and an even smaller number completed the doctoral requirements and graduated. Though students met the same requirements for admission, achievement, and graduation as did other doctoral students in this institution, substantive, scholarly knowledge in nursing was not encompassed in the course of study. A doctoral seminar in nursing provided opportunity to discuss nursing's problems but the need for pursuit of a body of theoretical knowledge in nursing was largely unrecognized.

By the 1950's stirrings of educational change in nursing, long in the brewing, began to be felt. Baccalaureate degree programs in nursing were increasing in number and community college programs in nursing (to replace hospital schools) were initiated. Federal monies in support of graduate education in nursing became available, setting in motion a sharp escalation in the numbers of nurses enrolling in master's degree programs.

As the same time that these changes were taking place the Division also embarked on the long-range task of trying to identify and develop a body of scientific knowledge specific to nursing. Faculty committees, workshops, and seminars were instituted. Three doctoral candidates, in a joint effort, focused their dissertations on trying to evolve principles of nursing with two outcomes. First, they all secured their doctoral degrees and second, it was evident that the approach which they used (an approach which interestingly enough was also being suggested by nurses in other places) would not provide the theoretical base nursing sorely needed.

Many blind alleys were explored. Difficulties in thinking in terms of broad principles in contrast to nursing's tradition of dealing with facts and rules of procedure (not infrequently referred to today as process) sometimes blocked

Rogers, M. E. (1971, September). Ph.D. in nursing. In *Future directions of doctoral education for nurses.* U.S. Department of Health Education and Welfare, Public Health Service, National Institute of Health, Bureau of Health Manpower Education, Division of Nursing, U.S. Government Printing Office, DHEW Publication No. (NIH) 72-82. Bethesda, MD.

progress. Nonetheless direction was maintained and the bare bones of potentially productive ideas began to accumulate flesh and blood.

Before 1960 these ideas though still embryonic were already being incorporated into the doctoral program. Doctoral research began to focus on human beings rather than on nurses and their functions. Research findings began to appear that could later take on new and enlarged meanings as they would become lodged within an organized conceptual system.

A logical plan for incorporating nursing's emerging body of abstract knowledge into the instructional process was evident. Quite properly this had been initiated first in the doctoral program. The elaboration of a body of abstract knowledge is dependent on scientists and scholars, in whatever the given field, for its accomplishment.

A population from which to recruit doctoral students in nursing began to emerge. Doctoral student enrollments edged upward, in part because the habit of "going to school" had been established, in part because universities were beginning to bear down on nurses for proper "educational credentials" for university faculty membership and for other reasons. Only a few applicants recognized the doctoral degree as a symbol of scholarly, scientific learning having direct relevance to the improvement of nursing education and nursing practice. Only as these students became able to perceive nursing as a learned profession and to become immersed in the exciting task of participating in evolving and elaborating a body of scientific knowledge specific to nursing did their motivation for doctoral study begin to take on scholarly significance.

Monies in support of doctoral study by nurses, both from Federal and from private sources, was a further factor in making it possible for a larger number of students to engage in full-time study.

By 1965, 82 students were enrolled for doctoral study at New York University of whom approximately 47 percent were full-time students. This year 41 full-time and 60 part-time students are engaged in studying for the Ph.D. degree with a major in nursing. These students range from those who are enrolled entirely in course work to those who are completing their doctoral dissertations.

Students continue to meet the same requirements for admission, achievement, and graduation as do other doctoral candidates in this institution but, today, students have as the central core of their doctoral program substantive, scholarly knowledge in nursing; specifically the study of the theoretical basis of nursing. Cognate courses, tool courses, research design and methodology, etc., enhance and enlarge the student's program but justification for the program's existence lies in the science of nursing—a science of whole man.

Our arrival at this stage in the evolution of nursing in its transition from a pre-scientific field to a scientific field is an outgrowth of multiple influences, events, and struggles. The validity of higher education in nursing rests squarely on the identification of an organized body of abstract knowledge specific to nursing and arrived at by scientific research and logical analysis. By definition, nursing, as a learned profession, is both a science and an art. The engrossing task of evolving an organized conceptual system for nursing had been begun. A critical shortage of faculty qualified to engage in such an endeavor was a major problem. Such knowledge was needed to prepare faculty and concomitantly there needed to be faculty equipped to prepare new faculty.

The old tale of the chicken and the egg—which comes first?—loomed large. A boot-strap operation got under way.

A basic premise that nursing was a learned profession was in sharp conflict with nursing's traditional and pervasive anti-educationism and general failure to perceive nursing as a socially significant endeavor in its own right. Moreover, despite a small portion of nurses in the nation who recognized that knowledgeable and safe nursing practice required scholars and scientists in nursing for such achievement, there was limited awareness even among this group that theories cannot be developed in a field that does not have an organized conceptual system out of which to derive theories.

Lacking a concept of nursing as a learned profession and a philosophy of nursing as a science compounded by a critical "dependency syndrome" that was abetted by a range of interests outside of nursing, nursing moved to support a dead-end reliance on other fields to provide some sort of a mix that might be used to explain an assortment of technical skills and the fruits of practical experience. Nurse–scientist programs contributed to increasing the numbers of persons prepared in fields other than nursing but were a clear denial of nursing's scientific and professional responsibilities. The development of clinical doctorates in nursing by-passed the essentiality of an organized theoretical base in nursing and substituted a mix of facts from other fields coupled with observation and doing. The elaboration of a science of nursing languished in spite of fine intentions.

At New York University the Division of Nurse Education refused to be beguiled into treading the primrose path to a piece of parchment. We have had no reason to regret this decision and if students are any guide to the wisdom of our decision then we indeed made the right choice. The impact of the nature of research and practice evidenced by undergraduate and graduate students introduced to the science of nursing and the guiding principles derived therefrom is remarkable and effective.

Doctoral study in nursing at New York University is founded upon the belief that nursing is a learned profession (as is true for all of our programs). By definition, then, nursing is characterized by an organized body of abstract knowledge specific to nursing. The science of nursing is an emergent—a new product. It is not a summation of facts and principles drawn from other sources. Nursing's conceptual system is acquired by reasoning, by creative synthesis. It is a new mode of thinking.

Nursing's science is a science of man: synergistic man, a unified system possessing his own identity. Man is neither an operating collection of systems, organs, and cells nor is he a summation of biological, physical, psychological, and social behaviors. Man exists only in his wholeness. He cannot be described, explained, or understood by studying his parts or the behaviors of his parts. Indeed he cannot even be perceived when the parts are perceived. The conceptual model of man represents a matrix of ideas which in its wholeness symbolizes man. Basic assumptions underwrite its formulation; a synthesis of ideas for a new way of thinking makes of it a connected whole; hypothetical generalizations and unifying principles derive from it.

Education for nursing's scholars and scientists requires that doctoral programs have as their core the critical and creative study of the science of nursing. The elaboration of nursing's theoretical system is dependent on this foundation. The incorporation of nursing science into undergraduate and graduate curriculums of substance requires scholars of nursing for fulfillment.

Michael Polanyi once wrote: "The existence of animals was not discovered by zoologists, nor that of plants by botanists, and the scientific value of zoology and botany is but an extension of man's pre-scientific interest in animals and plants." This might be paraphrased to read: "The existence of man was not discovered by nurses, and the scientific value of nursing is but an extension of man's pre-scientific interest in human beings."

Escalating science and technology, space exploration, and accelerating evolutionary change are forcing new theories of life and the universe. Proponents of humanistic sciences vie with those who support mechanistic explanations of life. Consonant with a negentropic universe, diversity and heterogeneity grow. The complementarity of man and environment belies the modern day shamans who threaten dire effects of cholesterol, cyclamates, nicotine, radiation, etc. at the same time that amphetamines, tranquilizers, birth control pills, and fluoridation enjoy concurrent popularity. A so-called expanded role of nurses is equally an expanded role for medical doctors, dentists, bioengineers, clinical psychologists, etc.—an outgrowth of changing times, technological advances, and public demand for a nature and amount of health services neither available nor yet envisioned.

The need for scholars and scientists in nursing should be beyond argument. The nature of their preparation must be projected within the framework of an unknown future and must be characterized by imaginative and knowledgeable concern for people.

Professional education in nursing, as in other fields, begins with the first undergraduate professional degree. That the first undergraduate professional degree is, in some fields, built atop a general education baccalaureate degree does not change the undergraduate nature of the education. Moreover current trends and recommendations strongly support incorporation of professional education squarely within a baccalaureate curriculum but requiring more time than the traditional four academic years though significantly less time than is presently true for some fields.

Graduate education leading to master's and doctoral degrees has long been an established part of higher education in America. Within recent times there has been extensive mushrooming both in the nature and number of graduate degrees offered in the educational market-place. Medical educators have only lately begun to develop graduate programs of study in medicine that would qualify their members for master's degrees and for the higher doctorates. The Ph.D. degree is being subjected to close scrutiny. Suggestions are rife for a range of substitute academic and professional credentials, generally less demanding in their scholarly requirements than the Ph.D. degree.

Undergraduate, master's, and doctoral programs properly constitute a sequence of increasingly complex learnings. Though each level of learning has its own unity and completeness they also provide the foundation for further learning for those whose goals and abilities are in accord with the continuing pursuit of formal education. The distinguishing characteristics of professional education in any field is [sic] the transmission of theory—not a body of technical skills. This is not to deny the importance of technical skills but rather to make clear that it is nursing's body of abstract knowledge that makes explicit professional education in nursing. It is utilization of this knowledge in service to people that determines the nature of nursing services. It is this body of knowledge that encompasses nursing's hypothetical generalizations and unifying principles—the descriptive, explanatory, and predictive principles essential to professional practice. It is this body of knowledge that gives substance to nursing's scientific humanitarianism.

Except as some portion of nurses fulfill the rigorous requirements of doctoral study of stature directed toward the elaboration of nursing's theoretical base through pure research in nursing, applied research in nursing will have no source on which to found its examinations of the real world. The Ph.D. degree has long been deemed to represent completion of a theoretically oriented research program of study. It is the appropriate degree for the preparation of nursing's theoreticians and pure researchers. This is not a proposal that the Ph.D. degree is the only appropriate doctorate in nursing. It is a proposal that unless there are nurses prepared in nursing for the scholarly responsibilities symbolized by the Ph.D. at its best there cannot be substantive education in nursing at any level regardless of the degree awarded.

A doctoral program of study presumes that the individual brings with him a broad base of general education and a firm foundation in the area in which he proposes to pursue doctoral study. For nurses seeking doctoral study in nursing such an assumption cannot be made. In general applicants tend to be best equipped in the social sciences, moderately prepared in the biological sciences, and startlingly impoverished in the physical sciences. Mathematics, logic, and philosophy only rarely appear on a student's transcript of previous college work. Wide variations characterize applicants' undergraduate nursing majors (although this is less marked among recent graduates) and graduate majors though purporting to be in nursing on occasion are so narrow and technically oriented as to suggest that they more nearly approximate what should have been continuing education for nursing's technically prepared graduates of ADN programs and hospital schools.

In consequence each applicant must be viewed individually. Undergraduate areas of weakness must be shored up. Previous learnings and a student's educational and professional goals must be evaluated. All students are required to demonstrate scholarly competence in research and investigation. Course requirements are planned to meet these goals. Cognate courses are included in the student's course of study with special emphasis on philosophy. Additional course requirements are determined on an individual basis and may include independent study when this appears appropriate.

The Ph.D. foreign language requirement provides for three options, namely: (1) a reading knowledge of two foreign languages, or (2) a reading knowledge of one foreign language and a two semester course in graduate statistics, or (3) a two semester course in graduate statistics and a two semester course in computer science. All students who do not elect to take the two semester course in computer science must complete as a minimum a concentrated, non-credit introduction to computer science offered through the New York University Courant Institute of Mathematical Sciences.

The doctoral dissertation is a significant aspect of the doctoral program. Each student has a three member sponsoring committee appointed at the time the student is ready to initiate work on the dissertation. The chairman of this committee is a member of the faculty in the Division of Nurse Education who herself holds an earned doctorate and is competent to serve in this capacity. It may be of interest to this group to note that for the past two years the chairman of the all-school committee to review and evaluate doctoral research designs has been a member of the Division of Nurse Education faculty. Further, a study of doctoral research designs submitted for the 5-year period 1964–1969 throughout the school and which was undertaken by the Dean of Graduate Studies, revealed that on every dimension examined doctoral designs submitted by students in the Division of Nurse Education had been accorded quality scores superior to any other unit in the school.

Resources of the entire university are available to doctoral candidates in nursing. The undergraduate and graduate schools of arts and sciences are of particular value in providing a range of offerings relevant to nursing.

The present organizational placement of nursing within the administrative structure of the university is unfortunate. However, it is hoped that efforts to establish a School of Nursing coordinate with all other schools and colleges within the university may bear fruit in the not too distant future. Despite this problem the Division of Nurse Education does control its professional curriculums within the framework of the university thus making possible scholarly learning in nursing.

CHAPTER 16

Nursing Education: Preparing for the Future

Martha E. Rogers

A bit of ancient history seems appropriate to initiate these comments. Surely, all nurses were introduced to Hygieia and those other famous goddesses of health as early symbols of nursing. However, history reveals a somewhat different story than ones you may have heard or read. As a matter of record, Hygieia was a distinct personality by 600 BC (or perhaps earlier).[1] At least 200 years before Asklepios was introduced, Hygieia was a powerful and independent goddess responsible for maintenance of health. Her primary symbols were a serpent and an open hand. When Asklepios finally appeared he was only a hero, and heroes were not very important in ancient Greece. His function was to serve Hygieia and to do her bidding. He was very dependent on Hygieia, rarely appearing without her. Eventually (approximately another 200 years later), Greek males sought to overcome female dominance. Asklepios was promoted to a god and in time took the serpent for himself.

Masculine dominance continued in the Western world. In 1888, for example, Friedrich Nietzsche stated that "when a woman becomes a scholar there is usually something wrong with her sexual organs." Nor has chauvinism ended yet. A recent article in the *New York Times Magazine* noted that "interns do a lot of what they refer to as scutwork. 'Interns become great nurses,' as a surgery intern said."[2] Then why haven't they been sued for practicing nursing without a license? Florence Nightingale's comment that "medicine and nursing should not be mixed up; it spoils both" needs to be remembered.

---

[1]See Marie-Therese Connell, "Feminine Consciousness and the Nature of Nursing Practice: A Historical Perspective." Topics in Clinical Nursing (October 1983), pp. 5–7.

[2]Michael Harwood, "The Ordeal: Life as a Medical Resident," *New York Times Magazine,* June 3, 1984. p. 46.

Entry Levels and Licensure

Despite studies carried out ad infinitum and almost continuously throughout the present century, there has been very limited progress in support of an educationally sound and socially motivated system of higher education in nursing commensurate with changing times and human needs. The most significant change has been replacement of hospital schools with associate degree nursing programs. Concomitantly, valid baccalaureate degree education in nursing goes unlicensed and is only minimally differentiated from the associate degree and hospital school level of preparation. The field of nursing has long had three entry levels to practice, and licenses for only two of these levels: the practical nurse level and the registered nurse level, for which associate degree and hospital schools prepare. Nursing has never licensed for the baccalaureate level, although the baccalaureate level is the cornerstone of nursing's educational system.

The myth that because all graduates of hospital schools, associate degree programs, and baccalaureate degree programs take the same licensing exam, they are therefore the same, approaches the ridiculous. With such logic one might properly ask why MDs and physician's assistants are not licensed according to one examination, or dentists and dental hygienists, or engineers and engineering technicians, and so on. Licensure exists to safeguard the public. There is critical need for the addition of a new license for the baccalaureate level of practice. Public safety requires it and professional credibility with other learned professions demands it. A grandfather clause for this new license must be limited to persons holding a baccalaureate degree with an upper-division major in nursing approved at the time of the student's graduation.

An excellent baccalaureate nursing graduate is not the same thing as an excellent associate degree or hospital school graduate. In both instances excellence is determined by different criteria. Both groups should be equally excellent, but excellence will be manifest in different ways according to the nature and amount of knowledge each possess [sic].

Professional Education

Nursing's survival as a knowledgeable endeavor demands that the education of nurses be squarely within educational institutions. Valid baccalaureate education requires a strong liberal arts foundation, substantive theoretical knowledge in the science of nursing, and the opportunity for students to demonstrate their ability to use their knowledge safely and effectively in service to people. Multiple community resources provide a range of laboratory settings. I agree with the recent report of the National Institute of Education, which recommended extending undergraduate programs beyond the usual four years in most professional fields.[3] I believe that the first undergraduate professional degree in nursing requires five years.

Regarding the evolution of professional education in nursing, I would add some words of warning. Hospitals are not educational institutions. They are but one of many resources for laboratory study in nursing and are highly inadequate settings for the broad scope of nursing. Moreover, it seems likely

---

[3]Ezra Bowen, "Bringing Colleges Under Fire," *Time,* October 29, 1984. p. 78.

that in the future a decreasing percentage of baccalaureate and higher degree graduates will be working in hospitals. To those who would reinvent the wheel—beware! The historical accident that put nursing preparation in hospitals and outside the educational mainstream has been unfortunate for both nurses and the public.

It is imperative that we provide a valid baccalaureate education in nursing along with the degree. We must remember that our responsibility is to all people and is by no means limited to diminishing numbers of those hospitalized. Anti-educationism and dependency are untenable positions. Nursing is a learned profession—peer of other learned professions—unique in the phenomenon of its concern and in its substantive theoretical base.

Professional education in nursing is more than a piece of paper—it is located in and controlled by an institution of higher learning that includes a college of the liberal arts and sciences. It requires five academic years that include lower- and upper-division general education. The transmission of a substantive theoretical base in nursing science primarily at the upper-division level, with appropriate laboratory study in the art of nursing, gives identity to the student's major. And I would note that study in the physical, biological, and social sciences does not constitute study in the science of nursing. Rather, the liberal arts and sciences are requisites for all college students who seek to become educated people.

A qualified faculty prepared at the graduate level *in nursing* is essential if there is to be professional education in nursing. The possession of and the ability to transmit theoretical knowledge in nursing is indispensable. How one uses knowledge depends on the knowledge one possesses. Functions are not nursing; they are how one uses nursing.

In these days of emphasis on cost containment, excessive charges by medicine and hospitals, budgetary battles, and the like, the public is properly concerned. Nurses are responsible for cleaning up their own act in terms of a society that both needs and wants knowledgeable nursing services.

Nursing's professionally educated population must be committed to people. They must be risk takers. They must be characterized by a mutual respect for differences. They must be imaginative and creative, and above all, they need a good sense of humor.

Education for the Future

High technology is having a large impact on nursing, as it is on the other areas of life. Automation, robots, the information revolution, and like events are not going away. Chatter of "high tech versus high touch" is fallacious. Both are meaningful adjuncts of practice in today's world. They are tools of practice. In the long term, if we educate for the future more jobs will be created than are destroyed. But for those who would maintain the status quo, the future is dim.

Before the end of this century, nurses can expect to be working in moon villages and space towns. Inclusion of "extraterrestrial" matters is a "must" in today's curriculum. Approximately 40 percent of RNs do not work in hospitals, and the percentage can be expected to increase in the future, particularly for baccalaureate and higher degree graduates in nursing. As Fritjof Capra has written, "we are trying to apply concepts of an outdated world view to a reality that can no longer be understood in terms of those concepts."[4]

Autonomous nursing centers, independent nursing practice, nurse midwifery, birthing centers, outer space employment are emerging—and all without the fallacy of so-called medical backup. Only nurses qualified by baccalaureate and higher degree preparation in nursing are competent to provide the knowledgeable judgments necessary to public safety and to give appropriate direction to nursing's members with associate degree, hospital school, and practical nurse credentials. The direction of change makes imperative nurses' move toward scientific identity and social responsibility. Whatever the future of nursing may be, it will be within the context of rapid change, diversity, new knowledge, and new horizons.

---

[4]Fritjof Capra, *The Turning Point* (New York: Simon & Schuster, 1982).

CHAPTER 17

Nursing Science: Research and Researchers

Martha E. Rogers

'Research' is one of the most prestigious terms in the English language today. Third graders look up words in the dictionary and call it research. Clerks tabulate long lists of figures and call it research. Nurses collect multiple specimens of urine and call it research. Medical doctors substitute artificial organs and psychologists collect test scores and propose that these are research. The public views the technological wonders that speed man's journey, relieve his boredom, increase his comfort, and are purported to add years to his life and is unbelievably willing to support all manner of proposals providing they are clothed in the magic word 'research.'

Concomitant with the mad rush to get on this eminent (and often remunerative) bandwagon is a growing awareness that technology is not science and that gadgetry and how-to-do-it are not research. Overemphasis on utilitarian inquiries has prompted Blair Kinsman to state, "Someday, someone is going to compare the claims for practicality in the budget requests with the results in the final reports and we'll all starve."[4] Buckminster Fuller, in the November 12, 1966 issue of *Saturday Review* has noted, ". . . we have been overproducing the army of rigorously disciplined, scientific, game-playing, academic specialists who through hard work and suppressed imagination, earn their Ph.D.'s only to have their specialized field become obsolete or by-passed in five years by evolutionary events of altered techniques and exploratory strategies."[1] Rather they produce deluxe quality technicians who lack creativity; who concentrate on proven scientific formulas and experiments; who perpetuate obsolescence by repetition.

Just what is research? Who does it? What is its significance to nurses, to nursing, and society—the recipient of nursing services?

'Research' has taken unto itself a variety of modifying adjectives, perhaps hopefully designed to clarify some of the confusion arising from the term's

Rogers, M. E. (1968). Nursing science: Research and researchers. *Teacher's College Record, 69,* 469–476. Reprinted with permission.

exceedingly loose usage. So, today, research is not uncommonly referred to as 'pure,' 'basic,' 'true,' 'truly basic,' 'valid,' 'applied,' 'clinical,' etcetera.

The National Science Foundation has defined basic research as "that type of research which is directed toward increase of knowledge in science. It is research where the primary aim of the investigator is a fuller knowledge or understanding of the subject under study, rather than a practical application thereof." Interestingly enough, Robert S. Morison of the Rockefeller Foundation has noted that ". . . Basic research is now widely recognized as even more practical than applied, if we only lengthen our time scale a little."[9] Gerard Peil[5] has defined pure or basic science as "devoted to the advance of knowledge" and applied science or technology as "the exploitation of knowledge already established." Further, he states, "Thus, it is clear, there must be an advance before there can be application . . . the cycle of progress is maintained by an interaction between pure and applied science in which the two enterprises fructify each other." Basic research creates new knowledge. Applied research does not create new knowledge though efforts are continuous to lend plausibility to claims that it does.

There is demonstrable effort to rouse support for basic (or theoretical) research. But as a nation we are not really oriented toward theoretical concerns. Despite 'scholars in Washington' and growing college enrollments too much intellect is still held suspect. 'Idea men' are more often associated with Madison Avenue than with philosophy—and creativity is commonly confused with brainstorming, problem-solving, and resourcefulness. *Time* Magazine's "Essay" of January 13, 1967 refers to "the American tradition of inspired tinkerers."[11]

Nonetheless, basic research is on-going. New concepts are revolutionizing man's beliefs about himself and his world. Theories are being translated into technology and our whole way of life is being changed. Space travel, extrasensory perception, and U.F.O.'s have become part of man's reality. Value systems are shifting. The public is demanding social and health services of a nature and quality clearly beyond that currently available. Meanwhile automation threatens man's privacy. Millions of dollars are going to build a hospital in Georgetown[1] that, according to reports, will isolate acutely ill and critical patients in a scientifically obsolete and sadly inhumane environment of microbial and familiar sterility. The immorality of experimentation without consent of the individual has become a national issue.

Compassionate concern (and not so compassionate concern) for the future of man's health and welfare is forcing major revisions in the roles, responsibilities, and nature of the multiplicity of health disciplines that have mushroomed in recent years. There is heavy investment in dollars and time directed toward studying who does what and how—and with singularly feeble results.

In this maelstrom of confusion nurses are struggling to find their way through to more effective and meaningful service to people. Quite obviously the complexity of knowledge and skill required to safeguard the recipients of nursing services has made mandatory the identification of a nucleus of professionally educated nurses distinct from those whose preparation is technical or vocational in nature. Such a premise is readily supportable. Only the most uninformed and those endeavoring to maintain a long obsolete hierarchal control would propose that in today's world society is better served by ignorance than by knowledge. (Though as we know there are a range of uninformed and vested interests who, under many strange guises, are endeavoring to do just this). Since the discussion of nursing as a learned profession is not my assignment this evening, I will simply state it as a basic assumption and proceed on this basis.

Nursing as a learned profession has, by definition, a range of characteristics. Some of these have direct relevance for the topic under discussion and thus seem important to note. Professional education is characterized by the transmission of a body of abstract principles arrived at by scientific research and logical analysis—*not* a body of technical skills. This is not to propose that technical skills are unimportant but rather to identify that which distinguishes professional education. A given body of theoretical or abstract knowledge is specific to a given discipline and encompasses the discipline's descriptive, explanatory, and predictive principles which guide its practitioners. Nursing has two major dimensions, namely: 1) the science of nursing and 2) the utilization or application of nursing's science for the betterment of man—the practice of nursing. (And let me point out—one cannot apply what one does not possess). Nursing's body of scientific knowledge is the product of nursing's scholars and scientists. Without nursing science professional practice cannot exist. Moreover, nursing's professionally educated members are specifically and solely responsible for both the development of this body of knowledge and for its application within the context of society.

A profession exists for social ends. Its direct responsibility is to the people it purports to serve. This takes precedence over all other relationships. The nursing profession exists to serve society. It does not exist to serve the ends of any other group. Nursing as a learned profession has *no* dependent functions. Nor does one profession delegate anything to another profession. Nursing, like all other professions, has many collaborative functions—indispensable to providing society with a higher order of service than any one profession can offer.

Nursing is concerned with people—all people—of whom only a segment is ill. A nation's first line of defense in building a healthy society lies in promotion of health and in prevention of illness. Any society that concentrates its health dollars and health services on care of the sick will never be a healthy society. The A.N.A. position paper on Education for Nursing—a remarkable and long overdue but nonetheless highly significant document—falls short of comprehending both nursing's tradition and generally accepted criteria of a learned profession. 'Care, cure, and coordination' are narrow, technically oriented, unimaginative, and inaccurate substitutes for nursing's real responsibilities and scope. Maintenance and promotion of health are ignored. Coordination is a strange and ridiculous irrelevancy for professional practice. Coordination is a responsibility shared jointly with all professional disciplines. It is indispensable to good health services but it is not professional practice for any discipline. Professional education in nursing is as substantial as professional education in law, theology, medicine, engineering, etc. Professional practice is the use of nursing's science for human health and welfare.

Over the past decade there has been growing cognizance among at least a portion of nurses that a body of abstract knowledge, the science of nursing, is indispensable to nursing's evolution and to society's safety. Unfortunately, there has been very limited awareness that "theory cannot be developed in a field that does not have clear, unequivocal concepts."[2] In consequence, efforts to demonstrate nursing's scientific orientation have produced a multiplying number of trivial and mediocre papers parading as research. Not infrequently high praise and tax dollars have been and are awarded pedestrian investigators whose primary assets are enthusiasm and a questioning attitude. 'How-to-do-it,' gadgetry, and self-examination predominate.

Heard with increasing frequency in nursing is 'clinical' research. One suspects that this term, in part, grows out of an effort to differentiate between self-study and the study of human beings. It implies a clinical setting and narrow orientation, and is more suggestive of applied than of basic research. Possibly it reflects a struggle toward identifying nursing's central concern—people—as the focus of nursing research. But the nature of research itself or the knowledges, tools, and abilities essential to fulfilling research goals are vague and generally little understood.

Nursing is in grave need of both theoretical and applied research. But only a miniscule [sic] amount of theoretical research in nursing has appeared. Consequently, applied research in nursing generally lacks the substance of fundamental concepts. Researchers in other disciplines study nurses, ad infinitum, to test theories in their own fields but they are, of course, unable to develop and test theories in nursing. Only nurses, highly qualified and competent, creative and intelligent, can create the conceptual base, develop the ideas and theories, and implement scholarly, independent research in nursing. And let me point out again that one cannot share what one does not possess. Peer participation in interdisciplinary research (of increasing importance) demands that the participants be highly competent in research in their own field if they are to share in developing creative ideas which integrate the knowledges of a variety of fields.

Nursing is concerned with human beings. The hypothetical generalizations and principles of nursing's science describe, explain, and predict about human beings, specifically, the life process in man.

Human beings are more than and different from the sum of their parts. They are *not* a summation of biological, physical, psychological, social, etcetera, attributes, behaviors, and functions. A description of biological man no more describes the life process in man than a description of hydrogen describes water. The phenomenon at the center of nursing's purpose is a whole.

Although the idea of man as a unified system is by no means a new concept (see ancient Greeks) this idea was quite thoroughly buried in the emergence of modern science. Dichotomies, multiple in nature, split man in many different directions. Only recently has there begun to be renewed recognition of man as having his own unique system—indivisible and possessing its own characteristics.

The emergence of a unified approach to the study of man was stimulated by the development of particle-field theory in physics at the turn of the century. In the 1930's Burr and Northrop published their historic statement of biological field theory and Kurt Lewin proposed a psychological field theory. Atomic and cellular theories have become obsolete. An energy field has replaced the cell as the fundamental unit of living systems.

A new world of undiscovered knowledge lies in wait. The phenomenon at the center of nursing's purpose (MAN) demands scientists and scholars in nursing to develop the insights and to implement the elaboration of nursing's scientific principles about the life process in man. And a basic premise in the study of the life process is that normal and pathological processes be treated on a basis of complete equality.

Nursing's science—its system of concepts is acquired by reasoning and to quote C. Judson Herrick, "It is creative; and an original idea . . . is not built up by simple summation of factual data. It is an emergent, a new product."[3] Nursing science is *not* a summation of facts and principles drawn from the basic sciences and other disciplines. Nursing science is a new product. Moreover, a science is open-ended; constantly evolving; never finished. It undergoes continuous change, revision, elaboration.

If you ask a biologist "What is Biology?" and he responds "It is the study of the biological world" this answer might be less complete than you want, but neither would you expect him to give you a complete picture of biological science in a paragraph or even in a year. Moreover, you would no doubt be aware that biological principles of today may not hold true tomorrow. For example, the conventional meanings of concepts like homeostasis, adaptation, and steady-state are demonstrably antiquated.[7] New terms are being introduced such as homeokinesis.

The over-riding need in nursing today is for basic research *in the science of nursing:* 1) that furthers the formulation of nursing's system of concepts; 2) that results in synthesis of knowledges for new concepts; 3) that is characterized by the creative development of testable hypotheses. Basic research in nursing is directed toward advancing knowledge which can enlarge our understanding of man and the universe. It is concerned with ideas. It is not achieved merely by a process of arrangement. It seeks to push back the frontiers of knowledge and those who seek to push back frontiers must have come close to those frontiers themselves. This is not to suggest that one must know all the multiplicity of facts that have accumulated through the ages. As Jacques Barzun has pointed out, ". . . the difficulty today is not that science has uncovered more facts than one mind can retain, but that science has ceased to be, even to scientists, a set of principles and an object of contemplation."[8]

True research potential among nurses must be identified. The nature of preparation for research in nursing must possess high validity and must be made explicit. A college president has stated that ". . . researchers will either come out of higher education or they are not going to exist. They do not come out of attics."[9] Education for scholarly research, whether basic or applied, is at the doctoral level. While one may expect, and rightly so, that all professionally educated nurses (meaning no less than a valid baccalaureate education with an upper division major in nursing) will initiate and further the exploitation of knowledge for the enhancement of nursing practice, such persons possess neither the knowledge or tools necessary for true research. At the same time the creative, intelligent, independent, curious, skeptical, energetic, non-conformist student or practitioner, emotionally committed to her career and possessing superior conceptual capacity is likely to carry within her the germ of creative research. She must be encouraged and at times tolerated. Opportunities for her continued study must be provided. We have great need for nurses dedicated to the passionate search for new understandings—a hallmark of the true researcher. And as Claude Bernard, the French physiologist, noted a century ago, "Those who do not know the torment of the unknown cannot have the joy of discovery."

The nature of preparation for research in nursing is the subject of strange controversy. Failure to grasp the fundamental structure of nursing as a science and the [pursuit of] the tortuous path of creative endeavor plagues many of nursing's most able members.

My further comments on this point have led me to insert a story here which some of you may have heard. It concerns a bit of healthy humor that occurred when two boyhood friends met after a long separation. As classmates they had fought hard to outshine each other in everything, and, as they moved from success to success, each had kept the other's head from getting too large by periodically putting him in his place. After graduation, they went their separate ways. Each flourished in his chosen field, one becoming a slender and model senior admiral; the other a ranking bishop, now grown paunchy with the prolapsed belly of the old. Recently the bishop, in colorful ecclesiastical costume, saw the admiral, in resplendent military uniform, across the Concourse in Grand Central Station. The bishop walked over, tapped the admiral on the shoulder, and said, "Pardon me, Conductor, can you tell me when the next train leaves for Boston?" The admiral turned, looked the bishop up and down, and parried with an equally ungracious riposte: "Madam, in your condition you shouldn't be travelling."

Failing to conceive of nursing as a learned profession and lacking a philosophy of nursing as a science (and one might add, nursing's glorification of dependency on others) many nurses seek answers in methodology and in other fields. The dead-end aspects for nursing science (and ultimately public safety) of the would-be scientist and researcher in nursing whose doctoral study prepares her to be a psychologist or sociologist, a physicist or physiologist, or statistucuab [sic] are more than unfortunate. Such persons are severely handicapped by the narrowness and inadequacy of their preparation for productive research in nursing. They lack both the fundamental knowledge and the conceptual frame of reference for even comprehending nursing science. Nursing cannot afford the additional substantial learning and re-learning such persons must undertake if they would prepare themselves for scholarship and research in nursing. The elaboration of nursing science languishes in spite of fine intentions. The routines of scientific investigation can be learned by many. Junior high school students are happily gathering hypotheses for their science projects. Studying 'how to clean a thermometer' has engaged nurses for years. But the identification and testing of creative ideas essential to nursing science cannot be found in rules-of-thumb or in other fields. Knowledge about MAN—nursing's purpose—must be developed. The so-called Nurse-Scientist programs are tragic derogation of nursing's purposes. One seeks education in law if one expects to practice law and a fine education in engineering is not a substitute. Nor am I anxious to tread upon the bridge designed by a medical doctor. Substantial knowledge in the science of nursing identifies nursing's professional members.

Nursing is commonly referred to as an applied science. But as I noted earlier, the application of knowledge is rooted in the unifying principles and hypothetical generalizations growing out of basic research in nursing. At this point in time, it seems beyond argument that the need for basic nursing research far outweighs the need for applied research and gadgetry. Knowledgeable, imaginative, audacious research must be encouraged and supported. Creative, intelligent nurses must be prepared in *nursing* for the great task of pushing back frontiers. We must cease advising the unqualified that all nurses do or should do research. Not all nurses possess the capacity for creative conceptualization for the production of scholarly, independent research. But those who do will contribute far beyond their numbers and without their contributions nursing will not fulfill its responsibilities to society.

Investigations in the science of nursing add to nursing's theoretical structure and concomitantly provide the knowledge that can be translated into practice. Their significance is not only to nursing but to others concerned with people. Most important of all, today's investigations in nursing science foretell a future of scientific evolution in nursing that must underwrite our social responsibility—our commitment to humankind.

Many years ago Roger Bacon wrote: ". . . above all, if a man could succeed but in kindling a light in nature . . . a light which should in its ray rising touch and illuminate all the border regions that confine upon the circle of our present knowledge; and so spreading further should presently disclose and bring into sight all that is most hidden and secret in the world, that man would be the benefactor of the human race."

References

1. Fuller, Buckminster. "How Little I Know," *Saturday Review,* November 12, 1966. p. 69.
2. Griffiths, Daniel E. *Administrative Theory.* N.Y.: Appleton-Century-Crofts, Inc. 1959.
3. Herrick, C. Judson. *The Evolution of Human Nature.* Austin, Tex. The University of Texas Press. 1956.
4. Kinsman, Blair, "On Scholarship," *The Johns Hopkins Magazine,* Vol. XVIII, No. 1, Winter 1966. p. 2.
5. Piel, Gerard. *Science in the Cause of Man.* N.Y.: Alfred A. Knopf, Publ. 1961.
6. Rogers, Martha E. *Reveille in Nursing.* Philadelphia, F. A. Davis Publ. Co. 1964.
7. Shaefer, Karl (Ed), *Man's Dependence on the Earthly Atmosphere.* N.Y.: The Macmillan Co. 1962.
8. Toulmin, Stephen. *Foresight & Understanding.* N.Y.: Harper & Row, Publ. 1961.
9. Wolfe, Dael (ed). *Symposium on Basic Research.* Wash., D.C. American Assoc. for the Advancement of Science (Publ. No. 56). 1959.
10. Young, Warren R. "It's a Miracle That We Save Any of Them," *Life,* Vol. 61, No. 23, Dec. 2, 1966. p. 110.
11. Young, Warren R. "Time Essay," *Time,* Vol. 89, No. 2, Jan. 13, 1967. p. 19.

CHAPTER 18

Nursing Research in the Future

Martha E. Rogers

Nursing's evolution from a semi-science to a science is emerging out of accelerating change on all fronts. Scientific and technological wonders escalate. New world views multiply. Diversification marks the fields of business and industry. A cashless society is on the horizon. Space towns and moon villages are scarcely a decade away with galactic grocery stores, health services, recreational centers, and the like inevitable inclusions in a space bound world society. The liberal arts and sciences including extraterrestrial matters are essential bases for learned professional education in any field.

Nursing as a learned profession is both a science and an art. A science may be defined as an organized body of abstract knowledge arrived at by scientific research and logical analysis. The art of nursing is the imaginative and creative use of this knowledge in human service. Historically, the term nursing most often has been used as a verb signifying 'to do.' When nursing is perceived as a science the term nursing becomes a noun signifying 'a body of abstract knowledge.' The education of nurses has identity in transmission of nursing's body of theoretical knowledge. The practice of nurses is the use of this knowledge in service to people. Research in nursing is the study of unitary human beings and their environments.

The uniqueness of nursing, like that of any other science, lies in the phenomenon central to its purposes. Nursing's long established concern with human beings and the world they live in is a natural forerunner of an organized abstract system encompassing people and their environments. The irreducible nature of individuals as different from the sum of the parts and the integrity of man and environment coordinate with a universe of open systems identifies the focus of a new paradigm and initiates nursing's identity as a science.

The purpose of nurses is to help all people achieve maximum well-being within their potential, wherever they are. The future of nursing is within the

---

context of rapid change, growing diversity, new knowledge, and new horizons. For nurses to fulfill their social and professional responsibilities in the days ahead demands that their practice be based upon a substantive theoretical base specific to nursing. A science of unitary human beings basic to nursing requires a new world view and conceptual system specific to nursing's phenomena of concern. The continuing development of nursing's body of abstract knowledge requires both basic and applied research in the science of nursing.

Principles and theories derive from an organized abstract system. Basic research is directed toward an increase in knowledge in a given science. Applied research investigates the practical application of knowledge already available. Baccalaureate degree graduates in nursing properly possess beginning tools of inquiry and are able to exploit knowledge for the improvement of practice. Master's degree graduates in nursing possess more sophisticated tools of study, identify more complex problems, and design and implement applied research. Basic research requires doctoral study in nursing with a high level of scholarly sophistication and the ability to push back frontiers of knowledge.

There is a critical need to differentiate between the study of nurses and what they do and the study of nursing. No one would question that the study of biologists and what they do is not the study of biology. Certainly there is usefulness in studying nurses, nursing practice, nursing education, nursing history, and the like but these should not be confused with the study of nursing science. Moreover while research in fields other than nursing may be useful to such other fields it does not further knowledge in nursing. A further word of warning to researchers comes from Raymond Miles at the University of California at Berkeley who noted recently "we are training people who are very, very good at solving problems which turn out to be yesterday's problems."

A science of nursing means asking new questions and seeking new answers. There are incongruities and contradictions between holistic directions in nursing and the forms of inquiry used by nurses. Descriptive, philosophical, and qualitative research in nursing is increasing. There is critical need for new tools of measurement appropriate to new paradigms. A few such tools have been developed and more are in progress.

Applied research should replace the use of the phrase "clinical research." According to dictionaries the term clinical means "investigation of a disease in the living subject by observation as distinguished from controlled study," "something done at the bedside." These definitions are inappropriate and inadequate for the scope and purposes of nursing.

Research is the study of relationships. Science is open-ended. The findings of research support or do not support hypotheses. They do not prove anything. A statement of a theory is an abstraction. A statement of the problem is a practical statement of how one proposes to test a theory. Theory and problem statements precede methodology. Stephen Jay Gould writing in *Natural History* (February, 1977) noted: "New facts, collected in old ways under the guidance of old theories rarely lead to any substantial revision of thought. Facts do not speak for themselves; they are read in the light of theory."

Many nurses are making notable progress in tackling the mysteries of the abstract. An anonymous quote that I like goes thus: "It's easy to see the seeds in the apple but it requires imagination to see the apple in the seeds."

The future of research in nursing is based on a commitment to nursing as a science in its own right. The science of nursing is identified as the science of unitary human beings. The research potentials of nursing's abstract system are multiple. It is logically and scientifically tenable. It is flexible and open-ended. The practical implications for human health and well-being are already demonstrable.

Seeing the world from this viewpoint requires a new synthesis, a creative leap and the inculcation of new attitudes and values. Guiding principles are broad generalizations that require imaginative and innovative modalities for their implementation. A science of unitary human beings identifies nursing's uniqueness and signifies the potential of nurses to fulfill their social responsibility in human service. The future of research in nursing is infinite.

SECTION THREE

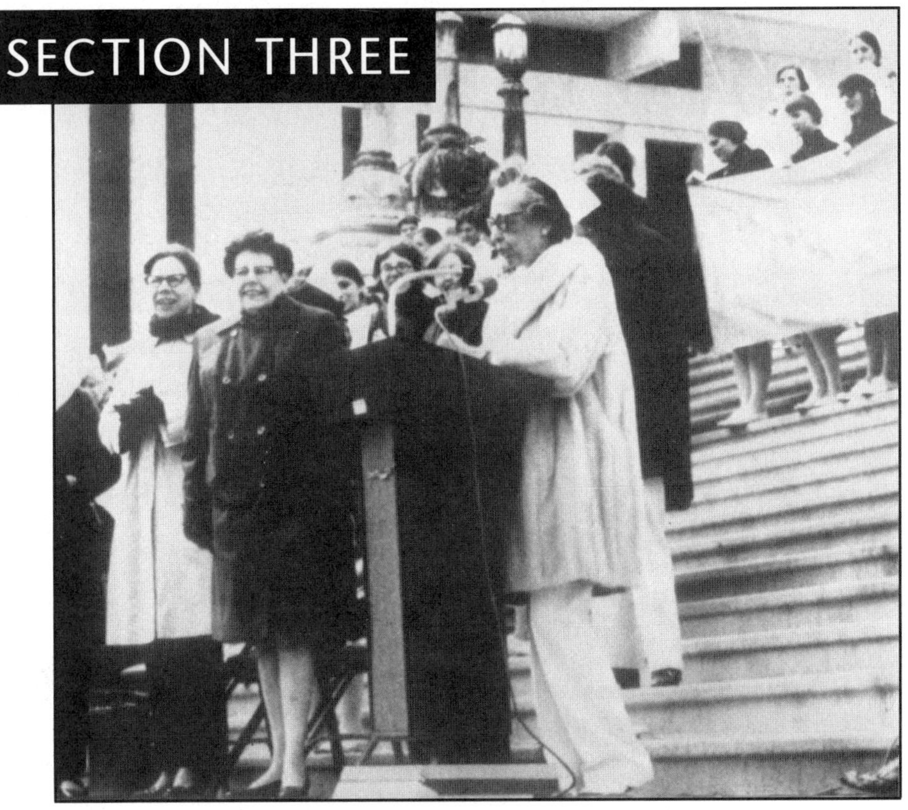

Martha Rogers at the March on Albany for Passage of the Revised Nurse Practice Act of New York State, 1970. (Photograph by Gean Mathwig.)

Professional and Political Issues

Section Editor
Elizabeth Ann Manhart Barrett

CHAPTER 19

Rogers' Professional Politics

Elizabeth Ann Manhart Barrett

Unity in nursing will only come about as diversity among nurses is recognized and valued. . . . The practice of nursing properly utilizes more than one entry level into nursing. . . . The future of nursing demands substantive nursing knowledge, social responsibility, professional commitment, a vision of the future, and the courage to implement one's convictions (Rogers, 1980a, p. 4).

Rogers will long be remembered as an eloquent and effective political statesperson for nursing. Rogers as politician has consistently, clearly, and loudly cried out her message that nursing is an autonomous profession with a substantive and unique body of knowledge. This political stance has changed nursing, leaving a legacy that has, albeit indirectly, had a pervasive impact on registered nurses and the public. Radical, highly controversial positions on the nurse-practitioner movement and licensure for entry into practice are courageously articulated in her writings on these and other issues faced by the profession in the past several decades.

The Professional Is Political

For Rogers, the professional was always political. Arriving in New York to assume responsibilities as chairperson of the Department of Nursing at New York University in 1954, Rogers wasted not a moment before becoming involved in professional organizations. Leadership in various nursing organizations remained a major commitment throughout her career. In 1956 she began serving 4 years as first vice-president of the New York State League for Nursing (NYSLN) and was elected president of NYSLN in 1960 (''Rogers Elected,'' 1960). During this time the foundation was laid for the greater autonomy required for the practice of nursing as an independent profession through, for example, the revision of the New York State Nurse Practice Act. More importantly, the foundation was laid for nursing to emerge as a science with a unique phenomenon of concern and a knowledge base different from other sciences. At the same time efforts to move all of nursing education into institutions of higher learning were accelerated.

From the beginning Rogers had a vision of nursing. She never said it would be easy to accomplish. In fact, in 1964 at the Michigan League for

Nursing convention, she admonished nursing colleagues that if nurses wanted to be professionals, they had better assume the responsibilities that go along with it. Mincing no words, which was always her style, she warned that studies revealed that nurses ranked manual skill high and thinking low and wanted to take orders rather than give them. Speaking about "new goals for the changing design of nursing," she noted, "There's no anesthesia for the pain we're going to have to go through to achieve this" ("Nursing Falling Short," 1964, p. 18).

Rogers was a charismatic leader! Throughout her career, she was an active, avid, accomplished politician and a powerful public speaker. As evidenced by writings presented in this section of the book, she used a variety of arenas to put forth her political positions relative to the nature, scope, and proposed direction of the nursing profession. Commitment to baccalaureate education as the first professional degree and to nursing as a basic science were continuous themes.

Arenas for publication of her professional and political postures included existing professional organizations (such as the newly formed New York State League for Nursing), professional journals with large circulations such as *American Journal of Nursing* (Rogers, 1975b) and *Image: The Journal of Nursing Scholarship* (Rogers, 1975a), publications not specific to nursing such as *Health-PAC Bulletin* (Rogers, 1978), and the newsletter of the Society for Advancement in Nursing (SAIN) (Rogers, 1979, 1980b, 1981), an organization she helped create to represent the interests of nurses holding baccalaureate and higher degrees in nursing as well as the consumer public.

These publications extended from the 1950s through the 1980s, with the 1970s probably representing the peak of Rogers' political activities. Rogers' first publications with a political bent were "Who Speaks for Nurses?" (Rogers, 1957) and "The Associate Degree Graduate Prepares for Professional Nursing Practice at the Baccalaureate Level" (Rogers, 1958). These were quickly followed by "Scope of Professional Nursing Practice" (1959) and "Nursing Science" (1959). While the latter two were printed without an author when published in *League Lines* of the New York State League for Nursing, they were noted to be written by her on her curriculum vitae and verified in personal communication (M. E. Rogers, personal communication, July 31, 1991). Rogers was chairperson of the editorial board of NYSLN *League Lines* at the time of publication.

Fiery rhetoric characterized Rogers' political modus operandi. This was nowhere better illustrated than in an article entitled "Cop-Out Compromises." In the article Rogers quoted President James Madison, who in 1788 commented: "I believe there are more instances of the abridgment of the freedom of the people by gradual and silent encroachment of those in power than by violent and sudden usurpation." After giving specific examples of what she considered cop-outs and compromises made by the American Nurses Association, state boards of nursing, American Academy of Nursing, American Nurses Foundation, National League for Nursing, and the federal government, she posed the following questions:

> Where is the commitment to social responsibility?
> Where is the commitment to nursing as a learned profession?
> Where is the commitment to providing society with knowledgeable nursing? (Rogers, 1979, p. 8).

Rogers fought throughout her career for those commitments. Indeed, they were the political drums for which she created the music for marching.

The Politics of Nursing Education

Rogers maintained that there is no such thing as "the nurse." She supported the concept of nursing as a "learned profession" and insisted that experience could not be equated with learning. She argued that nurses prepared for different careers in nursing; these careers were different from each other, not better or worse than one another.

In 1965 the American Nurses Association developed a position statement on nursing education that declared that all nursing education should take place within the mainstream of collegiate education. Further, there ought to be two types of nurses, "technical nurses prepared in two-year associate degree programs and professional nurses prepared at the baccalaureate level. When implemented nurses would no longer be prepared in diploma or hospital schools of nursing" ("Task Force Recommends," 1991).

In 1976 a legislative proposal was initiated by the New York State Nurses Association (NYSNA) "to provide for two categories of nurse licensure by the year 1985." This came to be known as the "1985 Proposal" ("Task Force Recommends," 1991).

In 1986 North Dakota was the first state to legally standardize the education required by two categories of nursing practice. In New York the NYSNA Entry into Practice Proposal was not enacted. In fact, a task force established by the NYSNA board of directors in 1990 issued a report to the board in 1991 supporting the current licensure process for all educational paths and further suggesting a new and additional credential be developed for nurses with a baccalaureate degree in nursing ("Task Force Recommends," 1991).

What came to be known as the Society for Advancement in Nursing (SAIN) Proposal is presented in this section of the book and contrasts with the NYSNA 1985 Proposal. This proposal was authored by the SAIN Governing Council (Resolution on Licensure, 1982). In fact, SAIN supported the coalition that was formed to defeat the NYSNA 1985 Proposal (New York State, 1985). Rogers, individually and as a leader in the SAIN licensure movement, insisted that separate licensure be required for professional practice by nurses prepared with the baccalaureate degree in nursing and that grandfathering into such a license was appropriate only for nurses who held a valid baccalaureate degree in nursing at the time of passage of such legislation.

The Politics of the Nurse-Practitioner Movement

Rogers was long involved in the fight for legal recognition of professional nursing's autonomy. She participated in the preparation, lobbying, testifying, and other activities that resulted in the eventual passage of the revision of the Nurse Practice Act in New York State in 1972. That act has served as a national model and a majority of states have since adopted similar legislation.

Considering her allegiance to autonomous nursing practice, it is no surprise that Rogers has opposed the nurse-practitioner movement from its inception in 1970, when the American Medical Association proposed that 100,000 nurses should be prepared as physicians' assistants in order to alleviate the physician shortage. As early as 1968, and no doubt long before, Rogers cried out that nursing has no dependent functions (Rogers, 1968). Rogers' position was that nurses were being recruited "out of nursing to be trained to work at a lower level—that of physician's assistant—in another field—that of medicine" ("Testimony of SAIN," 1977, p. 5). While Rogers affirmed medicine's prerogative to have assistants and nurses' right to change career goals, she questioned whether or not there was an issue of "social irresponsibility implicit in diverting nurses holding baccalaureate and higher degrees in nursing from providing those nursing services which can spell safety to the public" ("Testimony of SAIN," 1977, p. 5).

The Society for Advancement in Nursing (SAIN)

The Society for Advancement in Nursing, Inc., (SAIN) was born on January 11, 1974, in Greenwich Village, New York, to a group of leaders in nursing education (Hoexter, 1978). The organization was created to give voice to nurses who had earned at least a baccalaureate degree with a major in nursing. Established by Rogers and her colleagues, it continues to exist. Actively, for over a decade, SAIN was a strong political watchdog for the nursing profession and the consumer public. Never hesitating to vehemently speak out frankly and informatively, often taking a radical stance toward controversial health and social issues, and never intimidated by other nursing groups, political forces, or the medical-industrial complex, this organization provided a forum for addressing nursing issues, developing position papers, and preparing legislative proposals.

SAIN stood steadfast in its efforts to actualize nursing as a learned profession with various types of educational preparation, differentiated by the nature and amount of theoretical knowledge in nursing. Webster's 1960 *New Unabridged Dictionary,* second edition, defined "sain" as "to bless against evil influences and to heal." The organization adopted the Maltese cross as its logo (Hoexter, 1978).

With conviction not unlike crusaders, members were led by Rogers, who served as first president. Other members of the initial governing council were Joan C. Hoexter, first vice-president; Mary P. Kohnke, second vice-president; Erline P. McGriff, recording secretary; Patricia A. Moccia, corresponding secretary; Gean M. Mathwig, treasurer; M. Leah Gorman; and Pamela A. Price. Together they provided the leadership to address issues such as differences in nursing careers with separate licensure; recruitment, mobility, and continuing education of nurses; nursing malpractice; extending and expanding roles of nurses; nurses as physicians' assistants; institutional licensure; double standards of health care and professional education; racism in the health professions; misuse of pharmaceuticals; costs of health care; and the medical-industrial organization ("Issues to Be Examined," 1976).

Many of the issues of concern to SAIN are reflected in Rogers' writings in this section of the book. Many of these issues still loom large on the horizon of nursing education, nursing practice, and the health care system in this country and others. The political leadership role of nurses with baccalaureate and higher degrees as directed by Rogers and the SAIN crusaders remains as a foundation for formulating positions and acting on relevant concerns. More specifically, the objectives, expanded in 1983, of SAIN were as follows:

1. To differentiate between educational preparation and practice for professional and technical careers in nursing.
2. To initiate and support action directed toward new licensure for professional practice different from current registered nurse licensure.
3. To state positions on relevant issues in nursing and health.
4. To develop and implement strategies in support of positions taken.
5. To encourage all professionally educated nurses to endorse and support the philosophy and objectives of the Society for Advancement in Nursing ("Objectives," 1983).

Like Rogers, the founders and board members of SAIN were and continue to be strong women and men. Undaunted, unwavering, and often radical in her stance on issues, Rogers attracted other strong professionals to her leadership. Direct, clear, speaking out with the same voice regardless of the positions of the audience, the leaders of SAIN had an impact at state and national levels far beyond the power suggested by the numbers of their membership. The SAIN legacy was transmitted by means of publications, position papers, and perhaps particularly through the proposed act to amend the education law in relation to requirements for independent, registered, and practical nursing in New York State ("Proposed Act," 1983).

SAIN's position on licensure still stands and gives promise for the future. Indeed, many of SAIN's positions live on. History will reveal their impact on nursing education and nursing practice of the future.

Joan C. Hoexter served as SAIN's second president and Erline P. McGriff its third and current president. Current members of the governing council are: Ruben D. Fernandez, M. Leah Gorman, Joan C. Hoexter, Erline P. McGriff, Daniel J. O'Neal III, Shirley M. Robinson, Martha E. Rogers, Elizabeth Wagoner, and Beverly A. Warner. You may contact SAIN at the following address: SAIN, Inc., Box 307, Cooper Station, 11th Street and 4th Avenue, New York, NY 10003 (E. P. McGriff, personal communication, July 13, 1992).

Impact on the Profession of Nursing

Rogers, coming from a family of independent women, is perhaps a mid-century likeness of Lavinia Dock and Isabel Stewart, who earlier had marched with fellow nurses and women down Fifth Avenue in support of the rights of women and nurses. Rogers, dressed in a mink coat and a nurse's uniform complete with cap, marched with other nurses in Albany, New York, and made her famous speech on the steps of the capitol. For those who were there and for those who listened as her words echoed strongly throughout this country, there could be no doubt that as Martha Rogers spoke in favor of the 1972 Revised Nurse Practice Act of the State of New York, she spoke for autonomous nursing practice based on nursing as a scientific discipline independent and distinct from medicine. This theme of nursing as an independent scientific discipline spanned the lifetime of her career, beginning in 1937 as a rural public health nurse in Michigan and continuing in the 1990s as theoretician, educator, and political statesperson of national and international renown. Rogers is currently professor emerita, Department of Nursing, New York University.

Rogers has never considered herself a mentor since she believes that all nurses are fully capable of strong, independent action on their own and do not require mentors. She considers the roles of colleague and friend as more fitting. Nevertheless, many claim her as their mentor or inspirational guide.

In the 1970s New York University doctoral students sometimes mused that the discontented, the impatient, the intellectual rebels, and the renegades of the profession were attracted to and found a home at New York University and a leader in Rogers, whom they could respect. Who knows the extent to which this was true for the hundreds of doctoral students who have roamed the hallowed Shimkin Hall? Who knows the extent to which this influenced individual students' acceptance or rejection of Rogers' science and/or politics?

It is indeed difficult to estimate the magnitude of Rogers' impact, yet many nursing leaders in this country have been directly influenced in their professional, political, and/or scientific development by the leadership, scholarship, and yes by the personhood of Martha Rogers. Through her declaration of independence, accountability, and integrity for the nursing profession and its influence on the evolution of 20th-century nursing, it is even more difficult to estimate the indirect influence of Rogers on nurses as persons living a nursing career. Yet, it seems fair to propose that in some way what nurses know and do, whether it is in the educational, political, administrative, or practice arena, is more or less different because a particular registered nurse, Martha E. Rogers, born on the same day as Florence Nightingale, has knowingly participated in creating nursing. Rogers' rhythms have resonated throughout the nursing world and beyond. Her vision provides a guiding light for the future.

References

Dr. Martha E. Rogers elected NYSLN president. (1960, December). *League Lines, NYSLN,* p. 1.

Hoexter, J. C. (1978, June). SAIN—A brief history. *SAIN Newsletter,* pp. 2–3.

Issues to Be Examined from the SAIN Perspective. (1976, November). *SAIN Newsletter,* p. 13.

New York State Nurses Association's 1985 Resolution: Instant independent nurses and no more RNs via associate degree programs! (1985, Winter). *SAIN Newsletter,* pp. 1–2.

Nursing falling short, 200 at meeting told. (1964, October). *Detroit News,* p. 18.

Nursing science. (1959, May). *League Lines, NYSLN,* pp. 2, 5.

Objectives. (1983, February). *SAIN Newsletter,* p. 14.

Proposed act to amend the education law in relation to requirements for independent, registered, and practical nursing in New York State. (1983, February). *SAIN Newsletter,* pp. 1–11.

Resolution on licensure for entry levels to practice in nursing. (1982, October). *SAIN Newsletter,* pp. 2–4.

Rogers, M. E. (1957, December). Who speaks for nurses? *League Lines, NYSLN,* pp. 1, 4.

Rogers, M. E. (1958). The associate degree graduate prepares for professional nursing practice at the baccalaureate degree level. In *Yearbook of Modern Nursing 1957–1958* (pp. 275–279). New York: G. P. Putnam's Sons.

Rogers, M. E. (1959, November). Excellence is where you find it. *League Lines, NYSLN,* pp. 1, 8.

Rogers, M. E. (1968). Nursing science: Research and researchers. *Teacher's College Record, 69,* pp. 469–476.

Rogers, M. E. (1975a). Euphemisms in nursing's future. *Image: The Journal of Nursing Scholarship, 7*(2), 3–9.

Rogers, M. E. (1975b). Nursing is coming of age . . . through the practitioner movement, con (position). *American Journal of Nursing, 75,* 1834–1843.

Rogers, M. E. (1978). Peer review: A 1985 dissent. *Health-PAC Bulletin,* Jan-Feb, No. 80, 32–35.

Rogers, M. E. (1979, January). Cop-out compromises. *SAIN Newsletter,* pp. 4–8.

Rogers, M. E. (1980a, March). *The future of nursing.* Paper presented at the University of Louisville School of Nursing, Louisville, KY.

Rogers, M. E. (1980b, February). The umbrella that isn't! *SAIN Newsletter,* pp. 1–2.

Rogers, M. E. (1981, August). Unification: SAIN model. *SAIN Newsletter,* pp. 2–4.

Scope of professional nursing practice. (1959, May). *League Lines, NYSLN,* pp. 1, 2, 4.

Task force recommends bold new approach on entry: Supports current licensure process for all educational paths: Suggests new credential for nurses with BSN. (1991, July). *Report, New York State Nurses Association,* pp. 4–5.

Testimony of SAIN to New York State Assembly Higher Education Committee on issues concerning the health care field. (1977, May). *SAIN Newsletter,* pp. 3–6.

CHAPTER 20

Excellence Is Where You Find It

Martha E. Rogers

... Excellence is where you find it. I would extend this generalization to cover not just higher education but all education from the vocational high school to the graduate school. There may be excellence or shoddiness in every line of human endeavor. We must learn to honor excellence (indeed to demand it) in every socially accepted human activity, however humble the activity, and to scorn shoddiness however exalted the activity. There may be excellent plumbers and incompetent philosophers. An excellent plumber is infinitely more admirable than an incompetent philosopher. The society which scorns excellence in plumbing because plumbing is a humble activity and tolerates shoddiness in philosophy because it is an exalted activity will have neither good plumbing nor good philosophy. Neither its pipes nor its theories will hold water.

(From an address by John W. Gardner, President of the Carnegie Corporation, before the Association of Urban Universities in Nov., 1957).

The "trained nurse" as she was known and recognized a generation ago no longer exists. The scope of nursing practice has expanded and deepened. A body of knowledge, nursing science, is being identified. Diversification of workers within the nursing profession has emerged and concomitantly patterns of education for this diversity of workers have become clarified.

The health needs of people demand variety in nursing services. If society is to be served safely and adequately *respect for and recognition of the excellence of the contribution and the contributor regardless of level of practice* is essential.

We *cannot* afford to scorn excellence or tolerate shoddiness among any group of workers in nursing. A job well done; whether simple or complex, whether requiring minimal knowledge or extensive learning, is worthy of honor. Pride is what we are, what we know, and what we must do must replace insecurity, fear and low self-value. "Only when abiding conviction of social worth replaces lack of self-confidence, negativism, and carping comment will that climate of public opinion be created whereby nursing can move forward to greater selectivity of nursing personnel and to a level of nursing care that bespeak growth and development for the nurse herself and more and health service for society."[1] Only when nurses can respect the differences in preparation and responsibilities of the several kinds of nurses and at the same time maintain a feeling of high self-worth in their individual areas of competence can nurses achieve that level of nursing service that characterizes professional responsibility to society.

Regardless of the level of preparation the primary aim of all educational programs in nursing, from practical nurse programs through doctoral study, must be to prepare nurse practitioners.* Nurse practitioners will differ according to the knowledge and skills which are brought to bear on the health of society. The value the nurse places on herself and others will affect significantly the effectiveness of her practice.

Excellence is where you find it. Respect for excellence in all areas of human endeavor is an essential ingredient of dynamic nursing services.

---

[1]Brown, Esther Lucile, Nursing for the Future, Russell Sage Foundation, N.Y., 1948.

*Editors' note: The term *nurse practitioner* is used here to describe, in a general sense, practitioners of nursing. It is not to be confused with the meaning of the term after 1970 to indicate a particular role of "nurse practitioner."

CHAPTER 21

Accountability

Martha E. Rogers

Around this planet of people many persuasions, many beliefs—from the least knowing to the most scholarly; from the least advantaged to the most advantaged; from grim clingers to the past to avid probers of the future—all are confronted with a world whose dimensions have already undergone massive change and within which new values and growing complexities flow and ebb with ephemeral speed. Technological realities that only a short time ago were science fiction, in even the most technically advanced nations, today present ethical problems of, not only unresolved, but commonly unrecognized, magnitude.

Old ways of knowing and doing are no longer relevant. A decade ago George Counts noted that "as our feet tread the earth of a new world our heads continue to dwell in the past." Today Alvin Toffler's book, *Future Shock,* makes explicit confrontation with a tomorrow that is already here.

As new world views strain to emerge from the chrysalis of time-hardened traditions, probabilities for better achieving human health and welfare increase. Man's advent into outer space marks an era of accelerating evolution perhaps unequaled in the history of this planet. Science and technology, social complexification, and growing awareness of man's interrelatedness with nature testify to a negentropic universe of escalating innovation and diversity. Humanitarian advocates vie with machine disciples while the horizon pimples with evolutionary emergents full of surprises for the future.

The manifestations of "crisis of our times" are multiple and take many forms. Reactionaries of the right and left struggle to polarize the middle of the roaders. Civil rights organizations, Women's lib, peace movements, legislation to prevent human experimentation without informed consent of the individual, school and housing desegregation movements, among others, speak loudly to man's far too embryonic concern for human rights and the dignity of people.

Rogers, M. E. (1971, June). *Accountability.* Convocation address presented at the University of Utah College of Nursing, Salt Lake City, UT.

Vested interests, blind to social need, seek to maintain antiquated hierarchies and to beguile legislators and commissions with misinformation, negativism, and strange promises. Self-serving obsolescence is manifest by those who engage in monolithic efforts to deny the intent of national health insurance, community-based health centers, and socially responsible health services. And profits soar.

The witch doctors of yore have their present-day counterparts in fear mongerers who threaten dire effects of cholesterol, cyclamates, nicotine, mercury, radiation, and so on at the same time that amphetamines, tranquilizers, and birth control pills enjoy widespread popularity. And in neither instance is there scientific evidence rooted in a philosophy of synergistic MAN that would give substance to a modern-day "shaman's" claim either for or against these and multiple other drugs.

Shortsighted, narrowly conceived modifications of established practices parade under semantic banners proclaiming novelty. Home care services and health maintenance and promotion, initiated by nursing a century ago and continued without interruption to the present, are now solemnly proclaimed by medical doctors as a new creation of their own making.

Health careers multiply without regard for human safety. It is a sad travesty that registered nurses in hospitals spend one half their time in nonnursing activities while unskilled and semiskilled persons are assigned to nurse. Even more dangerous is an obsolete system that commonly denies society the knowledgeable judgments of nursing's professionally educated graduates of baccalaureate degree programs and the further safeguard of professional nurse direction for nursing's very important technically prepared graduates of associate degree programs, hospital schools, and practical nurse programs.

Computer technology is invading the privacy of individuals with active distress on the part of many. Genetic manipulation is moving the androids of science fiction into the real world. A perception of man's planet-bound past is beginning to give way to realization of his space-directed future.

But beyond the turmoil that shatters old securities and forces confrontation with a new world, there lies an evolutionary future of unequaled promise. Growing diversity presages new freedoms. Growing complexity speaks to a transcendence of man's present state. The "crisis in our time" is of a clearly different order from previous crises in man's evolutionary history.

To actively and creatively participate in realizing the future, whatever it may hold, demands unparalleled vision, a greatly expanded human compassion, the capacity to enjoy uncertainty, and courage to stand up and be counted; to initiate; to set direction that mankind may benefit. There is vast promise for those of wisdom, imagination, and daring whose social concern transcends personal gain and whose integrity does not vacillate.

Just as the world about us is undergoing sweeping changes, so too is nursing moving rapidly out of its prescientific era into its scientific era. Nursing's social significance achieves new dimensions of human service as knowledge melds with "commitment to people" and "courage to implement that commitment" knowledgeably, wisely, creatively, humanistically, and with vision.

Human beings are at the center of nursing's purpose. Nursing is a humanistic and a humanitarian science directed toward describing and explaining man in his synergistic wholeness and in developing the hypothetical generalizations and predictive principles basic to knowledgeable practice. The science of nursing is a science of man—the study of the nature and direction of human development.

A perception of man as a synergistic whole is clearly different from the traditional particulate view of human beings as collections of cells, organs, and systems or summations of biological, physical, social, and psychological attributes. Unitary man possesses his own integrity and manifests characteristics different from those of his parts. Just as detailed descriptions of the harmless metal, sodium, and that toxic gas, chlorine, do not predict the nature of everyday table salt, neither do detailed descriptions of parts of man predict the nature of synergistic man. The distinctive properties of man come into view only as the parts lose their identity.

Nursing is concerned with people, all people—well and sick, rich and poor, young and old—wherever they may be—in home, hospital, nursing home, clinic, school—at home, at work, at play. The phenomenon which nursing seeks to describe, explain, and predict about is clearly different from phenomena which are of primary concern to other health fields. It is this knowledge which nursing brings to the joint collaborations of a range of health professions and which adds new dimensions to human safety and to human service. Nursing is solely responsible for its own acts. It is further responsible for sharing equally with others in the great task of building a health society. No discipline today is even safe to practice alone. Only out of mutual sharing and mutual respect between health disciplines can there arise a nature and level of health services no single discipline is able or competent to provide.

The distinguishing characteristic of professional education in nursing is the transmission of nursing's body of abstract principles arrived at by scientific research and logical analysis—not a body of technical skills. This is not to deny the importance of technical skill but rather to make clear that it is nursing's theoretical knowledge that identifies nursing as a profession. It is the utilization of this knowledge in service to people that determines the nature of nursing services. It is this body of knowledge that makes possible a fulfillment of nursing's scientific humanitarianism.

Nursing exists to serve society. Nurses are directly responsible to the people they purport to serve. The nursing profession does *not* exist to serve the ends of any other profession. Nursing, as a learned profession, has *no* dependent functions. Nursing, like all other professions, has many collaborative functions—indispensable to providing society with a higher order of service than any one profession can offer. Nor does one profession delegate anything to another profession. Each profession is responsible for determining its own boundaries within the context of social need.

Nursing is concerned with human beings, only some of whom are ill. A nation's first line of defense in building a healthy people lies in maintenance and promotion of health. Any society that concentrates its health dollars and its health services on care of the sick will never be a healthy society. There is critical need for a concept of community "health services" to transcend the all too common concept of "sick services." Current activity toward making community-based diagnostic and treatment centers readily accessible to people, while critically needed, is not really incorporating a concept of health maintenance and promotion. Nurses are needed to exercise aggressive leadership that can transmute such centers into true community health resources directed toward maintenance and promotion of health. In fact it is imperative that nursing take the leadership if it is to be done. This is not to suggest that care of the sick is unimportant. Rather the sick reflect our failures to promote and maintain health. The sick do need nursing services and in reality consume the largest number of nursing hours.

That there is critical need for professionally educated nurses coordinate with learned professional personnel in other fields should need no belaboring. Documentation and recommendations for its accomplishment abound. Public safety demands it and humanitarian values support it. Institutions of higher learning are indispensable to its achievement.

Baccalaureate degree education in nursing is the cornerstone of nursing's educational system. Its *one* essential tie is with the college of arts and sciences in the institution of higher learning in which the college of nursing is located. The central focus of baccalaureate education in nursing is direct nursing services to people—all people wherever they may be. Baccalaureate degree graduates constitute nursing's hard core of professional practitioners. Higher education has a large responsibility for providing society with professionally educated nurses, as it has for preparing lawyers, medical doctors, theologians, engineers, basic scientists, and so on.

Nursing not only needs professionally educated personnel but it is also in great need of that large body of registered nurses possessing equally excellent preparation for technical practice. Technical education is not the first part of professional education. It is complete in itself. It prepares for a career worthy of honor in itself. Its products are entitled to respect for the knowledge they possess, the judgments they are prepared to make, and the services they are equipped to render. But baccalaureate degree graduates are no more interchangeable with hospital school and associate degree graduates than are dentists with dental hygienists.

A critical shortage of both professional and technical nurses is reported widely in numerous studies and is substantiated by employing agencies and by the public. It is indeed strange then to find that under a thin pretense of social concern, large sums of money are being spent in a morally reprehensible move to recruit nurses out of nursing and into medicine—with large amounts of misinformation and fallacious arguments.

The proposal to prepare physicians' assistants, though worthy in itself, has been distorted into a thinly disguised, socially irresponsible effort to increase even further an already acute shortage of nurses. Moreover, nursing's professionally educated personnel are being recruited to function at a lower level in medicine—an unbelievable human waste. Nursing's professionally educated personnel are the peers of medical doctors, dentists, engineers, lawyers, and so on. It would be equally appropriate for nursing to recruit medical doctors out of medicine and into associate degree programs in nursing as to recruit baccalaureate graduates in nursing into physician's assistant programs. Moreover, modifications of terminology are but subterfuges (ie, pediatric assistants, etc.).

The so-called expanded role of nurses is a further fallacy—designed to mislead and distort; partner to the "physician's assistant" gimmick. An expanded role for nurses is equally an expanded role for medical doctors, dentists, bioengineers, psychologists, and multiple others—an outgrowth of changing times, technological advances, and public demand for a nature and amount of health services neither available not yet envisioned. Not only is there nothing sacred about machines, but they are obsolete almost as soon as they are out.

The public is demanding active participation in determining health services and the public is entitled to factual information on which to base their participation and proposals. For as Bernard Baruch has noted, "Every man has a right to his opinions but no man has a right to be wrong about his facts." A Pandora's box of critical problems is opening up to the light of day. People are no longer willing to accept the rulings of self-appointed authorities.

Nurses carry a signal responsibility for exercising strong creative leadership in evolving health services commensurate with the needs of people in the days ahead. Nursing is the only health field that—today and throughout its history—has as a major purpose the maintenance and promotion of health. Disease prevention is a clearly different concept. Disease prevention is directed predominantly toward categorical diseases and even when not specifically categorical is nonetheless pathologically oriented and negative in its concern. And, in fact, prevention of disease is impossible of achievement if one accepts a theory of creative evolution.

Nursing is in a unique position to exercise courageous, visionary direction and leadership in proposing, initiating, and implementing interdisciplinary action toward creative community health services of a nature and amount vastly different from that which currently exists.

The future of human health and welfare requires of nurses a level of commitment and a degree of courage well beyond earlier demands. Contemporary nursing is a major social force. It is continually molding and being molded by the culture in which it exists. Man's capacity for initiating change is also the capacity of nurses for envisioning the future and determining sound direction in the great task of building a healthy society.

There is a story of an old and very wise teacher in early Athens. There was no question the teacher could not answer. There seemed to be nothing in life the old man did not understand. And finally, one of his students hit upon a way to defeat the old man's wisdom.

The student determined that he would catch a bird and hold it concealed in his hands. He would ask the old man to guess what he was holding. If the old man guessed it was a bird, then the boy would make him say whether the bird was alive or whether it was dead. And if the teacher guessed that the bird was dead, the boy would open his hands and let the bird go, free and alive. But if the wise man guessed that the bird was alive, then the boy would crush out its life and open his hands to reveal a dead bird.

And so it progressed, just as the boy had planned, until he asked the wise man: "Is the bird alive or is it dead?" And the old man said, "My son, the answer to that question is in your hands."

References

1. Counts, George S. "The Impact of Technological Change," *The Planning of Change.* New York: Holt, Rinehart, and Winston, 1962. p. 21.
2. Ehrenreich, Barbara and John. *The American Health Empire.* New York: Random House, 1970.
3. Gardner, John. *Excellence.* New York: Harper and Brothers, 1961.
4. Rogers, Martha E. *An Introduction to the Theoretical Basis of Nursing.* Philadelphia: F. A. Davis Company, 1970.
5. Toffler, Alvin. *Future Shock.* New York: Random House, 1970.

CHAPTER 22

Nursing's Expanding Role and Other Euphemisms

Martha E. Rogers

Harry Truman when told "Give 'em Hell" used to answer "I don't give them hell. I just tell them the truth and they think it's hell."

The topic to which I have been asked to address my remarks this afternoon is indeed timely. A euphemism is defined as a term alluding to an offensive thing by an inoffensive expression. The naivete with which many nurses have succumbed to seemingly harmless words is one measure of our gullibility and—interestingly enough—a contradiction of the "public advocacy" this Convention purports to be about. And, to the euphemistic jargon of "expanding role," must be added the sweetly sounding "pediatric associate," "family health practitioner," "nurse practitioner," "episodic and distributive," "Primex," "extended scope," and, let us not forget, the anomalous "physician's assistant" as well as other equally misleading words and phrases.

Nearly two hundred years ago President James Madison noted "I believe there are more instances of the abridgement of the freedom of the people by gradual and silent encroachments of those in power than by violent and sudden usurpation." More recently Lavinia Dock and Isabel Stewart warned against "influences that sap (nurses) independence and integrity." Are nurses to be taken in by dubious flattery—sometimes defined colloquially as soft soap (prime ingredient lye)? Or will we reaffirm nursing's social significance and fulfill our accountability to human health and welfare?

For more than a hundred years the scope of nursing has encompassed broad based concern for the health of people. Nightingale's claim that the art of health nursing was as important as the art of sick nursing has been made explicit in nursing's century old continuous and uninterrupted development of family health practice, community and home based health maintenance and promotion, and national and international leadership in designing and initiating public health measures—with care and rehabilitation of the sick and

Rogers, M. E. (1972). Nursing's expanding roles and other euphemisms. *Journal of the New York State Nurses Association, 3*(4), 5–10. Reprinted with permission.

disabled a constant concomitant of nursing's efforts to maintain and promote health.

Nursing is moving rapidly in its transition from a prescientific to a scientific field of endeavor despite attempted inroads by vested interests and anti-educationists both in and out of nursing. Professional and technical careers in nursing are explicit. Direct accountability to the public is a legal fact.

All manner of change is taking place. To speak literally, honestly, and without subterfuge of an expanding role for nurses is also to speak of an expanding role for medical doctors, dentists, social workers, clinical psychologists, engineers, lawyers, teachers—and so on ad infinitum. The term "expanding" is global and meaningless. New knowledge, new functions, new roles, new practice skills, new technology—are revolutionizing multiple fields and continuing education to "stay in place" has become a must for all.

Social revolution, radical revisions in values, new cosmologies, scientific upheaval, technological innovations, and rousing public demands for "health" services as well as for a thorough cleansing of the Augean stables of contemporary sick services are beginning to penetrate the walls of blind adherence to a non-existent status quo. Evolutionary acceleration is manifest in human development. Man's advent into outer space adds fuel to the capacity of life forms to transcend themselves. Humanists vie with machine disciples and the androids of science fiction move in to the real world. Fear mongers, ad nauseam, threaten all manner of dire outcomes which lack both philosophic and scientific validity. Proposed federal legislation has reached new heights of the ridiculous in a bill that would expand a law that prohibits cancer-causing substances in food and would then "essentially ban all food ingredients and most foods."[1]

A massive power struggle is underway with public demands pitted against major inequalities, incompetence, and over-charging by a so-called health system dedicated to self-serving obsolescence. The National Academy of Sciences assails the nation's emergency system.[2] The Health Policy Advisory Center decries Medicaid Mills and describes the lucrative misuse of medicaid monies by medical doctors, bankers, and real estate speculators.[3] New York's Health and Hospital Corporation is attacked for mismanagement and increasingly poorer services in the city's hospitals.[4] Ralph Nader rocks everybody's boat. Medical doctor charges go up far in excess of cost of living increases. Hospitals are picketed and store front health services are established. National Health Insurance Plans are proposed—and buried. Malpractice suits increase postulating an iceberg of even more errors hidden from legal action beneath the mighty waves of a strange complicity. And one wonders how much legislation has really stopped human experimentation without informed consent of the individual?

Nor is an angry public alone in the struggle to bring health to people. A range of health professions are rising up in opposition to medical chauvinists claiming an all-powerful control over multiple health fields in which the medical profession has neither knowledge nor competence. Efforts to deny society a range of knowledgeable health services are explicit in the A.M.A.'s and A.H.A.'s proposals for institutional licensure. An already acute shortage of nurses is worsened by efforts to get nurses to leave the field of nursing for the field of medicine. Practices established decades ago by nursing are being "discovered" by medical doctors, proposed as creations of their own making and then "delegated" back to nurses. For example the recent publication "Extending the Scope of Nursing Practice: A Report of the Secretary's Committee to Study Extended Roles for Nurses" is clear evidence of the last statement. This committee was chaired and co-chaired by medical doctors with the apparent support of nursing—i.e., the Staff Director of this Committee was a nurse. Why did a nurse deny nursing's accountability? Why did a nurse seek people from another field to tell nurses what to do? Who decides for nursing? Nightingale's statement—"Experience teaches me that nursing and medicine must never be mixed up. It spoils both"[5]—should be a warning to those who seem not to know the difference between placating a self-appointed authority and cooperative endeavor between identifiably different fields. And *now* the ancient Chinese art of Acupuncture is avowed to be the prerogative of the American medicine man.[6] What next!

That the American health and welfare system is in a crucial state is well recognized. Modifications of tradition and an obsolete status quo are unlikely to be tolerated much longer by an irate public. Nor will changing the sick care system be enough. People want to maintain their health and to become healthier. And do not confuse disease prevention with health maintenance and promotion. These are not the same things. Disease prevention is a narrowly conceived, negative, pathologically oriented approach rooted in past fallacies. Maintenance and promotion of health are positive developmental goals integral and unique to nursing and to nursing history. Nor will the jargon of "expanding role"—a cover-up for how to delegate medical tasks and get rid of nursing—give comfort to a society in sore need of knowledgeable nursing services.

What then is nursing's problem and nursing's task? Nursing is committed to serving human health and welfare. The scope of nursing was set in motion many centuries ago. It took on new dimensions of knowledge, artistry, and identity with Florence Nightingale. Today, nursing's traditionally broad scope has renewed credibility as an organized body of scientific knowledge specific to nursing evolves. The broad scope of nursing has not altered but the nature of nursing knowledge and nursing practice is changing rapidly in concert with changing times. Nursing has traditionally concerned itself with maintenance and promotion of health and habilitation and rehabilitation of the sick and disabled. Young and old; rich and poor; farmer, townsman, and metropolitan dweller—in home, school, business; hospital, clinic, nursing home; store front, ghetto, and country club; summer camp and student dormitory—all fall within the scope of nursing. Nursing's knowledge and the principles which guide nursing practice add a signal and unduplicated dimension to a much needed interdisciplinary approach to health.

Differing careers in nursing provide a range of personnel equipped in varying ways to evolve and provide creative nursing practices responsive to human needs. Confrontation with the reality of professional and technical careers in nursing is long overdue. Without such confrontation accountability and public advocacy are hollow claims. Vulnerability attacks our cowardice.

Perhaps it should not be surprising that, in a period of unprecedented escalation in knowledge and technology and of sweeping social change, we are so little able to take cognizance of John Gardner's plea for respect for individual differences and for recognition that 'equal' does not mean 'identical.'[7] Old securities are badly shaken. Many nurses are asking "Who am I?" in the health conglomerate. The term 'professional' has been misused so long in nursing that its real meaning is lost to many nurses—if it was ever known. Instead 'professional' for many is measured in hair length,[8] earrings, and uniform starch. But a learned profession by definition is characterized by an organized body of abstract knowledge arrived at by scientific research and logical analysis and used for social ends. It has *no* dependent functions. It has many collaborative ones. It is *not* identified by a body of technical skills. This in no way derogates the importance of technical skills. However it does make clear that it is not such skills that identify a learned profession. Hall and Thompson have noted that "In medicine, law, or engineering practitioners possess skills not held by laymen, but possession of scarce skills is not enough to distinguish professions from other occupations. The master plumber, or printer, the watchmaker, and the airline pilot possess skills not generally held by laymen, but they are seldom regarded as professions. What distinguishes the obvious professions from other skilled occupations is that the skills of the professional are derived from abstract knowledge of—relationships, or theory."[9]

Nursing is a learned profession. This does not mean that all who nurse are or need be professionals. On the contrary the jobs to be done require nursing personnel with different abilities, knowledges, and career goals. One is not better or worse than another. But they are different. And the difference lies in the nature and amount of knowledge each possesses and the intellectual skill in using that knowledge for human betterment. Professional education requires no less than a full college program of study leading to a baccalaureate degree with an upper division major in nursing. Baccalaureate degree graduates in nursing are no more interchangeable with registered nurse graduates of associate degree and hospital schools and practical nurses than are dentists with dental hygienists, medical doctors with physician's assistants, or engineers with engineering technicians. Society needs both kinds of nurses and both professional and technical careers in nursing are equally worthy of honor and respect. But technical education is not the first part of professional education and the panaceas proposed by career ladder dreamers do not change the reality. (Though some honest recruitment might.) A technical career is a career worthy in itself. It is not second rate nor do its practitioners need to apologize for the career they have chosen, the job they do, or the nature of the judgments they are prepared to make. And neither does the professional practitioner need to apologize because she went to college. But without identity the nursing technician is left in limbo and the professional practitioner is denied identity. And so it is that the September 10, 1972 *N.Y. Times* Crossword Puzzle makes "Hospital Aide" synonymous with R.N.

Despite the 1965 ANA Position paper on the Education of Nurses, federal differentiation as a basis for financial support, and multiple other items of readily documented evidence—nursing's failure to clearly and unequivocally differentiate professional and technical careers is explicit: 1) in misleading and not infrequently fallacious recruitment materials, 2) in absence of professional licensure—manifestly an ignoring of nursing's accountability for human safety, 3) in derogation of the rights of the professional practitioner to provide professional practice and the rights of people to receive professional nursing services, and 4) in the deception inherent in ambiguous statistics that treat types of programs and titles as a further means of avoiding confrontation.

In contradiction potential students and their parents do expect a difference between baccalaureate degree education in nursing and junior college and hospital school preparation. Admission requirements are different. The nature and amount of knowledge to be transmitted in each is different. The nature and range of job opportunities for which each is prepared are different. Salary differentials are a reality. Nor do short courses, workshops and institutes, or the misleading promises of training programs to prepare some anomalous family health practitioner to be hand maiden to medical doctors change one's career orientation.

There is no such thing as "the nurse." Nor does the generality "nursing practice" have meaning. There is professional practice and technical practice. But those who speak glibly of extending and expanding nursing practice do not really mean nursing—professional or technical. Rather the intent is to diminish and subjugate all nurses and nursing practice—to drain nursing personnel off into medicine's technical jobs of submissive posture in the high hope that nurses and nursing may be gotten rid of altogether. Legislative proposals to provide for alternate licensure in which nurses might call themselves R.N.'s *or* Physician's Assistants speak loudly and set the groundwork for getting rid of the R.N. in the next step.

Nonetheless efforts to deny society professional nursing practice do not stop it going on. Numerous nurses around the country are engaged in private professional practice—direct, autonomous services to people. A range of top leadership positions in governmental and voluntary health agencies are held by nurses. Nurses initiate social action and give top leadership to health planning.

The contradictions between what people think *is* are extreme. But a 'head in sand' philosophy more appropriately calls forth Whitehead's statement that "When attainable knowledge could have changed the issue, ignorance has the guilt of vice." I would further recommend Bernard Baruch's comment that "every man has a right to his opinions but no man should be wrong about his facts." Society needs and has a right to both professional and technical nursing services. Nurses have a right and a responsibility to practice according to the career they have chosen. Society has a right to be guaranteed minimal safety in professional practice as well as in technical practice and the need for differentiating licensure is critical and acute. And nursing does *not* license a professional worker. This has been pointed out—quietly it is true—by legal counsels federally and in a range of states including New York State some years ago.

Why have I spent so much time on clarifying careers in nursing? What does this have to do with the title of this paper? I would propose that it has everything to do with the topic. Its resolution is integral to nursing's future. And euphemistic labels are escapist sell-outs of the public we claim to care about.

The contradictions that plague nurses' perceptions of nursing would make a schizophrenic look healthy. Primary care by nurses is decades old but there are many nurses who cling desperately to dependency on other fields. The family health practitioner was initiated a century ago by nursing but this year's federal legislation to put tax dollars into preparing a "novelty," the family health practitioner, derogates such history, ignores accreditation requirements (for two decades all accredited baccalaureate programs in nursing have been doing this as a condition of accreditation), by-passes legal precedence, discredits educational preparation in nursing (both professional and technical), and disparages nursing practice—by denying recognition and support of the reality. Home care services are as old as modern nursing but there are many nurses whose awareness does not reach beyond hospital walls. Those who believe there is something to know in nursing and who are diligently engaged in the elaboration and transmission of nursing's body of scientific knowledge that people may benefit are little understood by nursing's anti-educationists still caught up in standards of doing and dependency. Professional and technical careers in nursing are a fact but "the nurse is a nurse is a nurse" continues to parade ominously in nursing literature, statistical reports, and in such notorious works as the Report of the National Commission to Study Nursing. Nurses idealize "nursing practice" but ignore the knowledge it must be based upon and then set criteria for excellence that are meaningless. The existence of excellence then, in both professional and technical practice, goes unnoticed.

With such diverse perceptions it is little wonder that nursing provides fallow ground for ploughing by vested interests. The plough share is sharpened with the verbiage of fancy words, distorted facts, and fine promises. The come-on is in blandishments and dollars. Tom Sawyer's ability to get his fence whitewashed was nothing to the way some nurses are racing to add more manual skills that are not nursing but are delegated in and by a pseudo-aristocracy of another field.

The scope of nursing is not new but it *is* taking on new dimensions of understanding and credibility. It does possess the characteristics of a learned profession. It is undergoing dramatic and accelerating transition within the context of escalating change. Nursing as a learned profession is here to stay but only those who can reach beyond Toffler's *Future Shock* and whose courage and commitment to people transcend the empty security of obsolescence, dependency, and willingness to be duped by euphemists and euphemisms will move into nursing's future.

Society will be heard and society will seek those knowledgeable and responsive to people—those who are seeking truly creative ways to health in a world in which the speed of change continues to quicken. "We ain't seen nothin' yet." In whatever ways the practice of nursing may alter, expand, extend, and develop—it *will* be the practice of *nursing.* It will *not* be the carrying out of non-nursing functions under the aegis of another field. Those who choose to leave nursing—whether they practice under the euphemism of 'pediatric associate' and the like, or as 'physician's assistant,' or engage in the narrowly conceived, non-humanistic derogation of man's wholeness in the medically propagated physical examination—have a right to do so. But they do not have a right then to claim identity with nursing.

Continuing education in nursing will be commonplace for those who do not want to join the ranks of the unemployable. (And this does not mean getting a degree.) When I say "in nursing" I further refer to a critical need for updating knowledge in the science of nursing as an indispensable prerequisite for revising and improving nursing practice.

References

1. *Herald Traveler and Boston Record American,* Thursday, September 21, 1972, p. 4.
2. *New York Times,* September 20, 1972, Section 1, p. 1.

3. *Health/PAC Bulletin,* no. 43, July-August 1972.
4. P.H.A.N.Y.C., *Public Health Notes,* August 1972.
5. Cope, Zachary, *Florence Nightingale and the Doctors,* Philadelphia, J. B. Lippincott Company, 1958, p. 121.
6. *Time,* September 18, 1972, p. 55.
7. Gardner, John, *Excellence,* New York, Harper and Row, 1961.
8. *American Journal of Nursing,* Vol. 72, No. 8, August 1972, front cover and Vol. 72, No. 10, October 1972, pp. 1801–1802.
9. Hall, R. D., and Thompson, J. D., "What Do You Mean Business is a Profession?", *Business Horizons,* Vol. 7, No. 1, Spring 1964.

CHAPTER 23

Nursing: To Be or Not to Be?

Martha E. Rogers

Nurses who "leave nursing to become physician's assistants, pediatric associates, and the like . . . are no longer entitled to identity as nurses."

Efforts to stop nursing's march toward identity and the evolution of scientifically based nursing services have been continuous and diligent since Florence Nightingale set in motion modern nursing. Other methods having failed, a new approach—one aimed at the obliteration of nursing without noticeable concern for social need or human welfare—has been designed by those still paying obeisance to an obsolete hierarchy. Cliches such as "expanded role," "physician's assistants," "pediatric associates," and multiple other meaningless verbosities provide subtle and not so subtle come-ons for the naive—nonsensical nomenclature designed to gull registered nurses into leaving nursing in order to play handmaiden to medical mythology and machines.

The public is demanding a nature and amount of health services that are a far cry from today's so-called "innovative" tinkering with traditional sick services. Charges wildly outrun costs in the mad race between the medical-industrial complex, on the one hand, and public capacity (and willingness) to support so lavish an empire on the other.[1] Shamanistic claims to medical omnipotence wrack the trembling edifice of medical pretensions. Magical threats attend an ecological negativism rooted in outdated cosmologies, and people are frightened into compliance by authoritative-sounding pronouncements proclaiming danger on every side.

Nonetheless, despite advocates of the status quo and grim clingers to time-hardened tradition, potentials for better achieving human health and welfare are becoming increasingly evident. Man's advent into outer space marks an era of accelerating evolution perhaps unequaled in the history of this planet. Science and technology, social complexification, and growing awareness of man's interrelatedness with nature testify to a universe of escalating innovation and diversity. Humanitarian advocates vie with machine disciples while the horizon pimples with evolutionary emergents full of surprises for the future. Civil rights organizations, woman's liberation, peace movements, legislation to prevent human experimentation without informed consent of the individual, school and housing desegregation movements—all of them speak loudly to man's developing but still far too embryonic concern for human rights and the dignity of people.

Health careers multiply without regard for human safety. Vested interests endeavor to do away with registered nurse licensure and, at the same time, diligently engage in legislative activities directed toward indiscriminate licensing of disparate and nebulously defined populations, providing such populations are made subject to the control of some medical priesthood. The AMA and the AHA want to do away with registered nurse licensure and make public proclamations that are often in strange contradiction to the facts.[2,3]

So unrestrained has become the battle for "control" through licensure that in August 1971 DHEW Secretary Richardson recommended a two-year moratorium on legislation that would establish new categories of health personnel with statutorily-defined scopes of functions. The extent to which this recommendation may influence federal and state action is an open question. After all, such a moratorium does have the potential of putting a few cracks in the present monolithic medical power structure.

But even cracks can be plastered over. Unless organized nursing comes forth with a clear, unambiguous, and forthright stand on licensure of health care personnel and concomitantly moves vigorously to provide for licensure of professional registered nurses as well as the current licensure for technical practice, human safety is at risk. Overt and courageous action to underwrite nursing's accountability to the public weal is pressing. The time is past for squabbling over differences of no real substance.

Denials of the reality of professional and technical careers in nursing are not only fallacious, they are ridiculous. Nursing's anti-educationists have rope handles on their argumentative shovels, unfit for digging or for leaning on. Professional and technical practitioners are sorely needed by society. But baccalaureate graduates in nursing are no more interchangeable with associate degree and hospital school graduates than dentists with dental hygienists or medical doctors with physician's assistants.

Who's in Charge Here?

The battle for domination becomes explicit in those anomalous phrases, "physician's assistant" and "pediatric associate." On the surface, proposals to develop assistants to medical doctors are not without merit. However, when such proposals are distorted into a major effort to persuade nurses to leave nursing to enter another field—medicine—some careful examination is in order. The overall shortage of registered nurses is particularly acute in relation to graduates of baccalaureate and higher degree programs. To deliberately seek to make this shortage even more critical—to con and coerce these nurses away from nursing—is morally reprehensible and socially irresponsible.

Further, *professionally educated* graduates of baccalaureate programs in nursing are the peers of physicians, dentists, lawyers, and other recognized professionals. Many persons seem unaware of the fact that the M.D. degree is a first undergraduate professional degree and that a number of medical educators have for two decades been working toward incorporating the professional core of medical education firmly within the undergraduate framework. To attempt, then, to recruit professionally educated nurses out of nursing and, even more flagrantly, to propose that they function at a lower level in the field of medicine represents an unbelievable human and intellectual waste, as well as an effort to deny society knowledgeable nursing services. It would be equally appropriate to recruit medical doctors out of medicine and into associate degree and hospital school nursing programs. Vague promises of dollars and reflected "glory" (as some see it!) are but added insult.

The naivete with which some nurses fall victim to a mythological "status rainbow" and leave nursing for a nonexistent pot of gold is a strange anomaly. They may swallow in entirety proclamations of "new functions" that in reality have been integral to nursing practice for many decades. Moreover, many so-called "new functions" are really limited to the confines of medical knowledge and medical practice and to the manipulation of machinery.

For example, a physician at the University of Virginia is reported to have initiated a 4-month program to turn "nurses into nurse practitioners."[4] How remarkable! The real intent of the program—to gull nurses out of nursing—becomes clear when one notes that potential recruits are promised that they will join second-year medical students in classes in medical pathology and medical diagnosis. Nurses who elect this program may become fine helpers to physicians but they will have neither improved nor enhanced their practice of nursing. In fact, it is reasonable to deduce that their capacity to engage in knowledgeable nursing diagnosis and care will be reduced, as a result of ambiguities introduced by a discipline that is essentially concerned with physiological pathology in contrast to nursing's concern with unitary man. Medical knowledge, no matter how relevant to medical practice, is not a substitute for the nursing knowledge that is essential to nursing practice.

The right to change one's career goals is not at issue. But nurses who leave nursing to become physician's assistants or pediatric associates must realize that they *are* leaving nursing. They must refer health care consumers to properly qualified nurse practitioners if those consumers are to receive competent and safe nursing service as well as truly comprehensive health services. Medical practitioners are properly limited to the practice of medicine. They are not competent to practice in or exercise control over any other professional field. The provision of comprehensive health care demands the services of a range of disciplines for even minimal safety, and medicine is only one of such disciplines.

The Science of Nursing

Nursing is a learned profession. Professional education in nursing requires no less than a full college program of study with an upper division major in the given field. Nursing's boundaries have advanced through an earlier, prescientific era into an emerging, scientifically based, humanitarianism that promises new and expanded benefits to people and society. The science of nursing is *not* a summation of facts and principles drawn from other sources; it is a science of synergistic man—unitary man—characterized by an organized conceptual system from which are derived the hypothetical generalizations and unifying principles essential to guide practice.[5] And the art of nursing takes on new dimensions as practice becomes underwritten with substantive nursing knowledge.

Nursing is concerned with people, all people—well and sick, rich and poor, young and old, wherever they may be, at work and at play. The phenomenon which nursing seeks to describe, explain, and predict differs clearly from the phenomena that are of primary concern to other disciplines. It is *nursing knowledge* that nurses bring to the joint collaborations of a range of health professions; it is nursing knowledge that adds new dimensions to human safety and human service; and it is nursing's body of scientific knowledge that guides nursing practice.

Nursing is solely responsible for its own acts. It is further responsible for sharing equally with others in the great task of building a healthy society. Only out of mutual sharing and respect among health disciplines can there arise a nature and quality of health services that no single discipline can provide on its own.

Nursing exists to serve society, and nurses are directly responsible to the people they purport to serve. The nursing profession does *not* exist to serve the ends of any other profession, nor does one profession delegate anything to another profession. Each profession must determine its own boundaries within the context of social need. As a learned profession, nursing has *no* dependent functions but, like all other professions, has many collaborative functions that are indispensable to providing society with a higher order of service than any one profession can offer. Only professionally educated nurses are safe or competent to guide nursing practice and to make the complex judgments that require substantive knowledge and a high degree of intellectual skill.

Nursing is concerned with human beings, only some of whom are ill. The first approach toward building a healthy people lies in maintenance and promotion of health. Any society that concentrates its health dollars and services on care of the sick will never be a healthy society. There is a critical need for a concept of community "health services" to transcend the all too common concept of "sick services." Present efforts toward creating community based and readily accessible diagnostic and treatment centers, while critically needed, do not really incorporate a concept of health maintenance and promotion. It is imperative that nurses exercise aggressive leadership if such centers are to be transmuted into true community health maintenance and promotion resources. This is not meant to suggest that care of the sick is unimportant. Rather, the sick reflect our failures to promote and maintain health. The sick do need nursing services and consume the largest number of nursing hours at the present time.

The nature and delivery of present health services are critically inadequate and unsafe and notably obsolete. Concomitantly, only limited attention is being given to the nature of those who propose to deliver these services. It is a sad travesty that registered nurses spend approximately half their time in nonnursing activities, while unskilled and semiskilled persons are assigned to carry out many nursing tasks. Even more dangerous is an obsolete system (partially perpetuated by nursing's anti-educationists) that denies society the knowledgeable judgments of professionally educated nurses and the further safeguard of professional nurse direction for nursing's very important technical practitioners.

Short-sighted, narrowly conceived modifications of long existing practices parade under the semantic banner of "innovation." For example, physicians are now declaring that home care services and health maintenance and promotion, initiated more than a century ago by nursing, are a new creation of *their* making. Nightingale's proposal that health nursing was as important as sick nursing was derogated by the vested interests of her day, but Nightingale nonetheless initiated the health visitor role in nursing. Nationally and internationally, nursing has been in the forefront in proposing and implementing positive health measures of wide-scale critical import. The family health practitioner has existed in nursing for over a century.

Nursing's qualified family health practitioner has also long been a primary health care provider. Certainly, all registered nurses are not prepared to initiate and implement primary health care services. This was made explicit in the 1930's with passage of the Social Security Act that included provision for higher education in public health nursing to prepare nurses for responsible leadership in the broad field of community health. The "ideal" team proposed 40 years ago included a public health nurse, a physician, a sanitary engineer, and a secretary. But when communities lacked the financial resources to engage in a full-scale health program, the public health nurse was identified as the single most important person best equipped to initiate and implement a program of community health. For nearly two decades all graduates of accredited baccalaureate degree programs in nursing have fulfilled requirements for broad-based community health practice. That the intent may have exceeded the reality in some programs is no reason to deny the existence of primary health care providers and family health practitioners in nursing.

And so one arrives at the misleading and fallacious implications of a so-called "expanded role." An expanded role for nurses is equally an expanded role for physicians, dentists, bio-engineers, psychologists, and many others—an outgrowth of changing times, technological advances, and public demand for a nature and amount of health services neither available nor yet scarcely envisioned. But the activities commonly attributed to nursing's "expanded role" generally replace nursing practice with non-nursing functions (thereby decreasing nursing services to people) or constitute deformed and delimited responsibilities that, in a valid form, have long been taken for granted as integral to the broad scope of nursing practice and outside the realm of medical practice.

Technology in Perspective

Monitoring new machines (or old ones, for that matter) is a skill that must be learned by all who would use them, regardless of their particular field. Neither full college nor graduate education is needed to develop such skill. However, the assessments to be made about persons whose care involves the use of modern technological tools *do* require a substantial scientific base—one that is specific to the given discipline and gained through baccalaureate or higher degree education.

Safe nursing judgments can be made only by nurses with a firm base in the science of nursing, not by persons in other disciplines who lack this scientific base. In the joint deliberations of a range of disciplines lies the potential for more effective services. This is not a denial of knowledge which many groups may hold in common; indeed, the interrelatedness of knowledge is becoming more and more evident. But the hard core of scientific knowledge that characterizes each individual profession provides the frame of reference within which that profession practices.

Divide and Conquer

A growing number of nurses are recognizing the strange and muted motivations underlying an increasingly open attack upon the continued existence of nursing. "Divide and conquer," truism though it is, is manifest in efforts to prevent nurses from joining their professional organization (even going so far as to threaten loss of employment) and in setting up quasi-competing groups under the aegis of a controlling male paternalism (even going so far as to provide Caribbean cruises!). And we must add here the dollar decoys to nurses to become enslaved under the cacophonic, standardless title of "physician's assistant." The multi-million dollar ploy to get rid of nurses and nursing has a grim and foreboding pattern.

Thus, in New York State, the governor recently vetoed a bill—one proposed by the New York State Nurses' Association and approved by both houses of the state legislature—that would have up-dated the definition of nursing. And he vetoed this bill, in a statement rife with misinformation, without discussion with those who would have clarified the facts and have at least made possible an informed statement. True, the use of nonsensical nomenclature found its way into legislative halls but with much less public success than proponents anticipated. It would seem that the public believes that nursing is a socially significant endeavor and a field having a major contribution to make in its own right to human health and welfare.

Nonsense words continue to abound in any discussion of health or nursing care delivery. A massive sweep of stale air, for example, attends the jargon of "episodic" and "distributive" put forth in *An Abstract for Action,* the report of the National Commission for the Study of Nursing and Nursing Education.[6] How reminiscent this is of an outmoded identification of nurses according to place of employment (i.e., hospital and public health) and how contradictory it is to public demands and health needs of people. Are health services to be impoverished and human safety placed in growing jeopardy on a band wagon of double-talk? Will nurses permit construction of a monolith to "nothing to know in nursing?"

Nursing is by no means guiltless in its failure to come to grips with significant issues and in its adherence to a sad state of dependency fostered by too prolonged an isolation from the mainstream of higher education and social responsibility. Confrontation with the status quo can be a frightening experience, and uncertainty as to who one is in the shifting kaleidoscope of often contradictory proclamations and proposals adds to the difficulties nurses face in determining responsible self-direction. But to those who believe that nursing is a socially significant endeavor there is already recognition that steps to implement a philosophy of humanitarian concern and to make clear nursing's unique and signal place in the health care system are already dangerously overdue.

To the need for the assertion of nursing identity must be added equal needs for commitment and courage, and these in turn must be translated into strong, aggressive action that has as its goal the betterment of mankind. Nurses must not continue to let themselves be cast in the role of the foolish and gullible emperor in the old fairy tale of "The Emperor's New Clothes." The emperor *believed* what he was told, despite all evidence to the contrary. In such foolishness and gullibility there is also vulnerability.

Specific actions need to be taken immediately if nursing is not to find itself relegated to musty history books and if society is not to be denied nurses and nursing services. Differentiation of professional and technical careers and licensure for each are essential. Persons who chose to leave nursing to become physician's assistants, pediatric associates, and the like must find their identity in the new field they have chosen. They are no longer entitled to identity as nurses.

A Call for Unity

A national unified front of social concern and responsible self-direction must take precedence over splinter groups concerned with their own special interests. Efforts "to divide and conquer" through draining nurses off into subgroups of other disciplines must be boycotted. Joint endeavors with other disciplines are to be encouraged, but only on a basis of mutual respect for the peer professional contributions of each. Nurses must take leadership in evolving, planning, and implementing health care for all people. When this is best carried out in concert with members of other health disciplines, it does not diminish nursing's responsibility for leadership.

Nursing is in a unique position to exercise courageous and visionary direction in proposing, initiating, and implementing interdisciplinary action toward creative community health services of a nature and amount vastly different from those that currently exist. Such action, however, will require of nurses a level of commitment and a degree of courage well beyond earlier demands. Contemporary nursing is a major social force. Man's capacity for initiating change is also the capacity of nurses for envisioning the future and determining sound directions in the great task of building a healthy society.

References

1. Health Policy Advisory Committee. *American Health Empire,* by Barbara Ehrenreich and John Ehrenreich. New York, Random House, 1970.
2. American Medical Association, Department of Health Manpower. *Licensure of Health Occupations.* Chicago, The Association, 1971.
3. Engelston, E. M., and Kinser, Thomas. Licensure of health care personnel. *Hospitals* 44:35–39, Nov. 16, 1970.
4. Nurse practitioner course opens in Virginia (News) *Am. J. Nurs.* 71:2096, Nov. 1971.
5. Rogers, Martha E. *An Introduction to the Theoretical Basis of Nursing.* Philadelphia, F. A. Davis Co., 1970.
6. National Commission for the Study of Nursing and Nursing Education. *An Abstract for Action.* Jerome Lysaught, Director. New York, McGraw-Hill Book Co., 1970.

CHAPTER 24

Nursing Is Coming of Age . . . Through the Practitioner Movement, Con (Position)

Martha E. Rogers

"Stop the world! I want to get off. . . ." Futile words indeed. Not only is there no stopping but the speed of change continues to escalate. Diversity grows.

"Future shock" is a household phrase. Evolution accelerates. People sleep less and live longer. Proponents of doom and ecological negativists are contradicted by a seemingly unprecedented population explosion and incredible achievements in science and technology, even to outer space exploration. The paranormal is normal. Man struggles to extricate himself from no longer tenable world views, and utopian dreams of disease control flounder amidst out-dated concepts of homeostasis, adaptation, and causality.

Development norms of even 30 years ago no longer are valid. Evolutionary emergence can be identified in rapidly changing life styles and astronauts grow taller as they roam far beyond this planet.

Cancer and cardiac conditions may properly be hypothesized to illustrate life's many probings for new rhythms. Dwellers in outer space may soon have to have support systems in reverse to visit this planet. It is no longer enough to ask "Why?" We must dream the impossible and ask "Why not?"

It is within this creative frame of reference that nursing has moved from its prescientific period into its scientific coming of age and the practice of nursing is thus taking on renewed substance.

For more than a hundred years the scope of nursing has encompassed broad-based concern for the health of people. Nightingale's claim that the art of health nursing was as important as the art of sick nursing has been made explicit in nursing's century-old continuous and uninterrupted development of family health practice, community and home-based health maintenance and promotion, and national and international leadership in designing and initiating public health measures—with care and rehabilitation of the sick and disabled a constant concomitant of nursing's efforts to maintain and promote health. Primary care by nurses is as old as modern nursing. Professional and technical careers in nursing are explicit. Direct accountability of nurses to the public is a legal fact.

An expanding role for nurses is equally an expanding role for medical doctors, dentists, engineers, social workers, psychologists, lawyers, teachers, and so on, ad infinitum. New knowledge, new functions, new roles, new practice skills, new technologies are revolutionizing multiple fields, and continuing education to stay in place has become a must for all.

First and foremost in nursing's thrust to the future is the urgent and long overdue need for clear, unambiguous differentiation of nursing's professional and technical careers. Professionally educated nurses are a reality, and platitudinous denials do not change the facts. The multiple problems which nursing faces will not be resolved except as nursing ceases to wallow in its antieducationism and declares its recognition of career differences.

Society needs both professional and technical nurses, and both are equally worthy of honor and respect. Technically prepared nurses do not have to apologize for the career they have chosen, and neither do professionally educated nurses need to apologize because they went to college to prepare for a professional career. Failure to differentiate careers puts in limbo nursing's technical registered nurse practitioners and denies the existence of professional nursing personnel. It is little wonder that twice last year the *New York Times* crossword puzzles made "hospital aide" synonymous with "R.N."

Nursing's future—its very existence as an identifiable field of endeavor—is dependent on differentiation that values nursing's body of scientific knowledge and makes explicit nursing's social accountability through separate licensure of nursing's baccalaureate degree graduates. It is incredible that in today's world there should continue to be bickering over problems that are empty rhetoric based on false assumptions and mendacious declamations.

Baccalaureate degree education in nursing is neither a replacement for nor an upgrading of associate degree and hospital school programs. Its emergence is a manifestation of escalating knowledge, changing times, new values, and public demand for a nature and amount of health services not only not available but scarcely imagined. It adds a new dimension to nursing's past and declares nursing's accountability for human safety.

Although baccalaureate degree education for nurses has existed for 70 years, and was given added impetus with passage of the Social Security Act of the 1930's, it was Mildred Montag's epoch-making initiation in 1951 of associate degree nursing programs to replace hospital schools that accelerated nursing's move into the nation's educational mainstream and which forced baccalaureate degree programs to take on more of the characteristics of learned professional education. Federal monies in support of graduate education in nursing strengthened the numbers and quality of nursing faculty. Doctoral study stimulated nurses toward actualizing their intellectual potential in theoretical formulations indispensable to a learned profession.

Between 1962 and 1972 employed nurses holding baccalaureate and higher degrees increased by more than 118 percent. During the same period 48.7 percent more associate degree, hospital school, and practical nurse graduates were employed in nursing with associate degree graduates accounting for the largest proportionate increase accompanied by a decline in hospital school graduates. The ratio of practicing baccalaureate and higher degree graduates to associate degree, hospital school, and practical nurse graduates changed from 1 professional to 14 technical in 1962 to 1 professional to 9.9 technical in 1972.

The valid baccalaureate degree characterized by a substantive upper division major in nursing is the first professional degree in nursing and is comparable to the initial professional degrees awarded in medicine, dentistry, engineering, law, and the like, which also are undergraduate first professional degrees. The doctor of medicine and other equivalent degrees are not to be confused with the higher doctorates—Ph.D., Sc.D., et cetera. Although growing numbers of persons representing a range of health fields are engaged in a diversity of social and health services of professional and subprofessional nature, medicine, dentistry, and nursing have long constituted the primary resources for such services. A comparison of numbers of personnel and growth rates in medicine, dentistry, and professional nursing brings into focus some commonly overlooked realities [Table 1].

Between 1966 and 1972 the number of baccalaureate and higher degree graduates in nursing increased by 45.4 percent, whereas for the same period the increase in dentists was 6.1 percent and in medical doctors only 10.6 percent. In actual numbers added to the employment market, professionally educated nurses exceeded both dentists and medical doctors. Nonetheless, in 1972 professionally educated nurses and dentists, respectively, constituted only approximately 20 percent each of available personnel compared with 58.1 percent medical doctors.

As the number and proportionate representation of baccalaureate and higher degree graduates in nursing have increased, so too has the traditional power structure become increasingly threatened. The notably larger scope of nursing in comparison with the fields of medicine and dentistry in particular, and other health fields in general, has been explicit since the beginning of modern nursing.

Table 1. Licensed Nursing Personnel Employed in Nursing

Year	Graduates with Baccalaureate Degrees in Nursing (n)	Graduates with Master's Degrees in Nursing and Doctorates (n)	Total (n)	Graduates with Diplomas, Associate Degrees, and Non-Nursing Baccalaureate Degrees (n)	Practical Nurses (n)	Total (n)
1962	43,500	11,500	55,000	495,000	225,000	720,000
1966	64,500	15,300	79,800	541,200	282,000	823,200
1970	80,000	19,000	99,000	601,000	370,000	971,000
1972	101,912	18,366	120,278	644,045	427,000	1,071,045

Data from *ANA Facts About Nursing,* 1966, 1970, 1972. American Nurses' Association, Kansas City, MO.

Nightingale initiated family health practice and set in motion nursing's broad-based orientation to the significance of the man/environment relationship. The first prenatal care in the Western world by any field was initiated by the Instructive Nursing Association of Boston in 1901. Community nursing was established in the United States in 1877 and by 1893 "all the social, economic, and industrial conditions affecting the lives of those receiving services were considered integral to the practice of 'visiting nurses.'"[1]

For many decades, "nurses on horseback" were the sole health providers to the mountain people of Kentucky. The first United States Public Health Service officer to be decorated by two foreign governments was a nurse. Despite major obstacles, including a well-developed antieducationism among many nurses, the profession has long provided distinctive national and international leadership in both the health and welfare fields [Table 2].

Today nursing is a house divided in its search to determine new directions for the future. Failure to clearly and unambiguously differentiate professional and technical careers in nursing, legally and otherwise, denies reality, jeopardizes the public health, and leaves nursing vulnerable to the onslaughts of vested interests. An insidious, socially unconcerned, heavily financed, and well-planned conspiracy to take over nurses and nursing is approaching a climax.

The naive in nursing are victimized by euphemisms, glib promises, and false declarations put forth by power and profit propagandists. Legal subtleties are being introduced into governmental chambers, designed to turn R.N.'s (particularly those with baccalaureate and higher degrees in nursing) into physician's assistants by whatever euphemism. The *Richmond News Leader* of February 26, 1975 head-lined an article, "A Nurse is a Nurse is a Nurse—Unless She's a Practitioner."[2] They should have added "And Then She's a Physician's Assistant—Not a Nurse."

The American health care system is in a notoriously sad state, and millions of dollars are being spent to keep it that way. Despite heavy documentation of society's needs for both professional and technical nursing services, major efforts are on-going to recruit nurses out of nursing into medicine.

Although there are almost three times as many M.D.'s as there are professionally educated nurses, nonetheless medicine is striving diligently to diminish these numbers and to force these nurses to practice at a lower level in medicine. That society will thereby be denied sorely needed, broad-based health services different from and beyond the scope, knowledge, and compe-

Table 2. Active Professional Personnel and Percent Changes

Year	Medical Doctors (n)	Change over Previous Period (%)	Dentists (n)	Change over Previous Period (%)	Graduates with Baccalaureate and Higher Degrees in Nursing (n)	Change over Previous Period (n)
1966	300,375	—	98,670	—	79,800	—
1970	311,203	+3.6	102,220	+3.0	99,000	+24.0
1972	333,259	+7.0	105,400	+3.1	120,278	+21.4

Data from *ANA Facts About Nursing,* 1966, 1970, 1972. American Nurses' Association, Kansas City, MO, and National Center for Health Statistics, Bethesda, MD.

tence of the medical profession seems of little concern to these proponents of intellectual waste and transgressors of public rights.

Not all nurses have succumbed to the blandishments of euphemisms and the increasingly blatant perfidy spawned by such terms as pediatric associate, nurse practitioner, primary care practitioner, geriatric practitioner, physician extender, and other equally weird and wonderful cover-ups—designed to provide succor and profit for the nation's shamans. As naivete gives way to recognition of the real intent behind this con game, one can expect that those nurses who are committed to a body of knowledge in nursing, who are cognizant of nursing's broad scope and eminent history, who believe that people have a right to knowledgeable nursing practice, and whose integrity and courage transcend today's widespread chicanery in the health fields will return to nursing, dedicated anew to providing the human services specific to nursing and beyond the ken and scope of other health disciplines.

The future of nursing rests in the hands of those committed to knowledgeable nursing. Those nurses who leave nursing to be assistants to physicians under whatever title will soon find that their permission to practice anything will derive from medical doctor certification and legal licensure under laws perpetuated by medicine for physician's assistants. The rights of these nurses to change fields is unquestioned, but those who have done so or who will do so in the future can no longer claim membership in the nursing fraternity. Moreover, programs of instruction, leading to degrees or otherwise, now labelled nursing but in reality preparing physician's assistants, must forego their titular fraudulence, naive though it may be.

Any program or course of study that requires M.D. instruction, certification, and supervision is not preparing for nursing practice. M.D.'s are licensed to practice only medicine. They have neither the knowledge nor the competence (nor are they licensed) to practice or to supervise nursing. Potential students of nursing have a right to know honestly the career for which they are to be prepared.

Nursing is a learned profession though all who nurse are not and need not be professionally educated. Decades of using the term "professional" to mean "to work for gain" has blinded many nurses to the meaning of "professional" as a learned occupation. Differentiation of nursing's professional and technical careers derives from the nature and amount of knowledge possessed by each. Experience is not a substitute for learning, and functions do not, per se, identify career differences. What one does is determined by what one knows, coupled with the intellectual judgment necessary to translate that knowledge into practice.

The need to establish standards and to license for professional practice in nursing cannot be overemphasized. In its absence, nursing's professional personnel, graduates of full college and university programs which offer a substantive, upper division, theoretical base in nursing, are denied identity and opportunity to use their knowledge for human betterment. The public is victimized by persons granted baccalaureates in the absence of baccalaureate education in nursing. Graduates of associate degree, hospital school, and practical nurse programs are held liable for acts for which they are unprepared and which require professional direction for their safe execution [Table 3].

Licensure for technical practice in nursing is of long standing. Registered nurse and practical nurse examinations are used nationally. One examination

Table 3. Distribution of Active Medical Doctors, Dentists, and Nurses with Degrees* in Nursing

Year	Medical Doctors n(%)	Dentists n(%)	Professional Nurses n(%)	Total (n)
1966	300,375(62.9)	98,670(20.6)	79,800(16.6)	478,845
1970	311,203(59.1)	116,980(22.1)	99,000(18.8)	526,483
1972	333,259(58.1)	119,700(20.9)	120,278(21.0)	573,237

*Baccalaureate degrees and higher.
Data from *ANA Facts About Nursing,* 1966, 1970, 1972. American Nurses' Association, Kansas City, MO, and National Center for Health Statistics, Bethesda, MD.

(rather than the current two) for associate degree, hospital school, and practical nurse graduates would unite these groups, eliminate meaningless dichotomies, and give rational coherence to this significant and much-needed career in nursing. Some form of grandfather clause would be needed for practical nurses in this process. Students seeking a technical career in nursing should be directed into college-based associate degree programs rather than into hospital school and practical nurse programs.

Registered nurse licensure is long established. The letters "R.N.," are highly cherished by most nurses. They spell valued technical practice to the public. Human needs dictate continuation of this career, and human safety demands licensure for this level of nursing practice. Nursing's technically prepared personnel are not second-rate citizens. Nor are they half-baked professionals. They are prepared to practice in a career that is worthy of honor and respect in itself.

Nursing has never licensed a learned professional worker as this term has come to be understood in our society. Nursing's professional personnel are as different from nursing's associate degree, hospital school, and practical nurse graduates as medical doctors are different from physician's assistants, dentists from dental hygienists, and engineers from engineering technicians. Society needs both professional and technical workers. One is not better than the other. Rather, they represent identifiably different careers equally worthy of honor and respect.

Licensure exists to protect the public. Licensure for professional practice demands that all so licensed whether by examination or by initial exemption from examination (as new licensing laws are passed) must possess no less than a full college program of study with an upper division nursing major. Anything less would continue to deny society safety in nursing services.

Initial licensure for professional and technical practice is only the beginning. In a world of accelerating change, innovations and creative ideas multiply like rabbits. Continued learning for all who nurse is of serious import, but for nursing's professional practitioners mandatory continuing education is critical. Quite obviously, self-regulation, regardless of the profession concerned, is notoriously inadequate. Continuing education must become a recognized way of life if society is to be served safely. It will be commonplace for nurses who do not want to join the ranks of the unemployable in nursing. Moreover, continuing education must have as its core the ongoing, updating of knowledge in the science of nursing which is indispensable to revising and improving nursing practice. Licensing laws for professional practice must incorporate mandatory continuing education within them.

Employment practices must be revised to recognize that knowledgeable nursing leadership is a critical factor in safeguarding human health and welfare. Yet in 1972, only 16 percent of those nurses holding administrative positions in nursing services were educationally qualified for their responsibilities. An additional 22 percent were reported to hold baccalaureates, some unknown proportion of which were not in nursing.[3] While certain non-nursing administrative tasks do not necessarily require substantive nursing knowledge, responsibility for the care of people does. Despite a 38 percent increase in nursing administrators with master's degrees from 1967 to 1972, approximately two-thirds of those holding nursing service administrative titles in 1972 were not prepared at even the minimal level for professional practice in nursing.

A numerical shortage in qualified nursing personnel for administrative positions is a reality. However, a value system that denies differences is unlikely to motivate nurses or employers to recognize that public accountability demands substantive knowledge in those who would direct nursing's services. Arguments for continuing federal monies in support of preparing nurses for these significant responsibilities require nursing's commitment to knowledgeable leadership. Employment practices do not reflect such a commitment, and failure to differentiate careers gives a hollow ring to accountability.

The situation is particularly crucial when one considers that some portion of employed nurses holding baccalaureate and higher degrees are actually practicing as physician's assistants, further decreasing the amount of knowledgeable nursing services, to the public detriment.

Third-party payment for nurses' services constitutes another issue of grave concern. Safety to practice as an independent practitioner requires professional education, and nursing's professional practitioners bring to society a nature and scope of service not available from any other source. They are independent practitioners, whether self-employed or otherwise, liable for their own acts, and responsible for the acts of others as appropriate. They are as entitled to payment for the services they render as are comparable persons in any other field. Moreover, society is entitled to and desperately needs the knowledgeable services such payment would make available.

Resolution of the health care crisis is heavily dependent on the extent to which nursing provides aggressive, knowledgeable leadership in setting new directions coordinate with human needs and new knowledge. Nurses must develop innovations in the delivery of health services that are truly creative and genuinely responsive to public demand. In fact, one might propose that strong nursing leadership is indispensable to any rational resolution of the current health situation.

Today's health care crisis is a miasma of vested interests, obsolescence, malpractice, incompetence, and questionable social concern. While some groups may be more guilty than others, few can properly throw the first stone.

Organized medicine, in print and on national TV, has declared "there is no health care crisis in this country."[4] Legislators and other governmental personnel bicker over national health insurance proposals, all of which suffer from the subversive tactics of the socially irresponsible.

Bankers, insurance companies, drug houses, the legal fraternity, hospital economists, nursing home owners, and a wide range of others have been implicated in postulated public rip-offs.

Organized nursing is slow to take socially aggressive positions that contradict the power structure in fear of already demonstrable, though not always obvious, retaliations from the power-profit sector of the health establishment and its governmental cohorts. Everyone blames everyone else.

In view of such a picture the eternal optimist might note that man has survived for many decades in spite of the health professions, so surely there is hope for the future. And so there is if nursing fulfills the promise of its past and strives mightily to build a future rooted in humanitarian concerns and creative ideas.

The ratio of professional to technical nurses needed to serve society in the days ahead is problematical. However, a workable proportion toward which to strive can be proposed as one professional to three technical nurses.

Today's shortage of nursing personnel is clearly in the population holding baccalaureate and higher degrees in nursing. Those who are committed to nursing as a learned profession and who are dedicated to providing the unique services which only nurses are prepared to offer must be identified and supported. Ways must be developed to increase their numbers and to provide for vastly improved geographic distribution so that all people here and in other lands may be served. Better geographic distribution must be predicated on adequate numbers of both professional and technical personnel.

New technologies as well as new knowledge must be incorporated into the instructional process. Novel ways of providing health services must be introduced. Nurses are central figures in any multidisciplinary health center. Whether the nurse is top administrator of such a center or is a team contributor, the inclusion of positive health measures of broad scope requires the active participation and leadership of qualified nursing personnel for its planning and implementation. Emphasis on care of the sick is not enough. Maintenance and promotion of health must be incorporated into the warp and woof of such centers if there is to be a healthy society.

In the days ahead, nursing's century-old struggle to be heard that people might be served will continue to confront the committed in nursing. Vain promises, illusions of gain, and rainbows of dependency will undoubtedly plague those of faint heart and little vision. Some will leave nursing, as some already have, to be swallowed up in the maw of medical shamanism no matter how labelled. But the majority will hang in—eschewing the antieducationism of nursing's past, striving to fulfill the substantive social responsibility of nursing's commitment, and creating with zest a new world of human service.

References

1. Dock, L. L., and Stewart, I. M. *A Short History of Nursing from the Earliest Times to the Present Day.* New York, G. P. Putnam's Sons, 1920, p. 162.
2. Propert, Joy. A nurse is a nurse is a nurse—unless she's a practitioner. *Richmond News Leader* (Richmond, Va.) Feb. 26, 1975, p. 31.
3. Arnold, Pam. Nurse administrators profiled: big job, low pay. *Am Nurse* 7:2, Apr. 1975.
4. Hoffman, C. A. Balanced system in A.M.A.'s concern. *U.S. Medicine* Jan. 15, 1973, p. 29.

CHAPTER 25

Euphemisms in Nursing's Future

Martha E. Rogers

This paper is designed "to tell it like it is" and "like it is" is buried beneath a massive array of euphemisms perpetrated to deny a future to nurses and nursing. A euphemism is defined as a term alluding to an offensive thing by an inoffensive expression. Seemingly harmless words have mushroomed into a euphemistic jargon that includes such remarkable ambiguities, fallacies and obsolescence as "expanding role, pediatric associate, family health practitioner, primary care (Primex product)," and other weird and wonderful cover-ups for the finest euphemism of all—"the physician's assistant." I have the strange belief that what people need is professional and technical nursing services. In fact I am just enough of an optimist to believe that nurses are going to wake up from this euphemistic nightmare and declare an honest accountability for and advocacy of human rights to socially significant health services.

The American health care system is in a notoriously sad state and millions of dollars are being spent to try to keep it that way. But "little public squeals" are amplifying into "big public howls." Vested interest villainies are being exposed. Power, profit, and propaganda—despite their overriding prevalence—are not really socially acceptable motives. What are some of the realities with which nurses must come to grips in order to declare the nature and direction of their commitment? Will it be a commitment to the continuing development of nursing as a learned profession or will it be a cop out to euphemisms, anti-educationism, and denial of social responsibility? What is really going on?

Proposals to prepare physicians' assistants should not have surprised anyone really. In fact the amazing thing about the whole idea is its 'Johnny-come-lately' aspect. Nurses have had assistants for decades. So too have engineers, lawyers, dentists, master plumbers, electricians, and no end of other experts.

Rogers, M. E. (1975). Euphemisms in nursing's future. *Image: The Journal of Nursing Scholarship, 7*(2), 3–9. Reprinted with permission.

Actually almost everyone in contemporary society is busy trying to find himself or herself or itself an assistant. Assistants are very great things and surely assistants to medical doctors are particularly great things.

The economic value of P.A.'s to M.D.'s is especially notable. How the medical profession could have overlooked such a fabulous potential profit for so long seems very strange when one considers the wide variety of other highly productive, dollar producing enterprises in which M.D.'s engage. Just the little matter of raising medical charges well in excess of other Consumer Index Categories[1] leaves one a little breathless. And one can only admire the seeming foresight that established grossly increased medical charges ahead of the federal deep freeze, thus providing an advanced base for further increases in charges as federal controls were relaxed.[1] But after all the Internal Revenue Service has only recently gotten around to investigating the exceptional and inflationary prices in the medical-care field[1] so perhaps medical doctors should be forgiven for their delay in marketing a physician's assistant.

With a little thought and a few carefully selected references one can find additional reasons why potential profits to be accrued from the services of physicians' assistants may have taken a lower priority. In a truly team approach by some of those oriented to the novel and innovative 'team way' of providing health services some medical doctors, bankers, and real estate speculators have founded a lucrative business in Medicaid Mills.[2] Then, of course, there are the many prime, dollar producing investments sponsored by the medical-industrial complex—manifest in a spiralling, self-perpetuating, monopolistic outpouring of pharmaceuticals, equipment, and other products guaranteed to delight the most money-grubbing soul and requiring only the turn-table of interlocking participation to assure constant supply and demand—and the dividends roll in.[3]

Of course some of these recondite maneuverings by private and public resources are beginning to be questioned. Like a class action suit was filed in a U.S. District Court February 13, 1973 which links a "non-profit" hospital, nine of its trustees, six Washington banks, and savings and loan associations in a conspiracy to overcharge patients for their own benefit. Could a "class action" become a "mass action?" Could the proverbial "Philadelphia lawyer" end up busier than the proverbial "one armed paper hanger with nettle rash?"

The hospital business has done so well that hotels like Ramada Inn, Hyatt House, Sheraton, Holiday Inns and other such industries are already in on the act. And like so many great inventions "it was medical doctors, not management experts, who discovered hospital capitalism." In fact, proprietary hospitals will net about $90 million in 1973 on a $1.5 billion gross.[4] American Medical International sells for $45 a share and has split twice since it was first offered twelve (12) years ago. With only 4th grade Arithmetic and a pencil (blue of course) one finds that 100 shares of American Medical International bought 12 years ago for $225 is now worth $15,600.[5] One proprietary hospital netted $74,000 in the first 10 months of 1972 from their kidney unit alone and another netted $58,000 on their kidney unit for the same period.[5]

Naturally it isn't only the proprietary sector of the hospital industry that is financially plump. A few state legislative bodies have gathered their facts, mustered their courage, and garnered their votes to cast out the strangely inappropriate euphemism of 'non-profit' and 'charitable' so cherished by the monolithic non-proprietary hospital industry. And who knows—perhaps the taxes recovered by these states can be appropriated back into the hungry maw of some other euphemism—like something called a 'physician's assistant.' After all it was the famous Dr. Stead of Duke University who quite pointedly stated, "They (physicians' assistants) were set up to support the present system."[6]

In any event let us turn to the physician's assistant and examine this fine new career dedicated to aiding and abetting the medical doctor in his pursuit of prestigious prerogative and assumed privity to erudition. Why there are even some who purport to believe that man's potential for health is really known only to devotees of physiological pathology with a soupcan of psyche to season the soma. And now here comes a 'sorcerer's apprentice' to lead the Medical Doctor into an expanded role. Expanded roles are almost as well known as physicians' assistants but the expanded role for the medical doctor may have strange dimensions scarcely envisioned by P.A. proponents. In fact it seems likely that the medical profession is scarcely aware of the burgeoning social demands and escalating broad based knowledges and technologies that make expanded roles imperative for everybody these days. However the medical profession is a long established field of endeavor so perhaps it can afford to ignore the changes taking place in all directions. Dr. Stead apparently wants P.A.'s to maintain the status quo and in the January 15, 1975 issue of *U.S. Medicine,* Dr. C. A. Hoffman, A.M.A. president, writes, "I am convinced now that there is no health care crisis in this country."[7] So what are physicians' assistants all about?

The public knows there is a health care crisis. The news media know there is a health care crisis. Nurses know there is a health care crisis. In the last decade doctors' bills have gone up 130% and hospital charges have risen 217%. The average hospital patient pays $100 a day and on up to $175 a day is not uncommon. In the last two years New York City's Blue Cross plan has jumped 71% and the story is the same across the country.[8] But as bad as these figures are they relate to only a narrow segment of health care—that portion which is within the scope of medical doctors and hospitals. Society is demanding a wide range of health services that requires [sic] the knowledges and skills of a variety of professional fields and which are beyond the ken of medical doctors and hospitals. Could this mean that it is not a shortage of M.D.'s that plagues the nation but rather a shortage of professionally educated nurses and other personnel concerned with the real scope of health care?

But back to physician's assistants and a quick look at the monetary potential they hold for their creators. How can they be such an economic asset? Let me give you an example from Sadler, Sadler, and Bliss's 1972 chronicle of *The Physician's Assistant: Today and Tomorrow.*[9] This particular physician's assistant held a master's degree. For outstanding labors (18.8% more patients seen than two pediatricians had previously been able to manage together and with no more office time for the pediatricians) this P.A. received the munificent sum of $7,620 (37–46% more than R.N. salaries in the same office). There was no increase in overhead or space requirements. The poor pediatricians, after all expenses, managed to eke out a mere clear profit of $16,800.

Or let us take the case of a nurse[10] who found herself seated in a nationally sponsored meeting of M.D.'s tightly clasping her little tape recorder that she might preserve the plethora of learning she anticipated would emerge. And imagine her surprise when this erudite gathering directed its scientific acumen to pursuit of the nurse specialist. For the grandiose sum of $20,000 it was predicted any nurse would succumb and a four fold profit could accrue to the farsighted M.D. whose potency in the situation would go unquestioned. Needless to say rocks fell from on high in a mighty deluge upon the listening nurse and her little tape recorder when she returned to the hospital nest prattling of power, profits, and propaganda. Now silence shrieks through the corridors and the little tape recorder became a "self-destruct" in no time. But villainy will out—won't it!

Naturally nurses are high on the list to be seduced out of nursing to be physicians' assistants. After all a little learning is a dangerous thing and the professionally educated nurse with a master's degree in nursing is already a degree ahead of the M.D.—a ghastly threat to all sorts of self-images. To be able also to make a profit out of self-preservation is truly frosting on the cake.

Although nurses seem to be the real priority in this game-playing, the development of all kinds of physicians' assistants programs evolve apace. Economic advantages germinate on the home front and in governmental closets. Only the M.D. gets paid and with characteristic largesse he dispenses pennies to the hands and feet that give him time for ruminating upon the human predicament and the dog-leg on the sixth hole.

Economic advantage is not the only asset of the physician's assistant. The P.A. makes a declaration of dependency. His guru no doubt leads him through the intricacies of getting answers to simply worded and of course neatly printed questions on a form dedicated to 'history' and 'physical' data.

The P.A. may learn a range of 'procedural' tasks and to recall Alfred North Whitehead, a properly trained person can pick these up in no time. So it is little wonder that Sadler, Sadler, and Bliss do report a training period of one (1) to two (2) years in general for physicians' assistants.[9] One of the strange inconsistencies that seems to pop up here is that not uncommonly nurses are asked to train these workers. Since nursing is not a part of medicine (despite the eagerness with which nurses may be courted on occasion by the medical fraternity), the question of just what is being prepared arises. Can it be that this new worker is really a nurse's assistant? Such confusion! We should have listened to Florence Nightingale when she wrote, "Experience teaches me . . . that nursing and medicine must never be mixed up. It spoils both."[11] Perhaps physicians' assistants should be given the option of becoming licensed as *either* a P.A. or an R.N. At least these licenses would have one thing in common. They identify peer career levels. Both verify preparation for technical practice. Of course there would be the problem for the P.A.-R.N. as to when he would be accountable to the M.D. and when he would be accountable to the professional R.N.

After all a *valid* baccalaureate degree program in nursing prepares a professional peer of the M.D. (and the engineer and the lawyer and the social worker, et al.). Associate degree, hospital school and practical nurse programs graduate nurses who are on an educational par with physicians' assistants. Now what's wrong with that? These are all socially significant, equally respectable, first-rate careers so are they not equally worthy of honor? John Gardner[12] tried to make this point when he emphasized that equal did not mean identical.

But alas! How often people fail to respect differences. How could society ever get along without pecking orders? Well—why not? Chickens do it, cows do it, sheep do it. Even baboons do it. And if someone can locate a good zoologist it seems likely he could identify some more who do it. Let it never be said that people are different from other animals. But the question still nags! Is this an insoluble problem?

True, American shamans may have some difficulties. After all they are greatly burdened with making moral decisions for women who want abortions, declaring the ancient Chinese art of acupuncture their prerogative, countering growing numbers of malpractice suits, struggling to discontinue all health services except those pared to the scope of medicine, trying to discover practices initiated by nurses a century ago so they can delegate them back to some naive nurse, clinging gallantly laboring manfully to get rid of all other licensure—save that which they would certify as limited to the guru's narrowed goals, jousting bravely with national health insurance proposals, and coming to grips with a multitude of other equally important endeavors. No wonder they need assistants. Surely they have no time to know there is a health care crisis.

How could such diligent persons be expected to know that midwives existed long before obstetricians and that the first prenatal care in the Western world was initiated by the Instructive Nursing Association of Boston in 1901. Or that Visiting Nursing was established in 1877 and by 1893 "all the social, economic, and industrial conditions affecting the lives of those receiving services were considered integral to the practice of visiting nurses."[13] Or that all accredited baccalaureate programs in nursing for two decades have prepared family health practitioners. The scope of nursing is markedly larger than that of medicine. Someone really goofed when they coined the terminological inaccuracy of "expanding the scope of nursing." It's the wrong way 'round. It should read "expanding the scope of medicine." Now there's a challenge for someone!

But again, let us get back to the physician's assistant. How should he be viewed? One eminent medical reference states that P.A.'s look like physicians: they wear short, white lab coats and swing stethoscopes. Madison Avenue, beware! It must be the stethoscope that is critical, however, because high school students from coast to coast may be seen wearing short, white lab coats. I suppose one might perceive the physician's assistant as a short, white lab coat and a gyrating stethoscope. But surely this can't be all. No, of course not. They are members of the health team—well at least of the medical team (remember that oath of dependency).

Teams are very important. Check the walls of any hospital where personnel may gather. In big print it says here "You are a member of the ream" (or some reasonable facsimile thereof). Patients know all about teams too. Sometimes their rooms look like Grand Central Station at 5:00 P.M. on a Friday afternoon. Public health agencies have teams. Clinics have teams. Schools have teams. The team spirit is very essential. Nurses are experts on "team;" so are social workers and psychologists and occupational therapists and nutritionists and a whole horde of other workers. But there is one big difference. The physician's assistant takes an oath of dependency to the M.D. Nobody else does and fortunately so for the poor, downtrodden public. The range of knowledges and competencies needed today for even minimally safe health services are such that no one professional field is capable of directing or supervising the judgments and decisions of another professional field.

So there is "the team" and everyone says, "Let's collaborate." And it's just like the dictionary says—collaboration means working with the enemy. Then someone says, "Let's set up a committee to study the problem" (or in the days of R & D—"let's get money from Washington and we'll research it"). And someone else says "We have to get the educators and the practitioners together—that's the whole trouble." Then somebody asks "Shouldn't the community be represented in this?" Immediately everyone concentrates on the community. This is very popular. It also takes the heat off of everyone else. Besides "they" can pick the "right" community representative and internal combustion can proceed at its own pace with a minimum of interference and only a modicum of well regulated confrontation.

Strangely enough the public is beginning to show anger. Can it be that they think they're being done in by inequities, incompetence, and overcharging? Now really, why shouldn't the public have to wait three hours to be admitted to a hospital? Just because hotels can admit at least three (3) times as many people in a third of the time and collect as many signatures, check out as many credit cards, and validate room space all at the same time is really no excuse for public impatience with the health care system. Hospitals are for *sick* people. So the next time you have to sit fainting in a hospital lobby for three hours or lie bleeding in an emergency room for even more hours just remember—this is a hospital. Your team is waiting (probably in the coffee shop)!

Once ensconced in motorized bed (hotels and motels have motorized beds too—in fact hotels and motels even have water beds—and sauna baths—and swimming pools—and bar rooms—and ice buckets—and stationary bicycles to exercise on—and ad infinitum)—but back to being ensconced in bed—a nurse takes your blood pressure, an intern takes your blood pressure, a resident takes your blood pressure, your own doctor may show up to take your blood pressure, and now a short whitecoated, stethoscope swinging physician's assistant also takes your blood pressure. But do not complain if your arm is now paralyzed with a circulatory deficiency. Undoubtedly there is a biostatistician out by the nurses' station rapidly working a little hand calculator (latest model in mathematical, technological efficiency) to get a mean and standard deviation for all those blood pressures. Thoroughness is the order of the day.

In what I have been saying you may think I have been directing criticism at medical doctors and physicians' assistants, per se. Such an erroneous interpretation would be most unfortunate. Indeed it would only serve to obfuscate the issue. For the medical doctor and his assistant I have the profoundest respect. In fact the M.D. expects to be honored, to have doors opened for him, to be oblivious to the most obsequious of greetings from lesser folk when he is embarked upon the arduous demands of his job, to be waited upon, and to have all others assume a properly vertical position as he hovers into view. Of course these little evidences of the stern fiber of bygone days are diminishing rather rapidly. Physicians' assistants won't be able to add these fatuous behaviors to the white lab coat and stethoscope. Indeed Women's Lib is getting rid of all kinds of quaint customs.

The physician's assistant is here. So too has a seemingly unending multitude of health careers multiplied without regard for human needs or human safety or for the potential employability or market value of the products of these nameless occupations. The public is thwarted, their health jeopardized, and their pocketbooks depleted. A massive power struggle is underway with public demands pitted against a so-called health system dedicated to self-serving obsolescence. Social motivation for emergence of a physician's assistant is abysmally lacking. Nonetheless these anomalous physicians' assistants (when the dust has settled) may turn out to be a worthwhile addition to the public scene.

In today's career patterns physicians' assistants fit nicely into place alongside engineering technicians, dental hygienists, nursing technicians, dietitians and a host of other highly significant and socially esteemed persons. As a member of the medical team, the P.A.'s vow of dependency sets the limits of his practice. But dependency has its rewards.

Recruitment into this fine new career is a masterpiece of game-playing. Con game ingenuities are especially impressive. The potential victims of the con game are selected with great care. An R.N. license is a highly desired prerequisite and the con man who corners a degree(s) toting R.N. duly beams with excitement. Here propaganda can really win him power and profits, eliminate professional competition, and hopefully diminish public flak about medical inadequacies. Estimations of the potential 'take' in this game are very large indeed—well worth the efforts of any good, dedicated con man. Nurses and nursing would be dispensed with. Institutions could license but only shamans could certify. Con game victims would be caught in an iron clad grip without recourse to law or liberty.

Modifications of the old shell game, with words for beans, have been particularly popular as an approach to enticing nurses so that they will leave nursing to follow the drummers of another discipline. Euphemistic labels are the coinage used. Nurse clinicians, pediatric associates, family health practitioners, primary care providers (Primex products), child health associates, physician's associates (note that apostrophe 's'. It is an A.M.A. symbol for dependency[9]), and a growing number of other jargonistic tags have been stuffed indiscriminately into the con man's bag of tricks. Apparently this particular game is losing some of its appeal. Or else the proselytizers think they already have it made. So Sadler, Sadler, and Bliss[9] write, "In this book 'physician's assistant' is a generic term which includes a range of mid-level health workers variously named: physicians' associates (Duke and related models), medex, nurse clinicians (pediatric nurse practitioners), child health associates, etc." Alex Kacen[14] suggests that the appellation "physician's assistant" be used exclusively rather than such terms as "physician's associate," "nurse practitioner," "medex," "clinical associate," "practitioner associate," etc. Can it be that the con men are so imbued with the magnificence of their own image that they deem this confrontation as eminent flattery (sometimes defined colloquially as soft soap—prime ingredient lye).

Now these comments are not to suggest that nurses who want to leave nursing should not do so. Quite the contrary! Nurses who want to leave nursing to be subsumed under the rubric of "physician's assistant" should be helped to do so—whether they now travel under a euphemistic label of nurse clinician, pediatric associate, primary care provider (Primex product), family health practitioner or some other specimen of dubious nomenclature. In fact it should be a great aid to the poor misled public to simply call physician's assistants "physician's assistants." Such a step should be implemented as quickly as possible.

This would of course openly diminish to some unknown extent the numbers of nurses currently available to meet the crying needs of people. But then nursing could get about its real business of providing knowledgeable *nursing* services. Those committed to nursing and to the rights of people to receive broad based health services would get on with it. Professional and technical nurses committed to nursing are already moving to provide creative leadership in evolving a clearly new and innovative health system responsive to human needs and in which maintenance and promotion of health are equally significant with care and rehabilitation of the sick and disabled. Such nursing leadership might even allow for a little optimism on the part of the public.

Concomitantly if physician's assistants are the really fine things that their proponents purport to believe they are then certainly their numbers should be increased. Why does not medicine look to the great age of technology for means of multiplication? Do not the characteristics of these products (oath of dependency, short white lab coats, swinging stethoscopes, data storage, etc.) lend themselves to the machine age? With a few good models and a cloning machine an inexhaustible supply of physicians' assistants could be available on demand. If really well done the product might be almost indistinguishable from an M.D. thereby quieting any unruly member of the public who might object to paying M.D. charges for robot services. Of course on the other hand there might be those who believed the robot worth more moola than the M.D. (Just look at what computers have done for medical diagnosis).

The public is the real victim in all this game-playing. How long will they permit themselves to be sacrificed to the power, profit and propaganda of head-in-sand philosophers? If nursing's public accountability and public advocacy have any validity, then nursing must take steps to assure that the public is heard. If there is such a thing as human rights, then nursing's complicity in malpractice must cease. If there is anything to be said for the public's rights to health services, then nursing must take a stand on the widespread, rampant profiteering that affects the total public and is disastrous for middle and lower income groups. If experimentation without informed consent of the individual is immoral (it is already illegal) then nursing must inform.

The physician's assistant is a red herring. Where will it lead? Who knows? Where will nursing go? The future is ours to write.

References

1. "Fees for Health-Care Here Under Audit by the I.R.S.," *New York Times.* November 19, 1972.
2. Health-Pac *Bulletin* 43. July-August 1972.
3. Ehrenreich, B., and Ehrenreich, J., *The American Health Empire.* New York: Random House, 1970.
4. "Suit Claims Hospital Cost is Inflated," *Washington Post,* February 14, 1973.
5. Rapaport, Roger, "A Candle for St. Greeds," *Harpers.* December 1972, p. 71.
6. Health-Pac *Bulletin* 46. November 1972, p. 16.
7. Hoffman, C. A., "'Balanced' System is A.M.A.'s Concern," *U.S. Medicine.* January 15, 1973, p. 29.
8. "Your Health Care in Crisis," *A Health-Pac Special Report.* May 1972.
9. Sadler, A., Sadler, B., and Bliss, A., *The Physician's Assistant: Today and Tomorrow.* New Haven: Yale University Press, 1972.
10. Journalistic immunity claimed for this one.
11. Cope, Zachary, *Florence Nightingale and the Doctors.* Philadelphia: J. B. Lippincott Co., 1958, p. 121.
12. Gardner, John, *Excellence.* New York: Harper and Row, Publishers, 1961.
13. Dock, Lavinia, and Stewart, Isabel. *A Short History of Nursing.* New York: G. P. Putnam's Sons, 1920, p. 161.
14. Kacen, Alex, "A Social Viewpoint of the Physician's Assistant Movement, Part I," *Physician's Associate,* Vol. 2, No. 3, July 1972.

CHAPTER 26

Legislative and Licensing Problems in Health Care

Martha E. Rogers

The four Ps of today's health care field—power, profit, politics and propaganda—have been on the health scene for some time, and with little evidence of social concern and public responsibility. Certainly many sectors of society question the amount of public good taken into consideration in health care legislation and licensing proposals. Two past presidents of the American Medical Association (AMA) have flatly stated, in the media and on public television, that there is no health care crisis in the United States; but most people think there is a health care crisis. In order to look at nursing, the entire health sector needs some examination.

Health is the second largest business in the nation. Health care inflation is running more than 50 percent above the consumer price index. Expenditures—and these are directly related to inflationary charges, most of which go to hospitals and MDs—are doubling every five years. The health scene is a product in part of a corporate society of bureaucratic controls, of recognized and political forces that determine the cost structure.

The Changing Health Field

A wide range of changes have occurred in the health care fields. The traditional professions of medicine, law and theology have taken on an entirely different look. Professionals have expanded to encompass a large variety which some people may refer to as semiprofessionals, pseudo-professionals or new professionals. The idea of professionals as controllers of their own profession and as entrepreneurs is going out, coordinates [sic] with the growth of power in a corporate society and of bureaucracy. In a bureaucratic system specialization increases; people know less and less about more and more. This

Reprinted from *Nursing Administration Quarterly,* Vol. 2, No. 3, pp. 71–78, with permission of Aspen Publishers, Inc., © 1978.

is not only true of the health sector, it is part of a whole way of life in various areas of industry and business.

In connection with bureaucratic developments, there is also a move toward more unionization of professionals. Physician organization is very much on the rise—physicians' unions now claim at least 16,000 members.[1] Teachers and nurses are moving toward unionization in some areas. The American Hospital Association (AHA) is considering ways of dealing with unions, often including efforts to prevent people such as head nurses and supervisors from participating in union activities, even though these people may have little say in the administrative process. Efforts are directed toward diminishing organized action, whether through the Economic Security Program of the American Nurses' Association (ANA) or through unions. The AHA has published materials on how to handle labor union campaigns in health care institutions.

In the medical-industrial complex directorates commonly interlock with corporate control. These often involve large businesses in which the majority of the money is held by a small number of people. Businesses such as drug houses, real estate, private and commercial insurance companies, Blue Cross Blue Shield, hospitals, physicians and lawyers may be involved.

The "Business Roundtable" is a giant corporation business lobby in Washington, D.C., with an annual budget of $1.5 million. It has 158 corporate members who investigate legislation that might be distasteful to the large companies, and who have been very influential on several occasions in stopping legislation relevant to health.

Problems in the Health System

Deception

Deception is a major problem in the health system. Forbes Magazine, a very prestigious business journal, has called the drug industry "the biggest crap game in the United States." There are so many new drugs today that one often hears there are hundreds of drugs in search of a disease.

The battle over the use of brand names versus generic names was fought by a joint lobby of the AMA and the American Pharmaceutical Association, and a bill was not passed. When New York City was in a financial bind and had to come up with about $45 million by the first of December, 1976, had the bill relative to the use of generic names been passed, New York City would have saved approximately the amount of money needed to pay that December deficit. The savings would have been in the area of drugs used in the Medicare-Medicaid services for which the city was paying.

In 1976, thirty thousand to 60,000 deaths from drug errors alone were reported in the news media. In one study, 95 percent of prescriptions written in the United States were reported to have had one or more errors.[2] Huge profits have been made in nursing homes through excessive Medicare-Medicaid charges. Some people have gone to jail; however, there are members of society who receive minimal penalties. According to the news media, one physician convicted of Medicaid fraud and sentenced to four years in prison became eligible for immediate parole.

Overexpansion

The Federal Council on Wage and Price Stability has commented on excessive inflationary behavior by physicians and their colleagues, noting that they ignore and hinder efforts to control costs. One witness at the council's 1976 hearings testified that health insurance now accounts for a bigger part of an automobile's cost than steel. Overbuilding of hospitals is taking place across the country. Yet on any one day, 25 percent of the nation's hospital beds are vacant. Consumers pay for these empty beds with their Blue Cross insurance.

"Two sets of social forces have been instrumental in shaping hospital expansion: (1) the powerful interests controlling the hospital—trustees, administrators, and doctors—along with the hospital supply, construction and drug companies, and banks which together make up the medical-industrial complex; and (2) health beneficiaries, such as labor unions, the poor and the elderly. . . ."[3] The economics of hospitals can be found in government subsidies, third party reimbursements, depreciation payments and a range of hidden subsidies.[4]

Cost Accounting for Power/Profit

There is a proposal circulating in Washington, D.C., that perhaps there will come a day when there will be true cost accounting—cost accounting based on true cost. With regard to National Health Insurance, this proposal manifests major efforts on the part of a range of different groups to maintain the status quo as a power-profit structure. The proposal is essentially limited to medical services which actually include a very narrow part of health. (In fact, medicine and hospitals do not provide health services; they provide sick services).

In the Kennedy-Mills proposal, which does include commercial insurance companies, they made the point that their decision to retain the insurance company's role was based on recognition of that industry's power to kill any legislation it considered unacceptable, not on the basis of social need.[5]

Accreditation Struggles

The Bureau of Competition of the Federal Trade Commission has denied the Liaison Committee on Medical Education continued acceptance by the Office of Education as a nationally recognized agency to accredit medical schools on the basis of AMA influence on the Liaison Committee, and AMA's well-established function as a powerful trade association which vigorously advances the economic interests of its physician members. Notices of this action went out to all nationally recognized accredited agencies and associations. This has direct implications for nurses and for the ANA's accreditation efforts.

In 1977 officers and board members of the National League for Nursing held a ballot that forced a board membership of nurses, MDs and hospital administrators. There was only one person on that ballot who could be considered a consumer and educator, and there was no assurance that he would be elected. While MDs and hospital administrators are lay people when it comes to nursing, it would be difficult to call them the consumer public.

Ethical issues such as the right to die, living wills, freedom of information and informed consent continue to mount. We continue to argue over them, struggle over them, fight over potential bills. There may be more time spent on how to get around informed consent than in giving informed consent. Moreover, information is often given in such a way that even the people giving it may not really understand what they are saying. The definition of death may depend on whether the health care provider wants to do a transplant or prefers to try out new technology that may maintain vital signs beyond any hope of reversibility. Cloning and DNA recombinations, abortions, capital punishment—all these are real issues in health services.

Licensure Losing Its Focus

Licensure, which was presumably established to protect the public, has gotten out of focus. All too often, those who control licensure for a given field are concerned with their own self-interests rather than with the public welfare.

Licensure may be used to keep others out or to maintain whatever control there is.

If institutional licensure took place, it would control the mobility of workers and services and would encourage unionization of all workers. In 1976 a lot of monies were given for the congressional election campaign. Medical organizations were by far the largest special interest group donors. Presumably, something was expected in return. One may properly ask, "What?"

Occupational certification is a euphemism for institutional licensure. There are problems in licensure and certification because the vested interests aren't giving up. Reports on institutional licensure omit MDs and dentists, but all other workers are implicated. If nurses are going to be under institutional licensure, MDs and dentists should also be subject to institutional licensure.

Placing nurses under institutional licensure does not benefit anyone. In a bureaucratic system, the human being is lost. Nurses become nursing machines. In institutional licensing where each institution determines its own standards and patterns of employment, licensing becomes an economic concept—power, profits, politics and propaganda. Mobility of workers is denied, and standards disappear.

The subcommittee on health credentialing of the U.S. Public Health Service has released several reports concerning health manpower credentialing. Although it has been stated that the subcommittee included representation of each agency concerned with health manpower, nursing has not been identified as being on those committees.

Vice President Rockefeller in the spring of 1976, speaking before the National Leadership Conference on America's Health Policy, recommended that the government undertake experimental programs in institutional licensure: "If successful on a national basis, the law should be changed to permit licensing of individual health care institutions instead of the present detailed establishment of credentials for individuals."[6]

At the national level, it has been proposed that there is no need to stop financing nurse education in hospital schools through patient care costs.[7] Since nurses work in many places other than hospitals, why should hospitalized persons be penalized? Are not people entitled to knowledgeable nurses as well as to knowledgeable persons in other fields? Hospital control of nurse preparation may be another way of extending the paternalistic system as a further means of moving toward institutional licensure.

Problems in Nursing

Declining Quality of Hospital Care

The quality of health care in hospitals is poor. About 10,000 nurses responding to a questionnaire said they wouldn't be hospitalized in the place they worked.[8,9] I wouldn't want to be hospitalized. I had the misfortune last year of being hospitalized twice in two different parts of the country. Care was not good in either instance.

PSROs have been set up as a means of monitoring medical care. Self-monitoring in any field has not been notably successful. Perhaps nurses are making a better effort to look at themselves, but trying is not good enough.

Nurses have the capacity to give direction to nursing as a socially responsible and socially responsive, knowledgeable field of endeavor. Why then are nurses so often contributing to their own demise and, even worse, participating in the rape of the public's health? Nurses are their own worst enemies. They can point to the errors in other people and say, "They did it," but when the chips are down, nurses are the people who are responsible. They are the people who don't have to let it happen.

Anti-educationalism, dependency and gullibility are some of the big problems in nursing. Nurses don't like to admit that they've been had. But there comes a time when they should admit it and do something about it.

Expanded Role—A Euphemism

Expanded role is a euphemism which has many nurses conned. With escalating technology, scientific inquiry, etc., everybody has expanding roles these days. Expanded roles are not new, and they are not peculiar to nursing.

A national committee, set up recently to study the extended nursing role, had two MDs as chairman and co-chairman. The committee established what nurses should do, and there wasn't a thing on that list that nurses hadn't been doing since Florence Nightingale. The MDs claimed the activities and delegated them back to nursing. Why did nurses permit this flagrant derogation of nursing's responsibilities?

Expanded roles recently became known as extended roles. Then the term physician extender was introduced, which was what was meant in the first place. In New York, the State Board of Regents has recommended that the title "physician extender" encompass PAs and NPs with uniform curriculum standards, and to authorize the certification of NPs in the expanded practice, subject to appropriate medical supervision. The ANA has announced that 175 nurses were certified by the Joint Program of the ANA Division of Maternal and Child Health Nursing and NAACOG (Nurses' Association of the American College of Obstetricians and Gynecologists). Are not these physician extenders? Studies that have been going on for some time indicate that MD profits and released time increase as a result of physician extenders.

NP Programs Detrimental to Nursing

The so-called NP programs which are being supported by federal dollars are designed to remove nurses from nursing to practice as PAs under the control, legal and otherwise, of MDs. In 1975 *A Report to Congress—Progress and Problems in Training and Use of Assistants to Primary Care Physicians* identified assistants as nurse practitioners and physician extenders. "Physician extenders are referred to by a variety of names, including physician assistant, physician associate, community health medic, family nurse practitioner, Medex, child health associate and pediatric NP. However, the term physician extender refers generally to graduates of all the programs reviewed."[10]

NP programs admit any RN including individuals with hospital school diplomas, baccalaureate, master's or doctoral degrees. The program includes the same content as PA programs. The trainees do not learn nursing; they learn how to assist MDs.

HEW [the Department of Health, Education, and Welfare] reported in 1976 that 5,500 practitioners had been trained in 145 training programs at a cost of more than $50 million. The programs ranged from 36 weeks to 104 weeks, and trainee ages ranged from 26 to 33.[11] There is a clear difference between monies allocated for advanced nurse training and monies allocated for NP programs. Advanced nurse training programs prepare people for nursing practice. NP programs prepare people to leave nursing and to practice as PAs.

Nurses Threaten the Power Structure

There are many arguments about how physicians need assistance and how the public is suffering. The public is suffering from a lack of quality health services, but at the same time an oversupply of MDs by the early 1980s is predicted.[12,13] However, if one examines the number of physicians, dentists and nurses with baccalaureate degrees, one finds that, relatively, the percentage of MDs is dropping; the percentage of dentists is remaining about the same; and the percentage of baccalaureate nursing graduates is increasing. In other words, the number of nurses with the kind of foundation that will enable them to work on a peer professional level with other disciplines is increasing, which threatens the power structure.

Will Nursing Disappear?

For many years, the National Institute of Mental Health has provided monies for nurse preparation and for the preparation of psychiatrists, psychiatric social workers and various other groups. Interestingly, medical pressure groups recently proposed that no monies go to nursing; rather, they should go to psychiatrists who can "take care of everything and tell the nurses what to do."

The Robert Wood Johnson Foundation recently put $3 million into getting nurses out of nursing and into becoming PAs. They are giving scholarships to selected nurse faculty to learn how to be PAs so they can return and teach those in their nursing programs how they too can be PAs. There is a need for PAs, but there is also a great need for nurses. The question is, will nursing disappear?

At a recent panel discussion in New York which focused on nursing's political, legislative and licensing problems, a non-nurse representative of HEALTH PAC (a lay organization dedicated to bringing the truth about the whole health care system to the public) made this comment: "I really see no future for nursing. You sound like people rearranging the chairs on the decks of the Titanic." Unless nurses man the lifeboats, her observation could become reality. Manning the lifeboats has to be for a purpose considerably larger than self-preservation—it must stand for social concern. Nursing exists to serve people. It does not exist to serve the ends of any other group. Legislation and licensure should be properly directed toward the public good.

References

1. *Health Labor Relations Reports* 1:1 (October 26, 1976) p. 12.
2. *Public Health Reports* 90:6 (November-December 1975).
3. *HEALTH/PAC Bulletin* No. 64 (May/June 1975) p. 3.
4. Ibid. p. 16–19.
5. Navarro, V. "Health and the Corporate Society." *Social Policy 5:5* (January/February 1975) p. 46.
6. *Health Conference Proceedings.* The National Leadership Conference on America's Health Policy. Washington, D.C., April 29–30, 1976.
7. *People, Power, Politics—for Health Care.* National League for Nursing. Pub. No. 52-1647 (1976) p. 11.
8. Funkhouser, G. R. "Quality of Care," Part I. *Nursing 76* 6:12 (December 1976) pp. 22–31.
9. Funkhouser, G. R. "Quality of Care." Part II. *Nursing 77* 7:1 (January 1977) pp. 27–33.
10. Comptroller General of the United States. For the Congress. *A Report to the Congress—Progress and Problems in Training and Use of Assistants to Primary Care Physicians.* HEW, April 8, 1975.
11. U.S. Department of Health, Education and Welfare. *HEW News,* December 20, 1976.
12. *U.S. Medicine* 12:4 (February 15, 1976).
13. *N.Y. Times* (November 16, 1976).

CHAPTER 27

Peer Review: A 1985 Dissent

Martha E. Rogers

Dear Health/PAC:

As a person who is actively opposing passage of the New York State Nurses' Association (NYSNA) "1985 Proposal," I am of course glad to find others who are also opposed. However, I can find no merit in sharing the stump with the author of your article "Closing The Door on Nurses, New York Style" which appeared in the September-October 1977 issue of the Health/PAC BULLETIN. Mr. Jenkins seems to be an antieducationist, socially irresponsible, and frequently misinformed as are those persons who are supporting the NYSNA "1985 Proposal."

The evolution of nursing takes place within the larger framework of social change. The recipients of nursing services are as entitled to knowledgeable nursing services as they are entitled to knowledgeable services in medicine, dentistry, engineering, law, social work and the like. Licensure exists to safeguard the public, not the worker. Unfortunately both the NYSNA and Mr. Jenkins seem to ignore this point.

Nursing's educational system prepares persons for three clearly different levels of practice. Licensure to practice is provided for only two of these levels: specifically, (1) the registered nurse level (for which hospital schools and associate degree programs prepare) and (2) the practical nurse level. *No licensure is provided for the baccalaureate level* of practice although human safety requires the knowledgeable judgments afforded by valid baccalaureate education in nursing.

That baccalaureate graduates currently take the same licensing examination as do hospital school and associate degree graduates is no more valid than if dentists were licensed according to their performance on a licensing examination for dental hygienists or medical doctors according to their scores on a

Rogers, M. E. (1978). Peer review: A 1985 dissent. *Health-PAC Bulletin,* January-February, No. 80, 32–34. Reprinted with permission.

physician's assistant examination or engineers according to how they achieved as engineering technicians.

Further Mr. Jenkins' suggestion that to require a baccalaureate degree in nursing is discriminatory against nurses who got their baccalaureate in some other field is at best very strange. Would he suggest that the engineering technician who secures a baccalaureate degree in sociology is then qualified to practice as an engineer? Will a degree in psychology qualify the physician's assistant to practice as a medical doctor? Will a degree in biology for the dental hygienist create a dentist?

Failure to establish legal standards and to license at the baccalaureate level of practice in nursing *leaves the public to be victimized* by (1) persons granted baccalaureate degrees in the absence of a baccalaureate education in nursing, (2) unreasonable expectations of associate degree, hospital school, and practical nurse graduates and (3) a health care system that endeavors to deny persons holding a valid baccalaureate degree in nursing their rights and responsibilities to use their knowledge for human betterment.

Concomitantly, there is continuing need for licensure of nurse graduates of associate degree and hospital schools (as long as the latter shall continue). These graduates are prepared for a career in nursing that society values and needs—a career worthy of honor and respect in itself. These graduates do not need to be "upgraded" in order to be socially significant. The words "Registered Nurse" and the letters "RN" identify this population. These nurses make decisions within the scope of their preparation. Certainly *they function with appropriate direction from nursing's baccalaureate and higher degree graduates.* But to propose this is a unique role (as did the author of this article) is to deny that knowledge makes a difference.

Further Mr. Jenkins seems unaware that baccalaureate education in nursing prepares a general practitioner—a person who works directly with people, who gives direct nursing services, and who makes those intellectual judgments demanding substantive nursing knowledge. Equally the assignment of responsibilities to associate degree and hospital school graduates when said responsibilities require the knowledge base provided in a baccalaureate program can spell danger to the public.

The grandfather clause which Mr. Jenkins refers to as a myth is in reality a way of maintaining the status quo under new labels for years to come. Most seriously, the public would be faced with large numbers of people labelled as something they would not be and lacking the knowledge necessary to fulfill the responsibilities society would have the right to expect.

Grandfather clauses are appropriate means of protecting the rights of persons and in this instance *persons holding baccalaureate degrees in nursing acceptable at the time of their graduation should be grandfathered in under a bill that would license for the baccalaureate level of practice.* Mr. Jenkins seems quite confused as to the purpose of this legislation since he indicates that the grandfather clause "fails to assure jobs" for example. The purpose of licensure is not one of assuring jobs. The grandfather clause proposed by NYSNA does fail to protect the public, however, which is a derogation of the purposes of licensure.

Mr. Jenkins' reference to "faith healing" as representing an area of uniqueness in nursing knowledge seems to be a statement without foundation. I know of no accredited nursing program at any level which teaches or prepares their graduates to practice "faith healing." If Mr. Jenkins is referring to the work of Dolores Krieger, PhD, RN in the area of Therapeutic Touch he is indeed ignorant of both her research and its translation into nursing practice. Human touch has been a *sine qua non* of nursing from before Florence Nightingale introduced modern nursing. To provide a scientific base for this intimate caring function places touch squarely within the framework of nursing's therapeutic modalities. In an age of mechanistic proponents and technological overabundance, nursing's long established humanitarianism finds significant expression in the establishment of scientific principles to underwrite practice.

I would not argue with the need for critical concern in the area of opportunities for minority groups. However I would point out that this is a major issue that has to be dealt with on many fronts. To deny knowledgeable nursing to the public because we as citizens have not confronted and acted on the real issue serves neither society nor minority groups. The problem will not be solved by passage or non-passage of the NYSNA "1985 Proposal."

The economics of nursing as presented by Mr. Jenkins deserves criticism as well. In a period of marked inflation, salaries for multiple groups have risen dramatically, including those voted themselves by legislators and others. Is it not reasonable that persons with equivalent responsibilities should find these manifest in their pay checks? Is Mr. Jenkins proposing that if nurses want jobs they had better keep their salaries down? As for a shortage or non-shortage of nursing personnel, Mr. Jenkins reflects his own lack of information rather than reality. Gross numbers do not tell the story. There continues to be a critical shortage of nurses prepared at the baccalaureate and higher degree level. In the employment market there is approximately one baccalaureate and higher degree graduate to nine associate degree, hospital school, and practical nurse graduates. The field of medicine has three times as many practicing MD's as their [sic] are baccalaureate and higher degree graduates in nursing. If one summed up the total of persons working in the field of medicine it seems likely they would number more than the total number of those practicing in the field of nursing.

As a final point I would note that there can be no unity that does not allow for and value diversity.

I find it most distressing to find such an uninformed, inaccurate article in Health/PAC, an organization for which I have had considerable respect and to which I have referred many people. Many more comments relative to errors in the article could be made. Suffice it to say that this article is a disservice to nursing, to your readers, and to a public sorely in need of safe health services, a commodity which seems to be in short supply these days.

CHAPTER 28

The Umbrella That Isn't!

Martha E. Rogers

Among the many myths that plague nurses and nursing there is one so full of holes as to approach the ridiculous. Specifically this myth proposes that because all R.N.'s take the same licensing examination they are therefore the same. A "nurse is a nurse is a nurse" is confirmed. Breeding of this common denominator takes place in "types of programs," so labelled to further ensure equivalence of product in the eye of the beholder. These "types" are then proposed to constitute valid categories for comparing performance on the R.N. licensing examination and, ipso facto, to declare one "type of program" better or worse than another.

Interestingly enough proponents of R.N. similitude emerging out of these "types of programs" may also declare with vehemence massive differences between practical nurses and registered nurses. In explication of these differences length of program is often brought to bear. What is this like? In general ADN and hospital school programs are approximately one year longer than practical nurse programs. In fact since practical nurse programs are generally a year in length then ADN and hospital school programs may be said to be approximately twice as long as practical nurse programs. Certainly it is reasonable to expect that whatever is going on in that second year (or double the time) is making some kind of a difference.

But there is still a third "type of program" to be considered. Baccalaureate degree programs in nursing are approximately two years longer than ADN and hospital school programs. In fact B.S. programs are, in general, twice as long as ADN and hospital school programs. Indeed the difference in length of program between B.S. and ADN/hospital schools is twice as great as the difference in length between ADN/hospital schools and practical nurse programs. Logic then decrees that B.S. graduates must be twice as different from ADN/hospital school graduates as ADN/hospital school graduates are from practical nurse graduates.

Rogers, M. E. (1980, February). The umbrella that isn't! *SAIN Newsletter,* pp. 1–2. Reprinted with permission of the SAIN Governing Council.

Length of total program is not the only temporal argument in this strong debate. The number of hours in required clinical practice is often presumed to predict competence on the job after graduation. Recently the wheel has been reinvented and an all-frills trip proposed in the so-called unification model proclaiming the only teacher of merit is the PRACTITIONER-teacher. Not only must students often spend unconscionable hours "in doing" but faculty must declare their allegiance to service agencies through joint appointments, jointly paid salaries, and in known instances without their presence in the halls of academe and minus ready access to the sources of theoretical learning indispensable to the creative teacher of substantive knowledge in nursing. Emphasis is on doing by everybody. The more the better. The concept of "a nurse is a nurse is a nurse" has been extended to encompass the academe.

But let me return to that holey (or holy!) umbrella that isn't. The R.N. licensing examination is the culminating test for the would be R.N. However there are other tests to which students are subjected prior to their graduation. Among these are standardized achievement tests. These tests are developed under the same general aegis as are state board examinations. Here though, something different is going on. There are two sets of achievement tests: one for associate degree and hospital school students and another one for baccalaureate students. Obviously somebody discovered that achievement for one group was not the same thing as achievement for the other group. Eureka! Now why hasn't this remarkable insight found its way into state boards?

Licensing presumably exists for the public good. It is a way of guaranteeing society that someone is minimally safe to practice something. The some one and the some thing differ according to field of endeavor and according to the nature and amount of learning that precedes admission to this rite of passage. Certainly the diversity of licenses and licensing examinations could be decreased dramatically if medical technicians, physician's assistants and medical doctors all took the same licensing examination and received the same license to practice. Similarly, one examination could serve to qualify dental assistants, dental hygienists and dentists for a common license. As a matter of fact this approach could be introduced into a range of fields such as clinical psychology, law, engineering, social work and others. Whether this would affect the nation's tax structure is a moot point. But perhaps the tax structure isn't the real issue. If the above suggestion to cut down on the numbers of licenses is a poor one why are nurses still trying to do it? The people have no legal guarantee that any nurse is safe to practice at the baccalaureate level of preparation despite the reality that it constitutes the first professional degree in nursing. Where does social responsibility come in?

An excellent dentist is not the same thing as an excellent dental hygienist. Neither is an excellent baccalaureate nursing graduate the same thing as an excellent associate degree or hospital school graduate. In both instances excellence requires different criteria for its determination. All should be equally excellent but excellence will be manifest in different ways according to the nature and amount of knowledge each possess.

It is time that heads come out of the sand—the holey umbrella just doesn't hold water.

CHAPTER 29

Unification: SAIN [Society for Advancement in Nursing] Model Myth Versus Reality: An Overview

Martha E. Rogers

There is an old anecdote about the devil and his friend who were walking along the street together. The friend noticed a man pick up something from the gutter. The friend said to the devil, "Look at that man. Why is he looking so happy? What was it he picked up off the street?" The devil answered, "A piece of truth. He picked up a piece of truth but don't worry about it." The friend then asked the devil, "How can you be so complacent? Isn't that dangerous to you?" The devil grinned and said, "Not at all. When he gets home with that piece of truth, I'm going to help him organize it and apply it."

The nurse propagated euphemism of "unification model" might well be likened to one of those pieces of the truth the devil is busily organizing and applying. Fact and fiction, myth and reality combine to create confusion and to obfuscate the real issues.

Under the guise of consolidating all nurses into some common goal one finds instead a harkening back to "a nurse is a nurse is a nurse" with education, practice and research proclaimed as standard attributes of all. Concomitantly, the myth of "doing" is exploited and the reality that one cannot use what one does not possess is overlooked. Out of a strange conglomerate there emerges a jack of all trades and an expert in none.

Despite declarations to the contrary a pervasive anti-educationism among nurses is revealed. Fear of diversity stalks the market place. Jargon and tradition confound nurses and the public. Moreover debates about myths are no

Rogers, M. E. (1981, August). Unification: SAIN Model. *SAIN Newsletter,* pp. 2–4. Reprinted with permission of the SAIN Governing Council.

more valid than the tale of the funeral director who is supposed to have advertised that "Our coffins are lined with real silk. Our competitors' coffins are lined with a synthetic material that may cause skin irritation."

"Unification: SAIN [Society for Advancement in Nursing] model" is designed to examine myths and realities underlying an oft deplored lack of unity among nurses and to propose that high value for diversity is a significant unifying force. In a world of escalating difference growing heterogeneity marks the future. Equal does not mean identical. Nor does variety postulate adversary relationships.

Facts and fallacies abound. Some myths are so pervasive that they are mistaken for reality and may generate innumerable other myths that then may be used as evidence in support of some original myth. A fact writ large is anti-educationism. Claims that all R.N.'s are professionals do not make an R.N. learned. Neither do paper credentials without substantive knowledge validate excellence. Strangely enough anti-educationists in nursing are by no means limited to those who have had little or no exposure to the higher learning. Nurses who have been privileged to be exposed to graduate education may be even more anti-educationist about nursing than their less educationally favored brothers and sisters.

Listing the letters R.N. before academic credentials does not make the R.N. an academic credential. The R.N. signifies a license and correctly follows academic credentials. Calling physician assistants nurse practitioners does not make nurse practitioners practitioners of nursing.

A characteristic of Abraham Lincoln was that he insisted on facts when a case was being presented. One day a committee came to him on a matter of public concern. The case was built largely on "supposings." Abe asked, "How many legs would a sheep have if you called its tail a leg?" As he expected they promptly answered, "Five." "No," said Lincoln, "it would not; it would have only four. Calling a tail a leg doesn't make it one."

A major "tail" is that "a nurse is a nurse is a nurse" if she is an R.N. Support for the myth includes declaring that because all R.N.'s take the same licensing examination they are therefore the same. The reality is that nursing's educational system prepares persons for three entry levels to practice and licenses for only two of these levels: namely, (1) the practical nurse level (2) the registered nurse level. There is no licensure for the baccalaureate level of practice. Licensing dentists according to their performance on a dental hygienist examination would be equally valid.

Anti-educationism is further explicit in the not uncommon practice of omitting academic credentials other than the doctorate and lumping all others into one category of R.N. Inasmuch as a number of nurses have secured their doctorates in fields other than nursing such discrimination is at best dubious. Moreover those nurses who do hold baccalaureate and higher degree credentials in nursing are denied the recognition that would identify some expected level of knowledge and competence.

Continued use of the phrase "types of programs" coupled with statistics that by-pass the reality that valid baccalaureate education in nursing cannot be equated with associate degree and hospital school programs is still common. And when an eminent university admits to graduate study registered nurses with or without a baccalaureate degree the critical nature of nursing's educational dilemma is explicit.

Token salary differentials between registered nurse associate degree and hospital school graduates and baccalaureate degree graduates provides further testimony to nursing's anti-educationism.

The social irresponsibility inherent in proposals to con the public into thinking all R.N.'s are the equivalent of baccalaureate degree graduates by means of a grandfather clause is unlikely to enhance nursing's image with the public. (Although I would propose that generally the public thinks more highly of nurses than nurses often think of themselves.)

Registered nurses by virtue of in-service training or completion of programs anywhere from 2 months to 2 years in length identify themselves as clinicians, specialists, nurse practitioners, mid-wives and other titles as desired. Certification requirements may or may not include academic credentials and may or may not be the responsibility of qualified nurses.

The oft heard 'nursing is eclectic' (which has been defined by some as 'the layman's cult') contradicts nursing as a learned profession in its own right.

Claims of hospital school superiority because students work their way through the program while associate degree and baccalaureate students are unskilled is a mammoth distortion of reality. It is a fact that all approved schools regardless of level require laboratory and clinical practice in nursing as an integral part of the educational process. And it is worth repeating that one cannot use knowledge that one does not possess.

The myth of independence needs a good hard look. Despite claims that nurses speak for nursing it is a fact that nurses permit and often encourage others to speak for nursing. Nurses seek certification from persons outside nursing although it is a reality that persons outside nursing have neither the knowledge or competence to certify practice in nursing. The so-called extended role in nursing is in reality the encroachment of medicine into nursing's long established domain. Medical doctors are not licensed to practice nursing nor do they qualify for admission to the licensing examination. The M.D. is a first undergraduate professional degree in medicine just as the B.S. is the first undergraduate professional degree in nursing.

One might properly ask why nurses were upset by introduction of a worker labelled a physician's assistant. Nursing properly determines the need for nursing assistants. Surely if medicine wants assistants to the M.D. that is their right. It is also their responsibility to train such persons. It is not the responsibility of nurses to train them or to take orders from such a group. One profession does not delegate to another profession nor does one profession give orders to another. The much vaunted talk of the need for medicine and nursing to work together will not be fulfilled until there is mutual respect for the differences in the knowledge and skills of each.

Why aren't nurses practicing nursing? Why do nurses so often fail to seek the guidance and supervision of qualified nurses? Why do nurses so often place high value on that which is not nursing and those who are not nurses? Anti-educationism and dependency combine to support the low self-esteem which characterizes many nurses.

There are other myths. For example, the myth that hospitals are health centers although the reality is that they are sick centers. Then there is the myth that hospitals are the center of nursing practice although the reality is that people wherever they are are central to nursing practice. Another myth worthy of consideration is that *all* nurses are underpaid. Certainly there are many who are, and in a field that is predominantly women discrimination is a reality. But all discrimination or lack of it is not outside nursing. One must ask underpaid relative to whom? By what criteria?

Another myth that should be mentioned is the global statement of a critical shortage of nurses. There is a critical shortage of baccalaureate and higher degree graduates in nursing. There is a critical shortage of nurses generally who are willing to work in a paternalistic, hierarchal system ill suited to the needs of the public or of nurses.

Unification: SAIN Model requires that we learn to place high value on differences; that we value nursing as a learned profession, as science and an art; that we respect and value differences in career goals; and that we perceive and value nursing as a knowledgeable, socially responsible endeavor—peer of other learned professions.

CHAPTER 30

Obsolescence Revisited: The Doing Syndrome

Martha E. Rogers

Anti-educationism in nursing rides again. Some are calling it "Unification Model," others "Faculty Practice," and others label it "Joint Appointments." After decades of struggle to put a substantive knowledge base underneath the practice of nursing there is now a kind of move to deny that knowledge makes a difference and to proclaim the doer chief of the clan. Apprenticeship is praised, a feeble wheel is reinvented, and excellence in either teaching or practice is denigrated. Proposed product: a jack of all trades.

A return to the "good old days" may sound appealing to those nurses who are trying to balance budgets and to other nurses caught in a squeeze of understaffing by qualified nursing personnel. Concomitantly aping outdated models in other fields will not help public longevity. These proponents of the "old out-house" and "no central heating" would be well advised to note that as the ratio of M.D.'s to population increases so too does the death rate. Could it be they are doing something wrong?

Certainly in the development of nursing's educational system we have made many mistakes. For some years functional areas (i.e., teaching, supervision/administration, and consultation) pre-empted advanced knowledge in nursing. But this has been undergoing notable change over the past two decades. Graduate education in the science of nursing identifies graduate programs in nursing for all students. How the students may choose to use this knowledge is their option. Developing excellence as a practitioner is not the same thing as developing excellence as a teacher. Nor is a faculty role something buried beneath the ivy any more than a practitioner role is something buried beneath the bedpans.

Certainly college and university faculty in nursing should be qualified by education and experience for the responsibilities they are assigned. Certainly they are responsible for keeping up to date in their field and maintaining

Rogers, M. E. (1980, October). Obsolescence revisited: The doing syndrome. *SAIN Newsletter,* pp. 6–7. Reprinted with permission of the SAIN Governing Council.

competence for doing their job. And this can be done in many ways. But mandating that all faculty spend 12 hours a week in the school library is as irrelevant as mandating that all faculty be employed in a service agency for 12 hours each week.

Why is there continuing chatter about divisiveness between service and education? In graduate programs students planning to teach and students planning to provide service seem to get along quite well together. In fact they share courses, ideas and ideals, goals and problems, and even a bottle of vintage wine when someone can afford it. Does commencement decree an adversary relationship to follow?

"Unification" as a euphemism might be better recognized as a denial of academic freedom. Can one really legislate peace and good will to all? Will a committee create togetherness? Without mutual respect for the differences in knowledge, skills, and expertise that identify and differentiate educators, practitioners, administrators, and researchers there can be no growth or good will.

The public has a right to expect that they will not be sacrificed on the altar of 'nursing obsolescence'. Growing diversity is man's future. Let us look ahead!

CHAPTER 31

Resolution on Licensure for Entry Levels to Practice in Nursing

Governing Council of the Society for Advancement in Nursing

WHEREAS, There are currently educational programs in nursing which prepare for three different levels of entry into nursing practice, and
WHEREAS, Licensure to practice is provided for only two of these levels; specifically (1) registered nurse practice, and (2) practical nurse practice, and
WHEREAS, It has long been recognized that baccalaureate preparation is basic to professional practice, and
WHEREAS, No licensure is provided for the baccalaureate level of nursing practice, and
WHEREAS, Human safety requires the knowledgeable judgments afforded by baccalaureate level preparation in nursing,
THEREFORE BE IT RESOLVED, That the Society for Advancement in Nursing, Inc. initiate steps to introduce appropriate legislation that would provide for licensure of graduates of baccalaureate programs in nursing, and be it further
RESOLVED, That the registered nurse license be retained with full protection of the practice privileges, registered nurse status, and reciprocity procedures for licensure, of all individuals holding a Board approved associate degree in nursing or a hospital school diploma in nursing or the equivalent as prescribed by law and who fulfill all legal requirements for licensure as a registered nurse; and be it further
RESOLVED, That the practical nurse license be retained for all individuals who have completed a Board approved program in practical nursing or the equivalent as prescribed by law and who fulfill all legal requirements for licensure as a practical nurse.

Authored by the Governing Council of the Society for Advancement in Nursing (SAIN). (1982, October). Resolution on licensure for entry levels to practice in nursing. *SAIN Newsletter,* pp. 2–4. Reprinted with permission of the SAIN Governing Council.

CHAPTER 32

SAIN [Society for Advancement in Nursing] Perspective

Governing Council of the Society for Advancement in Nursing

SAIN, Inc. has examined the facts and has concluded that the only way to clear up much of the confusion in nursing is to differentiate between two careers in nursing. SAIN has not addressed the LPN [licensed practical nurse] in our proposal, other than to state that the legal parameters of practice are congruent with the knowledge base of the LPN. The LPN is considered one of three avenues to a dependent nursing career.

SAIN is concerned about legally differentiating between careers at the registered nurse level. Both the education literature and the nursing literature discuss how careers in an occupation are educationally derived. Based on this literature and on the goals of nursing programs, SAIN supports the need for two careers in nursing. One career is represented by the registered nurse practice that has traditionally been provided by registered nurse graduates from hospital programs (as long as they continue to exist) and graduates of community college programs in nursing. These registered nurses are prepared to practice in hospitals and other settings. The second career is represented by the registered nurse practice provided by registered nurse graduates of a baccalaureate and higher degree program with a content major in nursing. These nurses are prepared to practice nursing independently and as a peer member (equal in knowledge and accountability) of the professional health team in any setting, exercise a leadership role in formulating policy statements concerning nursing and act on relevant issues in nursing and health care. SAIN also supports the need for a new license for the already established group of nurses who have been professionally educated in baccalaureate and higher

Authored by the Governing Council of the Society for Advancement in Nursing (SAIN). (1977, January). SAIN perspective. *SAIN Newsletter*, pp. 4–6. Reprinted with permission of the SAIN Governing Council.

degree programs in nursing. This license for the independent nurse (IN) would provide in the law for such nurses to function independently.

Moreover, there are clear distinctions between the two careers in three areas: knowledge base, responsibility, and role.

INDEPENDENT NURSE	REGISTERED NURSE
Knowledge Base	**Knowledge Base**
1. Broad in scope.	1. Narrow in scope.
2. Primarily theoretical, and deals with a broad range of nursing problems and situations.	2. Deals primarily with technical tasks in nursing.
3. Enables the IN to make broad judgments dealing with a wide range of nursing problems.	3. Limits judgment to dealing with technical tasks and a narrower range of nursing problems.
4. Develops leadership for social action.	4. Curricular emphasis on strong social consciousness.
5. Is that of a professional degree with a strong emphasis on continuing education.	5. Curricula designed to be terminal rather than transfer in nature.
6. Provides a strong research orientation.	6. No research orientation.

INDEPENDENT NURSE	REGISTERED NURSE
Responsibility	**Responsibility**
1. Identification of problems of a broad nursing range.	1. To recognize problems of a technical nature.
2. Ability to do long-range, total planning.	2. To plan daily assignments.
3. Implementation of a total plan.	3. To implement daily assignments.
4. Evaluation and alteration of a total plan.	4. To evaluate and replan own tasks.
5. Ability to generalize and test from the collected data.	5. To collect and transmit data.
6. Ability to recognize deviations from health, changes in client's condition, and to predict from these.	6. To recognize, report, major deviations from health and changes in patient's condition.
7. Ability to evaluate and utilize research of others and to do research in nursing.	7. To develop a high degree of technical skill.
Role	**Role**
1. Assume leadership in nursing.	1. Work under supervision.
2. Collaborate with other professionals.	2. Assist the professional.
3. Direct the work of other nursing personnel.	3. Understand and utilize the services of the unskilled worker.
4. Serve the community in a leadership capacity.	4. Participate actively as a citizen in the community.

In essence, the knowledge base determines role and responsibility. Tasks do not define the kind of practice one offers. Some baccalaureate programs are offering courses in physical assessment and medical history taking. This is not substantive nursing knowledge; it is more sophisticated technical skills. These skills certainly do not professionalize a curriculum, and have little to do with *nursing* practice. Moreover, if these skills are used in the role of physician extender, then, they are technical *medical* skills. By definition, gathering medical observations and implementing technical medical tasks is vested in the realm of the medical profession. Medicine and nursing are two separate, autonomous, collaborative professions. Nursing is not, by definition, the extension of technical medical tasks. To include such technical medical tasks and skills in a baccalaureate nursing education curriculum is to decrease the time available to teach substantive nursing knowledge.

Nursing/Medicine: Autonomous/Collaborative Careers

Nursing is equal to medicine and independent nurses collaborate with other professional groups. This means that a person with a baccalaureate degree in nursing knows as much about nursing as a medical doctor knows about medicine. When a physician and an Independent Nurse (I.N.) collaborate concerning a client, the M.D. discusses medical assessment and the I.N. discusses nursing assessment. An I.N. has a valuable service to offer, separate from, independent of, the medical needs of the client. As a matter of fact, the client does not have to have medical needs to have nursing needs. The I.N. makes a judgment about a client based only on the substantive nursing knowledge base, on the legal definition of nursing practice, and on the assessment of the client. An I.N. can practice nursing in the *absence* of a medical diagnosis, physician's treatments and prescriptions, institution policy, nursing tradition or other I.N.'s The registered nurse finds these elements helpful guides to nursing practice, and is dependent on them for direction.

CHAPTER 33

Proposed Act to Amend the Education Law in Relation to Requirements for Independent, Registered, and Practical Nursing in New York State

Governing Council of the Society for Advancement in Nursing

The Society for Advancement in Nursing, Inc. proposes these changes in Article 139, Nursing, Title VIII, Education Law, New York State. (N.B.: New language is underlined. Deletions from current law are in brackets. Asterisks denote items to be negotiated.)

Article 139

Nursing

Section 6900 Introduction

Section 6901 Definition of practice of Nursing

Section 6902 Practice of Nursing and use of title "independent nurse" or "registered [professional] nurse" or "licensed practical nurse."

Section 6903 State Board for Nursing

Section 6904 Requirements for a license as an independent nurse

Authored by the Governing Council of the Society for Advancement in Nursing (SAIN). (1983, February). Proposed act to amend the education law in relation to requirements for independent, registered, and practical nursing in New York State. *SAIN Newsletter*, pp. 1–11. Reprinted with permission of the SAIN Governing Council.

Section 6905 Requirements for a license as a registered nurse
Section 6906 Requirements for a license as a licensed practical nurse
Section 6907 Limited permits
Section 6908 Exempt persons
Section 6909 Special provision
Section 6910 Renewal of license

S 6900 Introduction

This article applies to the profession of nursing and to the requirements for independent nursing, registered nursing and practical nursing. The general provisions for all professions contained in article one hundred thirty of this title apply to this article.

S 6901 Definition of Practice of Nursing

1. The practice of the profession of nursing as an "independent nurse" is defined as the utilization of substantive knowledge in the science of nursing requiring a prerequisite foundation in the liberal arts and sciences and an upper division college major in Nursing for the purpose of maintaining and promoting human health, preventing illness, diagnosing potential and actual health problems, caring for and rehabilitating the sick and disabled, achieving a dignified death, and such additional acts as are proper to be performed by an independent nurse. The "independent nurse" is directly accountable to the public for the judgments made and the services rendered.

2. The practice of nursing as a "Registered Nurse" is defined as performing tasks and responsibilities requiring general education and a nursing major of junior college level within the framework of maintaining and promoting human health, preventing illness, diagnosing potential and actual health problems, caring for and rehabilitating the sick and disabled, achieving a dignified death, and such additional acts not requiring the knowledge, judgment, and skill of the independent nurse and as are proper to be performed by a registered nurse. The registered nurse is responsible for implementing direct nursing services to people in a range of settings under the appropriate direction of an independent nurse and is accountable to the public for the services rendered.

3. The practice of nursing as a "licensed practical nurse" is defined as performing selected tasks and responsibilities within the framework of maintenance and promotion of human health, prevention of illness, care and rehabilitation of the sick and disabled, achieving a dignified death, and such additional acts not requiring the knowledge, judgment, and skill of an independent nurse or a registered nurse and as are proper to be performed by a licensed practical nurse. The licensed practical nurse is responsible for implementing direct nursing services in a range of settings under the direction of an independent nurse or a registered nurse and is accountable to the public for the services rendered.

S 6902 Practice of Nursing and Use of Title "Independent Nurse" or "Registered [Professional] Nurse" or "Licensed Practical Nurse"

Only a person licensed or otherwise authorized under this article shall practice nursing and only a person licensed under section sixty-nine hundred four shall use the title "independent nurse" and only a person licensed under section sixty-nine hundred five shall use the title "registered nurse" and only a person licensed under section sixty-nine hundred six shall use the title "licensed practical nurse."

S 6903 State Board for Nursing

A state board for nursing shall be appointed by the board of regents on recommendation of the commissioner for the purpose of assisting the board of regents and the department on matters of professional licensing and professional conduct in accordance with section sixty-five hundred eight of this title. The board shall be composed of not less than seventeen [fifteen] members, nine of whom shall be independent nurses and four [eleven] of whom shall be registered nurses and four of whom shall be licensed practical nurses all licensed and practicing in this state for at least five years. An executive secretary to the board shall be appointed by the board of regents on recommendation of the commissioner and shall be an "independent nurse" licensed in this state.

S 6904 Requirements for a License as an Independent Nurse

To qualify for a license as independent nurse, an applicant shall fulfill these requirements:

(1) Application: file an application with the department;
(2) Education: have received the minimum of a baccalaureate degree in nursing in accordance with the commissioner's regulations;
(3) Experience: meet no requirement as to experience;
(4) Examination: pass an examination satisfactory to the board and in accordance with the commissioner's regulations;
(5) Age: be at least * years of age;
(6) Citizenship: meet no requirement as to United States citizenship;
(7) Character: to be of good moral character as determined by the department; and
(8) Fees: pay a fee to the department for admission to the examination and for initial license of * dollars and for each re-examination * dollars, and for each biennial registration * dollars.

S 6905 Requirements for a License as a Registered Nurse

To qualify for a license as a registered [professional] nurse, an applicant shall fulfill [the following] these requirements:

(1) Application: file an application with the department;
(2) Education: have received a hospital school of nursing diploma or an associate degree in nursing in accordance with the commissioner's regulations, or completion of equivalent study satisfactory to the department in an approved program in independent nursing;
(3) Experience: meet no requirement as to experience;
(4) Examination: pass an examination satisfactory to the board and in accordance with the commissioner's regulations;
(5) Age: be at least ____*____ years of age;
(6) Citizenship: meet no requirement as to United States citizenship;
(7) Character: be of good moral character as determined by the department; and
(8) Fees: pay a fee to the department for admission to the examination and for initial license of ____*____ dollars; for each re-examination ____*____ dollars, and for each biennial registration ____*____ dollars.

S 6906 Requirements for a License as a Licensed Practical Nurse

To qualify for a license as a licensed practical nurse, an applicant shall fulfill [the following] these requirements:

(1) Application: file an application with the department;
(2) Education: have completed a program in practical nursing in accordance with the commissioner's regulations, or completion of equivalent study satisfactory to the department in a program conducted by the armed forces of the United States or in an approved program in registered nursing or in independent nursing;
(3) Experience: meet no requirement as to experience;
(4) Examination: pass an examination satisfactory to the board and in accordance with the commissioner's regulations;
(5) Age: be at least ____*____ years of age;
(6) Citizenship: meet no requirements as to United States citizenship;
(7) Character: be of good moral character as determined by the department; and
(8) Fees: pay a fee to the department for admission to the examination and for initial license of ____*____ dollars; for each re-examination ____*____ dollars, and for each biennial registration ____*____ dollars.

S 6907 Limited Permits

1. A permit to practice as an independent nurse or a permit to practice as a registered nurse or a permit to practice as a licensed practical nurse may be issued by the department upon the filing of an application for a license as an

independent nurse or as a registered nurse or as a licensed practical nurse and submission of such other information as the department may require to (i) graduates of schools of nursing registered by the department, (ii) graduates of schools of nursing approved in another state, province, or country or (iii) applicants for a license in practical nursing whose preparation is determined by the department to be the equivalent of that required in this state.

2. Such limited permit shall expire one year from the date of issuance or upon notice to the applicant by the department that the application for license has been denied. One renewal thereof for a period not to exceed six months may be issued in the discretion of the department upon submission of an explanation satisfactory to the department for the applicant's failure to become licensed within the original one-year period. Not withstanding, the foregoing provisions of this subdivision, if the applicant is waiting the result of a licensing examination at the time such limited permit expires such permit shall continue to be valid until ten days after the department notifies the applicant of the results of such examination.

3. A limited permit shall entitle the holder to practice nursing only under the supervision of an independent nurse currently registered in this state and with the endorsement of the employing agency.

4. Fees. The fee for each limited permit and for each renewal shall be ___*___ dollars.

5. Graduates of schools of nursing registered by the department may be employed to practice nursing under supervision of an independent [professional] nurse currently licensed [registered] in this state and with the endorsement of the employing agency for ninety days immediately following graduation from a program in nursing and pending receipt of a limited permit for which an application has been filed as provided in this section.

S 6908 Exempt Persons

1. This article shall not be construed:

a. As prohibiting the care of the sick by any person provided such person is employed primarily in a domestic capacity and does not hold himself or herself out, or accept employment as a person licensed [registered] to practice nursing under the provision of this article, or as preventing any person from the domestic administration of family remedies or the furnishing of nursing assistance in case of an emergency;

b. As including services given by attendants in institutions under the jurisdiction of or subject to the visitation of the state department of mental hygiene if adequate medical and nursing supervision is provided;

c. As prohibiting such performance of nursing students enrolled in registered schools or programs as may be incidental to their course of study;

d. As prohibiting or preventing the practice of nursing in this state by any legally qualified independent nurse or registered nurse or practical nurse of another state, province, or country whose engagement requires him or her to accompany and care for a patient temporarily residing in this state during the period of such engagement provided

such person does not represent or hold himself or herself out as an independent nurse or as a registered nurse or as a licensed practical nurse licensed [registered] to practice in this state;
e. As prohibiting or preventing the practice of nursing in this state during an emergency or disaster by any legally qualified independent nurse or registered nurse or licensed practical nurse of another state, province, or country who may be recruited by the American National Red Cross or pursuant to authority vested in the state civil defense commission for such emergency or disaster service, provided such person does not represent or hold himself or herself out as an independent nurse or as a registered nurse or as a licensed practical nurse licensed [registered] to practice in this state;
f. As prohibiting or preventing the practice of nursing in this state, in obedience to the requirements of the laws of the United States, by any commissioned nurse officer in the armed forces of the United States or by any nurse employed in the United States or by any nurse employed in the United States veterans administration or United States public health service while engaged in the performance of the actual duties prescribed for him or her under the United States statutes, provided such person does not hold himself or herself out as an independent nurse or as a registered nurse or as a licensed practical nurse licensed [registered] to practice in this state; or
g. As prohibiting the care of the sick when done in connection with the practice of the religious tenets of any church.

S 6909 Special Provision

1. Notwithstanding any inconsistent provision of any general, special, or local law, any licensed independent nurse or licensed registered [professional] nurse or licensed practical nurse who voluntarily and without the expectation of monetary compensation renders first aid or emergency treatment at the scene of an accident or other emergency outside a hospital [doctor's office] or any other place having proper and necessary medical equipment, to a person who is unconscious, ill or injured shall not be liable for damages for injuries alleged to have been sustained by such person or for damages for the death of such person alleged to have occurred by reason of an act or omission in the rendering of such first aid or emergency treatment unless it is established that such injuries were or such death was caused by gross negligence on the part of such independent nurse, or registered [professional] nurse or licensed practical nurse. Nothing in this subdivision shall be deemed or construed to relieve a licensed independent nurse or a licensed registered [professional] nurse or licensed practical nurse from liability from damages for injuries or death caused by an act or omission on the part of such nurse while rendering professional services in the normal and ordinary course of his or her practice.

[2. Nothing in this article shall be construed to confer the authority to practice medicine or dentistry.]

[3. An applicant for a license as a registered professional nurse or licensed practical nurse by endorsement of a license of another state, province, or country whose application was filed with the department under the laws in effect prior to August thirty-first, nineteen hundred seventy-one shall be licensed only upon successful completion of the appropriate licensing of all educational requirements is submitted to the department prior to September one, nineteen hundred seventy-seven.]

2. An applicant for a license as an independent nurse without examination must file an application within one year of the effective date of this act. Such applicant shall be currently licensed as a registered nurse and prior to the effective date of this act shall have graduated from a board approved senior college program of study with an upper division major in nursing in this state or any other state or province or country which program of study, at the time of graduation of such persons, required the satisfactory completion of a senior college program of study considered by the board to be equivalent to the minimum standards then in effect in New York state for a baccalaureate or equivalent graduate degree in nursing.

S 6910 Renewal of License

All applicants for renewal of license as an independent nurse or as a registered nurse or as a licensed practical nurse shall be required to furnish evidence of their participation in continuing education each year as established by regulation of the board.

S ____*____

This act shall take effect ____________*____________.

CHAPTER 34

The Need for Legislation for Licensure to Practice Professional Nursing

Martha E. Rogers, ScD, RN, FAAN

Nursing is a learned profession. Professional and technical careers in nursing are a reality. Graduates of valid baccalaureate degree programs that provide a substantive upper-division major in nursing are as different from nursing's technically prepared graduates of associate degree, hospital school, and practical nurse programs as medical doctors are from physician's assistants, as dentists are from dental hygienists, and as engineers are from engineering technicians.

Differentiation of professional and technical practitioners derives from the nature and amount of knowledge possessed by each. Experience is not a substitute for learning, and functions do not, *per se,* identify career difference. What one does is determined by what one knows and the intellectual judgments one makes in translating knowledge into practice.

Despite substantial antieducationism among nurses, evidence has been growing over several decades that there is a critical need for development of a clear, unambiguous identity for nursing's professionally educated practitioners. Reports of commissions and committees, federal and state attorney rulings, salary differentials (token though they may be), public consensus that full college programs of study are clearly different from associate degree and service agency programs, and a multiplicity of other factors combine in support of a need for honest confrontation with this critical problem.

Licensure exists to protect the public. Registration of nurses was initiated in the United States at the turn of the present century. However, at no time has nursing guaranteed society of any nurse's safety as a professional practitioner. Concomitantly, it is the professional nursing practitioners who must take re-

Rogers, M. E. (1985). The need for legislation for licensure to practice professional nursing . . . classics from our heritage. *Journal of Professional Nursing, 1,* 384. Reprinted with permission.

sponsibility for making knowledgeable judgments on issues beyond the ken of nursing's technicians but crucial to ensuring human safety.

Failure to establish standards and to license for professional practice in nursing leaves the public prone to being victimized by persons granted baccalaureate degrees in the absence of baccalaureate education, technically prepared nurses who have no professional preparation in nursing, and a health care system that denies professionally educated nurses the opportunity to use their knowledge for human betterment.

Professionally educated nurses leave nursing disappointed, disgusted, discouraged, and disheartened by the critical lack of social responsibility manifest in nursing's failure to openly recognize the identity and potential of professional practitioners. Euphemistic distortions of reality, misinformation conveyed through misuse of statistical data, and the public irresponsibility inherent in appeasement policies combine to diminish even further the provision of knowledgeable nursing practice.

Over 1,000,000 licensed nurses are currently practicing nursing today. Of this group, more than 100,000 possess baccalaureate and higher degrees. How many in this group of 100,000 can safely provide professional services to people? The public has no guarantee of safety. The potential student seeking a professional career in nursing has no guarantee that the program she or he selects will provide such preparation or that on graduation she or he will be able to practice as a professional.

Licensure for professional practice in nursing is long overdue. In its absence, human health is jeopardized, fraudulence in recruitment practices continues, and placement of a high value on ignorance is pervasive. Licensing laws for professional practice must be written and professional examinations must be developed. People are at stake.

SECTION FOUR

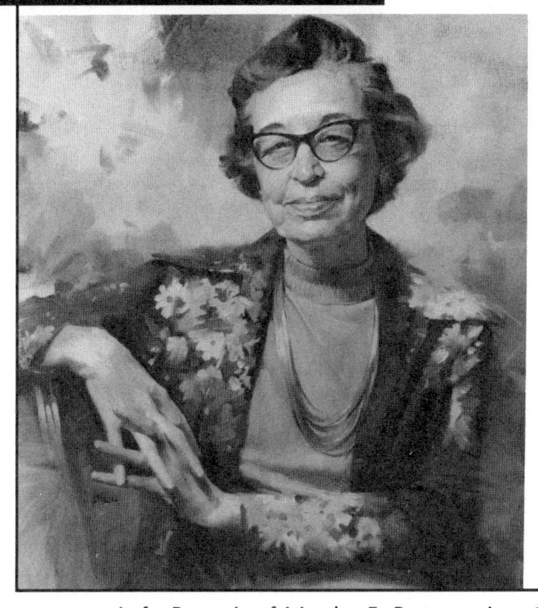

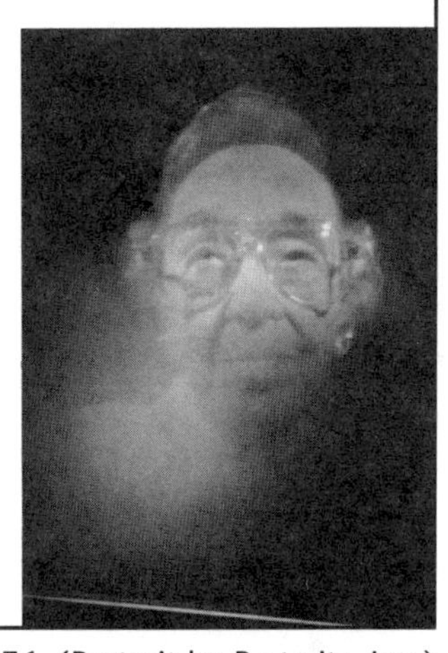

Left, Portrait of Martha E. Rogers, circa 1976. (Portrait by Portraits, Inc.) Right, Holographic portrait of Martha E. Rogers, 1992 (Portrait by Ana Maria Nicholson.)

Nursing Science: Evolution of the Science of Unitary Human Beings

Section Editor
Violet M. Malinski

CHAPTER 35

Highlights in the Evolution of Nursing Science: Emergence of the Science of Unitary Human Beings

Violet M. Malinski

Martha E. Rogers is one of nursing's foremost scientists. She is unique among the early cohort of nurse theorists for her insistence that nursing is a basic science and that the art of nursing practice can be developed only as the science of nursing is delineated. Whereas the majority of early theorists drew on knowledge developed in other disciplines to formulate theories for nursing, Rogers offered a new way of looking at people and their world, synthesizing what is now known as the Science of Unitary Human Beings. Rather than formulating her ideas around health and illness, Rogers identified the life process of the person and the person/environment mutual process as critical in understanding the phenomenon of concern to nurses: unitary human beings and their environment. The following chapters represent seminal writings in the evolution of this nursing science. Beginning with its early expression in the 1960s, moving to the publication of her landmark book in 1970, further elaborating the Science of Unitary Human Beings during the 1980s, and ending with the refinements of the early 1990s, readers can follow the evolution of nursing science in Rogers' own words. The following summary highlights key points in this evolution.

Rogers' (1961) first book, *Educational Revolution in Nursing,* presented an embryonic view of nursing science. She identified three postulates that provided, when synthesized, "a basis for a unified conceptualization of man and the universe" (p. 19):

1. "Through time and space man's continuous interaction with the universe moves him toward and away from multiple potential states of equilibrium" (p. 18).

2. "Man can initiate change and predict the subsequent series of changes within the limits of his own knowledge and a dynamic universe" (p. 19).
3. "Man is uniquely able to unite the past, present, and future in adapting to and changing with an evolving universe" (p. 19).

Rogers' (1964) second book, *Reveille in Nursing,* identified nursing as a learned profession with its own body of abstract principles from which to evolve the art of nursing. She wrote that nursing's purpose is "to assist individuals, families, and groups to achieve that maximum level of well-being which lies within the potential of each person" (p. 34). Rogers offered definitions of nursing science and nursing practice. Her early language reflected what she now sees as outdated or inconsistent concepts, including prediction, diagnosis, intervention, and interaction. The essence of her ideas, however, shines clearly through the terminology: the person is different from the sum of the parts, life is a process of becoming, and both "normal" and "pathological" processes are reflections of the life process. "Man is at the center of nursing's purpose" (p. 36), and "nursing science is directed toward understanding the life process in MAN" (p. 37). Rogers identified man as an open system, a complex electrodynamic field in constant interaction with the universe. These core ideas were amplified in her 1970 book, *An Introduction to the Theoretical Basis of Nursing.* Three chapters from that book are reproduced in this section.

In the 1970 book Rogers identified five basic assumptions of Rogerian science and what were then four principles of homeodynamics. Although the language is outdated and many of the original ideas have been modified, the book is historically significant as the foundation for this nursing science and for the links that Rogers drew to ideas emerging in other sciences. Using a variety of interdisciplinary sources, Rogers carefully supported the foundation she was building for nursing science. The ideas were her own, but she showed how they were similar to, expanded on, or offered new insights into emerging views in other sciences. The Rogerian scholar interested in what Rogers identified as both the contributions and limitations of systems theory and Einstein's view of space-time, for example, will delight in the earlier chapters of *An Introduction to the Theoretical Basis of Nursing.*

In Chapters 6 through 10, not reproduced here, Rogers presented the foundation for each of the following five basic assumptions of nursing science:

1. Chapter 6: "Man is a unified whole possessing his own integrity and manifesting characteristics that are more than and different from the sum of his parts" (p. 47).
2. Chapter 7: "Man and environment are continuously exchanging matter and energy with one another" (p. 54).
3. Chapter 8: "The life process evolves irreversibly and unidirectionally along the space-time continuum" (p. 59).
4. Chapter 9: "Pattern and organization identify man and reflect his innovative wholeness" (p. 65).
5. Chapter 10: "Man is characterized by the capacity for abstraction and imagery, language and thought, sensation and emotion" (p. 73).

These assumptions have since been modified; some are no longer accurate within the current formulation of the Science of Unitary Human Beings. For example, in later writings Rogers substituted "human being" for "man" and modified any wording that suggested a linear process (exchanging, unidirectional). The second assumption conveys an *interaction between* person and environment. Current language is different, reflecting Rogers' belief that the person/environment process is integral. While both the human energy field and the environmental energy field are different by definition, they are inseparable. There is no exchange of any kind, rather a continuous mutual process. She eliminated space-time because many readers interpreted it as Einstein's space-time concept. Rogers also replaced wording that suggested stasis (eg, "organization"), as continuous change is basic to this science. "Pattern" and "patterning" are now used rather than "pattern" and "organization."

Another word that appears in the 1970 book but was deleted at a later time is "repatterning." As a prefix "re-" conveys going back, recalling, or repeating something again, and this is not what Rogers intended to convey. Although there may be similarity, there is never sameness or repetition. Again the operative words in her current writings are "pattern" and "patterning" to convey continuous, creative, innovative change.

In 1970 Rogers introduced the term "homeodynamic" to describe the life process. She identified and discussed four principles of homeodynamics that provide hypothetical generalizations about this life process:

1. "Reciprocy is a function of the mutual interaction between the human field and the environmental field" (Rogers, 1970, p. 97). Reciprocy "postulates the inseparability of man and environment" (p. 97).
2. "Synchrony is a function of the state of the human field at a specified point in space-time interacting with the environmental field at the same specified point in space-time" (p. 99). Synchrony postulates that change "will be determined by the simultaneous interaction" (p. 99) of human and environmental fields.
3. "Helicy is a function of continuous innovative change growing out of the mutual interaction of man and environment along a spiralling longitudinal axis bound in space-time" (p. 101). Helicy "postulates an ordering of man's evolutionary emergence" (p. 100).
4. "The principle of resonancy postulates that change in pattern and organization of the human field and the environmental field is propagated by waves" (p. 101).

In the mid-1970s, reciprocy and synchrony were replaced with the principle of complementarity, defined as the mutual simultaneous interaction of the human and environmental energy fields. Rogers found that the words "reciprocy," "synchrony," and later "complementarity" were interpreted by readers according to their usage in other disciplines rather than as she intended them. She also realized that the ideas conveyed in the four principles could be condensed into three. Reciprocy and synchrony, therefore, only appeared in the 1970 work. The process of change, the nature of change, and the context of change are preserved in resonancy, helicy, and integrality.

Rogers also highlighted the importance of relationship and meaning to both theory development and research. She believed that nurses seek meaningful relationships to help describe, explain, and predict the life process as a phenomenon of wholeness. Rogers later eliminated prediction as a nursing goal. This is consistent with both the acausal nature of Rogerian science and the early emphasis on the importance of uncovering relationships in scientific endeavors.

Chapter 39 in this book presents a paper on the theoretical basis of nursing that Rogers delivered in 1971. She described the theory of accelerating evolution and examples of research questions it generated. She identified what she saw as misunderstandings of four-dimensional space-time and used the word "multidimensional" to describe the energy field.

The editors had access to Rogers' files and found another copy of the 1971 paper with penciled notations and changes that she used in presenting the material to her students at New York University in the 1970s. Notable among them are the refinements in language that reflect the mutual process of human and environment. For example, the sentence "Man and environment are contiguous and together equal the universe" was modified to "Man and environment are inseparable and together are coextensive with the universe." The first sentence reads as though two pieces of a puzzle are put together to form the whole, not what she intended. (Rogers later dropped "coextensive," for the same reason. This word still conveyed particulate rather than unitary phenomena.) Her notations described the four-dimensional energy field and substituted "energy" for earlier references to electrical (electrodynamic, electrical field potentials) in relation to field. In discussing the paranormal, Rogers ceased to refer to the senses, as in the evolutionary emergent of a sixth sense, and labeled the phenomena under discussion as (field) behaviors.

A period of 9 years elapsed before Rogers published another article on nursing science. During that time she was actively publishing in relation to various professional and political issues confronting nursing. Simultaneously she continued to develop and refine her ideas related to nursing science, presenting them to graduate and doctoral students at New York University and to audiences as an invited speaker at many conferences.

In her 1980 chapter in Riehl and Roy, reproduced here, Rogers called her work a conceptual system and identified the four building blocks of nursing science: energy fields, a universe of open systems, pattern and organization, and four-dimensionality. She no longer discussed the five assumptions presented in 1970. She presented the three principles of helicy, resonancy, and complementarity (later integrality). The wording was slightly different from later definitions but conveyed the same ideas. Rogers pointed out that the principles have meaning only within the context of this conceptual system. She saw complementarity as subsumed within helicy but chose to present it as a separate principle both for clarity and to emphasize the significance of mutual simultaneity, with its inherent contradiction of causality. She identified three theories: the theory of accelerating evolution, paranormal events, and rhythmical correlates of change, emphasizing with the latter that she meant field rhythms not biological or psychological rhythms.

In *Science of Unitary Man: A Paradigm for Nursing,* Rogers (1981) (not reproduced here) referred to her work as a paradigm rather than a conceptual system and deleted "mutual simultaneity" in favor of "continuous, mutual process." Rogers found that "simultaneity," with the implication of two or more things happening at the same time, was particulate and thus did not convey her meaning, better captured in continuous, mutual process. This changed the definition of complementarity from "the interaction between human and environmental fields is continuous, mutual, simultaneous" (Rogers, 1980, p. 331) to one that emphasized "the continuous, mutual process between human and environmental fields in contradiction to highly cherished causality" (Rogers, 1981, p. 1721).

In 1983 Rogers (1983) contributed a chapter to *Family Health: A Theoretical Approach to Nursing Care* (not reproduced here). She continued to call her work a paradigm; reiterated the building blocks and principles of resonancy, helicy, and complementarity; and introduced some of her proposed correlates of the developmental process that she had introduced to her students in the 1970s (eg, longer rhythms, shorter rhythms, seems continuous; time drags, time races, seems timeless). These are postulated to describe the process of change in what she was then calling unitary human development (and later became unitary human change). Rogers emphasized the difference between the unitary human (irreducible) and the holistic human (sum of parts). The family, as the focus, becomes "an irreducible, four-dimensional, negentropic family energy field" (p. 226) in continuous mutual process with the environmental field. She acknowledged the diversity of family forms as encouraging a positive view of change and of a family's capacity to participate knowingly in change.

Digressing from the chronology for a moment, Rogers (1989c) again elaborated on the concept of family field in *Rogerian Nursing Science News.* A reader submitted questions concerning the mother/fetus mutual process, whether they were two fields or one during pregnancy and after birth, and how bonding and attachment fit within the context of energy fields. Dr. Rogers responded:

> Energy fields are infinite. One identifies the fields one wishes to study. Maternal and fetal fields may be perceived as a single irreducible field or they may be perceived as separate fields. If perceived as a single field, it is irreducible and is in continuous process with its environmental field. If they are perceived as separate fields, each is integral with his/her environmental field.
>
> At birth these are two individual human fields. The infant is not a fetus. The infant and the mother are each integral with their respective environmental fields. If one wishes to perceive the infant and mother as *one* irreducible field, they would then be perceived as a group, just as one would perceive a family field or any other group field. The group field is irreducible and is integral with the environmental field of the group.
>
> The concepts of bonding and attachment do not refer to irreducible human and environmental fields.
>
> Re-examine the Principles of Homeodynamics. Describe the human and environmental field manifestations of field pattern. All manifestations emerge out of the continuous mutual process of human and environmental fields. (p. 3)

In Rogerian nursing science, the human energy field can be conceptualized as an individual, a family, or a group in terms of the nurse's focus.

Rogers next appeared in print in two edited works (Rogers, 1986; Rogers, 1987), with chapters highlighting similar content. The 1986 chapter is reprinted here. By this time she had eliminated "organization" and referred to "pattern" alone, now defining it "as the distinguishing characteristic of an energy field perceived as a single wave" (1986, p. 5) rather than as "a mosaic of waves" (Rogers, 1983, p. 222). She renamed the third principle "integrality" for greater clarity and accuracy and revised the wording of all three to make them clearer and mutually exclusive. Rogers also highlighted the importance of pattern as a key concept in the principles of homeodynamics.

In a 1988 article in *Nursing Science Quarterly* (reprinted here) Rogers expanded on accelerating evolution and space exploration. She reiterated that "nursing is integral with the rapidly changing world" (p. 99) that she described. Earlier Rogers had discussed Therapeutic Touch, meditation, and imagery as examples of noninvasive therapeutic modalities congruent with the new worldview she presented. She now introduced humor, sound, color, and motion.

The conceptual system, paradigm, or abstract system became the science, specifically the Science of Unitary Human Beings. Rogers has been consistent in referring to nursing as a science, specifically a basic science. Others have referred to Rogers' theory of nursing, but Rogers herself disagrees with the designation of her work as either a theory or a conceptual model. Rather she has explained consistently that her work reflects the science of nursing and that multiple theories can be derived from the postulates and principles of the science. In the 1988 article she provided a list of definitions of specificity relevant to the Science of Unitary Human Beings, defining science as "an organized body of abstract knowledge arrived at by scientific research and logical analysis" (Rogers, 1988, p. 100).

In 1989 Rogers (1989a) contributed a chapter to the third edition of Riehl-Sisca's *Conceptual Models for Nursing Practice* (not reprinted here). The content was similar to what she had written earlier. However, she did provide examples of manifestations of relative diversity in field patterning (formerly called correlates):

lesser diversity		greater diversity
longer rhythms	shorter rhythms	seem continuous
slower motion	faster motion	seem continuous
time experienced as slower	time experienced as faster	timelessness
pragmatic	imaginative	visionary
longer sleeping	longer waking	wakefulness

(Rogers, 1989a, p. 185)

These are postulated to express the continuous, creative change in the flow of human/environment field patterning.

In Barrett's book Rogers (1990a) updated her science, calling it the Science of Unitary, Irreducible Human Beings. She deleted the term "four-dimensional," replacing it with "multidimensional"; the definition remained unchanged. Again, Rogers had used "multidimensional" back in 1971. She was never sure it was the appropriate word, as "multi-" means many or multiple and seemed to her to imply adding dimensions. She introduced "four-dimensional" in 1980, but was never sure that this adequately conveyed her intent, either. People often assumed that Rogers and Einstein were talking about the same phenomenon (ie, four-dimensional space-time). She adopted "multidimensional" again for a brief time, as reflected in the 1990 definitions.

The manifestations of field patterning remained unchanged. A major change was her deletion of probability from the system in favor of unpredictability, which she saw as more consistent and supportive of the view of change presented in the principles. The wording of the principles was changed to reflect this perspective. She reiterated that this nursing science is applicable both to individuals and to groups, whether family or other type of group.

Rogers also wrote of the difference between "holistic," a word she had long since abandoned, and "integral." "The irreducible nature of individuals is different from the sum of the parts. The integralness of people and environment that coordinate with a multidimensional universe of open systems point to a new paradigm: the *identity of nursing as a science*" (Rogers, 1990a, p. 6).

The following may better illuminate the difference between integral and holistic. In another 1989 issue of *Rogerian Nursing Science News,* Rogers (1989b) responded to a second question from a reader concerning vital signs (blood pressure, pulse, respiration) and their role in Rogerian science-based practice. Rogers wrote that facts can only be understood in the context of theory:

> . . . So-called "vital signs," whether measured in home, hospital, work place, at the beach, or elsewhere are merely facts. They are commonly used as indicators of biological systems and are interpreted in the light of a closed system, 3 dimensional, entropic, causal model. Numerical norms are often deemed sacrosanct. Interpretation of these facts does not focus on unitary human beings nor can one generalize from a part to a whole. Moreover, a summation of such facts is equally invalid as a predictor of the whole. Numerical values as such are inadequate and often dangerous. . . . All characteristics, attributes, behaviors, and the like are manifestations of the whole, of the energy field pattern. A synthesis of manifestations of field pattern is one of growing diversity, continuously innovative rhythmicities, and a range of multiple observable data to provide continuously evolving profiles of individual fields. The Principles of Homeodynamics postulate the nature of change and serve as probabilistic guidelines.
>
> Overuse, misuse, and reliance on numerical values for whatever facts are potentially dangerous. Hypochondriasis is generated and outcomes could be lethal. Outdated world views provide a poor basis for nursing practice.
>
> Therapeutic modalities in nursing focus on irreducible human beings and are directed toward promoting maximum well-being. Individualization of services is a must. (p. 6)

In Parker's book Rogers (1990b) (reprinted here) presented the space-age paradigm for nursing and the new worldview that encompasses both earthkind and spacekind. She proposed that a new species, *Homo spatialis,* will evolve as changes occur during the experience of space travel. Rather than manifestations of pathology, these changes are manifestations of human and environmental field process. Future nursing practice on earth and beyond will include Therapeutic Touch, imagery, meditation, relaxation, color, taste, sound, fragrance, humor, laughter, mood, and attitude.

The last article that appears in this section was published in 1992. Here Rogers included one major change, replacing the word "multidimensional" (formerly "four-dimensional") with "pandimensional," conveying union. Again, the definition remained unchanged. She presented her four postulates (no longer called building blocks) of energy fields, pattern, pandimensionality, and openness, as well as the principles, manifestations of field patterning, and theories she derived from the science (accelerating evolution/change and paranormal). She discussed the importance of the new worldview represented by this science for nursing and the space age.

Rogers has consistently espoused her view of nursing as a basic science whose aim is to promote health and well-being for all persons wherever they are, in the home and community, in the clinic or hospital, and in space. Her love and respect for people shine through as she highlights unitary, irreducible human beings and their unitary, irreducible environments as the phenomena of concern to nurses. Her respect and regard for nurses shine through in her recognition of a unique knowledge base in nursing and the call for autonomous practice whereby nurses can use that knowledge for the betterment of humankind.

Perhaps one of the greatest stumbling blocks for those interested in Rogerian nursing science is the fact that Rogers' last book was published over 20 years ago. The tendency to seek out the book as the definitive source rather than more current articles and/or chapters has often meant that nurses have used outdated assumptions and concepts in developing a Rogerian theoretical framework for their own work. Hopefully the chronological evolution of Rogers' ideas which follows in this section will assist both the neophyte and the more knowledgeable Rogerian nurse. Readers are invited to embark on their own exploration of nursing science through the following chapters.

References

Rogers, M. E. (1961). *Educational revolution in nursing.* New York: Macmillan.

Rogers, M. E. (1964). *Reveille in nursing.* Philadelphia: Davis.

Rogers, M. E. (1970). *An introduction to the theoretical basis of nursing.* Philadelphia: Davis.

Rogers, M. E. (1971). *The theoretical basis of nursing.* Paper presented at the University of Illinois School of Nursing, Chicago, IL.

Rogers, M. E. (1980). Nursing: A science of unitary man. In J. P. Riehl & C. Roy (Eds.), *Conceptual models for nursing practice* (2nd ed.) (pp. 329–331). New York: Appleton-Century-Crofts.

Rogers, M. E. (1981). Science of unitary man: A paradigm for nursing. In G. E. Lasker (Ed.), *Applied systems and cybernetics* (pp. 1719–1722). New York: Pergamon.

Rogers, M. E. (1983). Science of unitary human beings: A paradigm for nursing. In I. W. Clements & F. B. Roberts (Eds.), *Family health: A theoretical approach to nursing care* (pp. 219–228). New York: Wiley.

Rogers, M. E. (1986). Science of unitary human beings. In V. M. Malinski (Ed.), *Explorations on Martha Rogers' science of unitary human beings* (pp. 3–8). Norwalk, CT: Appleton-Century-Crofts.

Rogers, M. E. (1987). Rogers's science of unitary human beings. In R. R. Parse (Ed.), *Nursing science: Major paradigms, theories, and critiques* (pp. 139–146). Philadelphia: Saunders.

Rogers, M. E. (1988). Nursing science and art: A prospective. *Nursing Science Quarterly, 1,* 99–102.

Rogers, M. E. (1989a). Nursing: A science of unitary human beings. In J. P. Riehl-Sisca (Ed.), *Conceptual models for nursing practice* (3rd ed.) (pp. 181–188). Norwalk, CT: Appleton & Lange.

Rogers, M. E. (1989b). Questions for Dr. Martha E. Rogers: Dr. Rogers' Answer. *Rogerian Nursing Science News, 1*(3), 6.

Rogers, M. E. (1989c). Questions for Dr. Martha E. Rogers: Dr. Rogers' Response. *Rogerian Nursing Science News, 2*(1), 3.

Rogers, M. E. (1990a). Nursing: Science of unitary, irreducible, human beings: Update 1990. In E. A. M. Barrett (Ed.), *Visions of Rogers' science-based nursing* (pp. 5–11). New York: National League for Nursing.

Rogers, M. E. (1990b). Space-age paradigm for new frontiers in nursing. In M. E. Parker (Ed.), *Nursing theories in practice* (pp. 105–112). New York: National League for Nursing.

Rogers, M. E. (1992). Nursing science and the space age. *Nursing Science Quarterly, 5,* 27–34.

CHAPTER 36

The Aims of Nursing Science

Martha E. Rogers

The central aims of science are . . . concerned with a search for understanding—a desire to make the course of nature not just predictable but intelligible.

—Stephen Toulmin

The science of nursing is an emergent—a new product. The inevitability of its development is written in nursing's long commitment to human health and welfare. With today's rapid and unprecedented changes, new urgency has been added to the critical need for a body of scientific knowledge specific to nursing. Only as the science of nursing takes on form and substance can the art of nursing achieve new dimensions of artistry. Knowledgeable nursing services are indispensable to public safety. Humanitarian values add a further imperative to the search for understanding man and his world.

The predictive principles needed to guide nursing practice emerge out of nursing's conceptual system. Science seeks to make intelligible the world of man's experiences. Nursing science seeks to make intelligible knowledge about man and his world that has special significance for nursing. The phenomenon central to nursing's conceptual system is the life process in man. A conceptual model of the life process in man [see Chapter 12] provides the base from which relevant theories may be derived and tested.

Science is concerned with meanings rather than with facts. A conceptual frame of reference is an indispensable prerequisite to the ordering of knowledges and to the formulation of meaningful propositions. An organized system of concepts further provides a repository for experimental observations which can enrich the conceptual system in the continuing search for systematic relationships among a range of phenomena. Concomitantly, it must be kept in mind that "the accuracy of an observation does not, in itself, make it valuable to science."[1]

Rogers, M. E. (1970). The aims of nursing science. In M. E. Rogers, *An introduction to the theoretical basis of nursing* (pp. 83–88). Philadelphia: F. A. Davis. Reprinted with permission.

A conceptual system is characterized by an interrelated set of postulates having relevance for some central phenomenon. Out of the conceptual system, theories emerge directed toward achieving further understanding of the real world. Theories are abstractions. They underlie the development of testable hypotheses and, in the testing, may be supported or refuted.

Every scientific statement does not have to be tested before it is accepted, but it must be capable of being tested.[2] History provides many examples of notions found highly useful long before being subjected to experiential verification. This is not to propose that testing may not be necessary, but rather to point out that theories may be quite significant even before they have been tested. The generation of theory is the outgrowth of abstract thought and abstraction is clearly different from concrete behavior. The formulation of theories is concerned with relationships. The capacity to envision new ways of perceiving phenomena and to propose meaningful explanations for these perceptions is a characteristic of theoretical formulation. "Observation and experiment do not provide the conceptions without which inquiry is aimless and blind."[3]

The emergence of a science of nursing demands a clear, unequivocal conceptual frame of reference. This is not to propose that nursing's conceptual system is either static or inflexible. Quite the contrary. In its evolution it is properly subject to reformulation and change as empirical knowledge grows, as conceptual data achieve greater clarity, and as the interconnectedness between ideas takes on new dimensions. Nursing's abstract system is a matrix of concepts relevant to the life process in man. Postulates integral to the system are asserted and testable hypotheses derive from the system.

Nursing is an empirical science. As with other empirical sciences, its purpose is to describe and explain the phenomenon central to its concern and to predict about it. The life process in man is a phenomenon of wholeness, of continuity, of dynamic and creative change. The multiplicity of events, both actual and potential, that may attend its becoming provide the experiential data of nursing research. The identification of relationships between events provides for an ordering of knowledges and for the development of nursing's hypothetical generalizations and unifying principles.

If the process of life is to be studied and understood, normal and pathological processes must be treated on a basis of complete equality. Health and illness, ease and dis-ease are dichotomous notions, arbitrarily defined, culturally infused, and value laden. The life process possesses its own unity. It is inseparable from the environment. The characteristics of the life process are those of the whole. As the life process in man is understood, its multiple manifestations lend themselves to explanation and to prediction.

A concept of the life process in man that views the notions of normal and pathological as invalid bases for studying man may not be readily perceived by those who have been imbued with the idea that health and sickness are discrete entities, each subject to its own independent study. But health and sickness, however defined, are expressions of the process of life. Whatever meaning they may have is derived out of an understanding of the life process in its totality. Life's deviant course demands that it be viewed in all of its dimensions if valid explanations of its varied manifestations are to emerge. Predictions, the keys to knowledgeable intervention, will be no better than the extent to which they arise out of an increasing understanding of life's innumerable potentialities.

The all-too-common perception of man as predominantly subjected to multiple negative environmental influences with pathological outcomes denies man's unity with nature and his evolutionary becoming. A man-environment dichotomy is presumed, rather than recognition of the complementary nature of the man-environment relationship. The well documented negentropic qualities of life require a positive approach for their understanding.

The development of a science brings with it the need for a language of specificity.[4] The language of everyday life is filled with ambiguities. The word "field" may be used to refer to a cotton field, a baseball field, a magnetic field, an airport, or a sphere of influence. For one person the word "nuts" may conjure up visions of an edible delight while for another there may arise an image of small metal blocks with threaded holes in them. To someone else "nuts" may represent an exclamation of disgust or scorn. Semantic confusion is not an uncommon problem among people. Generally one determines the meaning of a word within the context of its usage and does not pursue exactness of meaning with the user. While this kind of generality seems to serve reasonably well for much of day-to-day living, it is highly inadequate for scientific use.

The development of a scientific language evolves out of the general language. Terms in everyday usage are given precise and unambiguous meanings. They are then so understood by all members of a given scientific discipline. Development of such a language is directed toward achieving simplicity and clarity. Depiction of reality attains greater accuracy. Symbolic representation of relationships becomes possible. On occasion it may be necessary to invent a new word in order to secure adequate precision and clarity. That a new word may have to be coined is not a "carte blanche" for a rash of new terminology. Nor is a scientific language properly developed for the purpose of covering up a pseudoscientism (not an unheard-of feat). Jargon, one of Langer's[5] "Idols of the Laboratory," is more of a pretense toward technical sophistication than it is an expression of ideas.

Description, stated in general language terms, attends the early stages of development of a science. With growth of a particular science there arises the need for more precise terminology in which to state generalizations and to communicate the abstract formulations of the science. The furtherance of scientific inquiry in nursing requires a technical language of specificity. Translation of nursing's body of scientific knowledge into meaningful service to man demands that explanatory and predictive principles possess clarity and exactness.

Nursing aims to assist people in achieving their maximum health potential. Maintenance and promotion of health, prevention of disease, nursing diagnosis, intervention, and rehabilitation encompass the scope of nursing's goals. Nursing is concerned with people—all people—well and sick, rich and poor, young and old. The arenas of nursing's services extend into all areas where there are people: at home, at school, at work, at play; in hospital, nursing home, and clinic; on this planet and now moving into outer space.

The science of nursing aims to provide a body of abstract knowledge growing out of scientific research and logical analysis and capable of being translated into nursing practice. Nursing's body of scientific knowledge is a new product specific to nursing. Concomitantly, the science of nursing does not arise out of a vacuum nor are the knowledges encompassed by nursing science necessarily of meaning only to nurses.

Nursing is a humanistic science. As such, the methods of classical science have a number of limitations for applicability to nursing research. Reductionism, representative of an atomistic world view in which complex things are built up of simple elements, is contrary to a perception of wholeness. The subjective world of human feelings must be incorporated into so-called "objective science" to provide a more comprehensive epistemology relevant to the study of man. Dubos has written: "Science does not progress only by inductive, analytical knowledge. The imaginative speculations of the mind come first, the verification and the analytic breakdown come only later. And imagination depends upon a state of emotional and intellectual freedom which makes the mind receptive to the impressions that it receives from the world in its confusing, overpowering, but enriching totality."[6]

Maslow[7] decries what he calls desacralization of science and points out "that 'cool' perceiving and neutral thinking" are not the only ways for discovering truth. Such experiences as pain, joy, redness, etc., create major difficulties for investigators seeking "rigorous definition" as a method of concept formation. Peering through a microscope is deemed an acceptable means for securing objective knowledge, but one must question the validity of human beings as proper subjects for microscopic detachment. The real world encompasses observer and observed, with both contributing their measure to any ascribed situation. New methodologies must be devised to supplement, enhance, and transcend traditional approaches to the search for understanding.

A body of scientific knowledge is clearly different from the uses to which that knowledge may be put. The science of nursing is prerequisite to the process of nursing. The science of nursing must be incorporated into nursing's instructional programs. Concomitantly, students must have opportunity to test the validity and reliability of theory in the real situation—the laboratory of human life. Broad principles are put together in novel ways to help explain a wide range of events and multiplicity of individual differences. Action, based on predictions arising out of intellectual skill in the merging of scientific principles, becomes underwritten by intellectual judgments. The distinctive nature of professional practice in nursing is spelled out in nursing's unifying principles and hypothetical generalizations.

The education of professional practitioners in nursing requires the transmission of a body of scientific knowledge specific to nursing. This body of knowledge determines the safety and scope of nursing practice. The imaginative and creative use of knowledge for the betterment of man finds expression in the art of nursing. Education opens the doorway to developing the art of practice. The purpose of professional education is to provide the knowledge and tools whereby an individual may become an artist in his field. It is not to prepare the skilled practitioner. And as Robert Hutchins has noted, ". . . the most practical education is the most theoretical one."[8]

Nursing's abstract system is the outgrowth of concern for human health and welfare. The science of nursing aims to provide a growing body of theoretical knowledge whereby nursing practice can achieve new levels of meaningful service to man. A conceptual model of man is at the base of nursing's abstract system and provides a frame of reference from which guiding principles may be derived.

References

1. Polanyi, Michael, *Personal Knowledge,* Chicago: The University of Chicago Press, 1958, p. 136.
2. Popper, Karl R., *The Logic of Scientific Discovery,* New York: Harper Torchbooks, 1965, p. 48.
3. Nagel, Ernest, "The Philosopher Looks at Science," *Medicine and the Other Disciplines.* New York: International Universities Press, Inc., 1960, p. 24.
4. Hempel, Carl G., *Fundamentals of Concept Formation in Empirical Science,* Chicago: University of Chicago Press, 1952, p. 1.
5. Langer, Susan, *Mind: An Essay on Human Feeling,* Volume I, Baltimore: The Johns Hopkins Press, 1967, p. 36.
6. Dubos, René, *The Dreams of Reason,* New York: Columbia University Press, 1961, p. 122.
7. Maslow, Abraham H., *The Psychology of Science,* New York: Harper and Row, 1966, p. 121.
8. Hutchins, Robert M., *The Learning Society,* New York: Frederick A. Praeger, Publishers, 1968, p. 8.

CHAPTER 37

Nursing's Conceptual Model

Martha E. Rogers

. . . the molding of a system of concepts means nothing less than the creation of a new language, a new mode of thinking.

—F. Waismann

A system has been defined as "an assemblage of facts or ideas that is adjusted and regulated to form a connected whole."[1] The interrelatedness of ideas that gives wholeness and unity to nursing's conceptual system is built around the life process in man. As ideas become organized into a meaningful frame of reference, there emerges a conceptual model of the life process in man, which can then provide a base for theoretical operations pertinent to continuing study and elaboration of the conceptual system.

A conceptual model is an abstraction. Such a model is not real but is instead a *representation* of the universe or some portion thereof. A model of the life process in man is an imaginary construct which provides a way of perceiving the life process and serves as an aid to thinking. Revision and change occur as emerging empirical evidence points up inconsistencies and inadequacies in the proposed model. The theoretical nature of the model does not free it of the need to take into account the real world. Concomitantly, it is in the abstractness of the model that facts and observations are transcended and meaning emerges.

For purposes of this chapter, the terms "man," "life process," and "life process in man" are used interchangeably. "Model" is used to mean a "conceptual model of the life process in man." The model to be proposed represents a matrix of ideas which in its wholeness symbolizes man. Moreover, man is an integral part of the universe. Man and environment are complementary systems, not dichotomous ones. In consequence a model of man must affirm the unity of nature.

Nursing's conceptual model rests upon a set of basic assumptions which have been discussed in Unit II [*An Introduction to the Theoretical Basis of*

Rogers, M. E. (1970). Nursing's conceptual model. In M. E. Rogers, *An introduction to the theoretical basis of nursing* (pp. 89–94). Philadelphia: F. A. Davis. Reprinted with permission.

Nursing]. These assumptions constitute statements of fact postulated to be true and describe the life process in man as characterized by wholeness, openness, unidirectionality, pattern and organization, sentience and thought. These are characteristics that underlie and must be taken into account in the development of the model.

An energy field identifies the conceptual boundaries of man. This field is electrical in nature, is in a continual state of flux, and varies continuously in its intensity, density, and extent. It may be likened to fields of the physical world in its capacity to demonstrate the presence of electrical charges and their correlates. Theoretically, electrical fields extend to infinity. Concomitantly, for practical purposes they may be deemed bounded according to selected criteria. The human field is postulated to have its boundary contiguous with the boundary of the environment. The environment is, itself, an energy field electrical in nature. The interaction between the human field and the environmental field takes place across the conceptual boundaries of these two fields which together are coextensive with the universe.

The human field extends beyond the discernible mass which we perceive as man. The concentration of energy, having a nature and density which is visible to the human eye, encompasses only a portion of the individual's identity. Multiple irregularities characterize the boundaries of man's energy field. At times the field may extend farther into the environment and at other times retreat in the direction of man's visible core. The nature and intensity of the man-environment interchange across these fluctuating boundaries varies both between individuals and for given individuals at different points in time.

Numerous colloquialisms suggest corollaries between such postulated energy fields and the observed world. For example, persons may be referred to as magnetic, forceful, moody, withdrawn—observations consistent with a concept of fluctuating field intensities and dimensions. The great actor, with capacity to enthrall an audience, penetrates the environmental boundary and his energy field, like a giant pseudopodium, reaches out to engulf a portion of the outer world, receding only when the drama ends.

The human field possesses its own identifiable wholeness. Despite its dynamic nature and its continuous interaction with the environment, it maintains identity in its ever-changing but omnipresent patterning. Pattern and organization of the field express themselves in a wide range of ways, all of which have relevance for the integrity of the field. Pattern evolves with kaleidoscopic uncertainty coordinate with the nature of the man-environment energy exchange taking place through space-time. Growing complexity of organization is an outgrowth of the multiple interactions occurring along the continuum of life. When pattern and organization no longer exist, the integrity of the human field is destroyed and death ensues.

Death is postulated to represent a transformation of energy. In whatever way one may perceive events subsequent to death, relevant testable hypotheses are yet to be proposed. At the same time the passing of a human life has its own objective reality. At death the human field ceases to exist, and identity as a living human being is gone. The process of dying may be of long or short duration. It is a period of transition in which the integrity of the human field, as such, diminishes and dies.

Envision the human field embedded in the curvature of space-time. The life process is the expression of the rhythmical evolution of the field along a

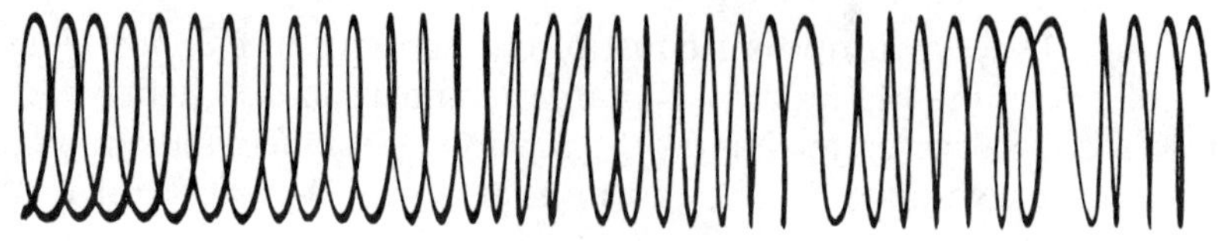

Figure 1.

spiralling longitudinal axis, bound in the four-dimensional space-time matrix and ever shaping and being shaped by the environment. The human field occupies space, extending in all directions. The field projects into the future as well as into the past. The creativity of life emerges out of the man-environment interaction along life's continuum. The human field is continually adding new dimensions of growing complexity, evidenced in life's negentropic qualities.

The communication of concepts is sometimes helped by the use of concrete illustrations. The reader is no doubt familiar with the child's toy known as "Slinky." (There is also a "Junior Slinky"—smaller but perhaps more effective as an aid to understanding the proposed model.) The life process lacks the evenness and regularity of this interesting toy, but with a little effort the "Junior Slinky" can be twisted, its spirals stretched or shortened, its intervals between spirals narrowed or widened. Larger spirals of "Slinky," itself, may be superimposed upon the spirals of the toy. Visualize "Slinky" as embedded in space and its sequence of spirals as coordinate with the passing of time.

Imagine the life process moving along the "Slinky" spirals with the human field occupying space along the spiral and extending out in all directions from any given location along a spiral. Each turn of the spiral exemplifies the rhythmical nature of life, while distortions of the spiral portray deviations from nature's regularities. Variations in the speed of change through time may be perceived by narrowing or widening the distance between spirals [Figure 1]. (For example, compare 20 turns of the wire per inch to 5 turns per inch.) Energy exchange between the human field and environment is a constant concomitant of the evolving life process. Sentience and thought arise out of this interaction and give further evidence of the wondrousness of life. This is not to be interpreted as a mechanistic design. Rather, it is proposed as an aid to perceiving life's realities and potentialities.

The limitations of a concrete example to illustrate an abstraction are multiple. "Slinky" is proposed as a stimulus to ways of perceiving man. It is not a representation of man. The basic assumptions presented in Unit II [*An Introduction to the Theoretical Basis of Nursing*] underlie any extrapolation of ideas emerging out of examination of "Slinky." Nursing's conceptual model derives from a synthesis of ideas which then form a unified and meaningful system.

Man is a unified whole having his own distinctive characteristics which cannot be perceived by looking at or describing the parts. Nor does a summation of parts add up to man. The fundamental unit of the living system is an energy field. It is this field which gives unity to the concept of wholeness. The human field interacts as a whole with the whole of the environment. Changes taking place in the human field and in the environment are holistic in nature. Pattern and organization give identity to the field and are themselves field phenomena. Alterations in pattern and organization are continuous and reflect the unitary nature of the life process. Man evolves as a totality.

The most difficult construct to comprehend in nursing's conceptual model appears to be that concerning the wholeness of man. When man is perceived, the parts, whether cells, organs, or systems; biological, physical, or psychological; disappear from view. The whole and the parts cannot be perceived simultaneously. The identity of man exists only in his wholeness. This wholeness is central and indispensable to nursing's conceptual model.

The life process is an evolutionary emergent. The capacity of life forms to transcend themselves is an expression of the advancing differentiation and complexity which characterizes both man and environment in their concomitant and interrelated evolution through space-time. The life process evolves along the curvature of space-time. Events along the continuum are unique. Events do not come again or repeat themselves. Similarity between events cannot be construed as repetition of events. Human behavior does not revert back to earlier stages—the path of life is unidirectional.

Sentience and thought arise out of life's complexifying, probabilistic goal-directedness. Consciousness is a facet of man's becoming and in its emergence reflects man's expanding awareness of the world about him. In the process of evolution, man's search for meaning takes on new dimensions and his capacity for understanding grows. Ontogenesis and phylogenesis evidence a lengthening of conscious awareness (the waking state) through time. Coming into awareness is postulated to represent new levels of complexity with correlates in the ongoing development of cognition and feelings. The capacity to experience one's self and the world and to make sense out of one's experiences is an emergent along life's longitudinal axis.

Human behavior is synergistic.* Behavioral manifestations of the life process are symphonic expressions of unity and cannot be dichotomized as objective or subjective, as internal or external, as mental or physical. They are unique to the whole and their identification in the real world provides evidence of consistency in the interrelatedness of ideas which form the structure of nursing's conceptual model.

The model of the life process in man basic to nursing's abstract system may be postulated to be represented by an energy field embedded in the four-dimensional space-time matrix and becoming increasingly complex as it evolves rhythmically along life's longitudinal axis. Pattern and organization are maintained amidst the constant change attending the continuous interaction between man and environment. Nursing's principles of homeodynamics, discussed in the next chapter, derive from this model.

Reference

1. Stulman, Julius, *Fields Within Fields Within Fields,* New York: The World Institute, Vol. 1, No. 1, Spring 1968, p. 7.

---

*Synergy is defined as the unique behavior of whole systems, unpredicted by any behaviors of their component functions taken separately.

CHAPTER 38

Homeodynamics: Principles of Nursing Science

Martha E. Rogers

. . . the existence of harmonies which foreshadow an indeterminate range of future discoveries.

—Michael Polanyi

Descriptive, explanatory, and predictive principles give substance to nursing's conceptual system and make possible knowledgeable nursing practice. Principles derive from the imaginative synthesis of available data. General patterns and regularities characterizing the phenomenon under study are identified and provide a means for systematically anticipating future events.

Principles are stated as hypothetical generalizations and theories. They are provisional. The degree to which a principle approximates reality increases as confirmation grows and greater precision is attained. Supplementation and modification of a principle may become necessary in order to encompass exceptions and to more faithfully represent the real world. To the extent that a principle possesses universality, its potential for usefulness increases.

Formulation of a principle opens the way to a range of investigations of conditions under which a particular principle holds. As evidence of the validity and reliability of a principle accumulates, its value as an empirical tool is enhanced. Commonalities between events come into view. The significance of a principle may take on new dimensions of meaning beyond those envisioned by the formulator of the principle. Principles are symbolic. They are representations of the real world and must be tested against actuality to verify their correctness.

The formulation of scientific principles basic to nursing derives from the conceptual model discussed in Chapter 12. Facts and ideas are synthesized to present a coherent pattern consistent with the known world. Unifying princi-

Rogers, M. E. (1970). Homeodynamics: Principles of nursing science. In M. E. Rogers, *An introduction to the theoretical basis of nursing* (pp. 95–102). Philadelphia: Davis. Reprinted with permission.

ples are proposed and are stated as hypothetical generalizations about the life process in man.

The life process is homeodynamic. An energy field, the fundamental unit of the living system, portrays the dynamic nature of life and is basic to the derivation of nursing science principles. The principles of homeodynamics enunciated and discussed in this chapter are four in number, namely: principle of *reciprocy,* principle of *synchrony,* principle of *helicy,* and principle of *resonancy.* These principles postulate the way the life process is and predict the nature of its evolving. These are broad generalizations which are deemed to conform to experiential data and to lay a foundation for developing testable hypotheses potentially fruitful in furthering nursing's understanding of the life process in man.

The theoretical basis of nursing is expressed in its guiding principles. Thus, the establishment of connections between events is made possible and technological application is permitted. Further occurrences are subject to prediction, and intervention directed toward achieving specified changes becomes practicable.

Fundamental principles are properly characterized by generality and precision. Description, couched in everyday language, may serve in the early stages of development of a science. However, explanatory and predictive effectiveness requires the evolving of a language of specificity with potential for symbolic and mathematical representations. Definitions take on increasing clarity and exactness.

A principle is a theoretical formulation. Facts, like pieces of a jigsaw puzzle, fall into place and achieve meaning within the framework of theory. Nursing's principles of homeodynamics provide a way for describing, explaining, and predicting a wide range of events having direct relevance for the professional practice of nursing. Let us proceed to a discussion of these principles.

Principle of Reciprocy

The principle of reciprocy is predicated upon the basic assumptions of wholeness and openness and the dynamic nature of the universe. The life process in man is deemed to be characterized by an energy field which then may be specifically identified as the human field. The environment is defined as all that which is external to a given human field and is thus stated to be the environmental field. The human field and the environmental field are continuously interacting with one another.

The relationship between the human field and the environmental field is one of constant mutual interaction and mutual change. The mutuality of the man-environment interaction process specifies that man and environment are to be perceived simultaneously. These are reciprocal systems in which molding and being molded are taking place in both systems at the same time. The concept embodied in this principle is contrary to an older view of man adapting to multiple environmental forces. Rather, it is the man-environment interaction process that portends the future, not the flexibility of man in adjusting to environmental changes. The human field and the environmental field are continuously repatterned. With each repatterning, subsequent interaction is revised and new patterning in both man and environment emerges.

This principle provides a basis for explaining the creativity of life. It furnishes a conceptual approach to understanding why all persons exposed to a given disease do not become ill. Unanticipated outcomes associated with extensive use of D.D.T., the unpredicted reversal in purportedly diminishing tuberculosis and venereal disease rates, and emergence of the "battered child syndrome" become less surprising when viewed from the perspective of reciprocy.

The principle of reciprocy postulates the inseparability of man and environment and predicts that sequential changes in the life process are continuous, probabilistic revisions occurring out of the interactions between man and environment.

This principle may be stated in symbolic form thus:

$$R = f\,(M_1 \rightleftarrows E_1)$$

in which R stands for Reciprocy
M stands for the human field
E stands for the environmental field

and can be read as "Reciprocy is a function of the mutual interaction between the human field and the environmental field."

Principle of Synchrony

The principle of synchrony may be stated as follows: Change in the human field depends only upon the state of the human field and the simultaneous state of the environmental field at any given point in space-time.

The life process evolves unidirectionally along the space-time continuum and is bound in the four-dimensional space-time matrix. Space-time binding enunciates the contemporaneous nature of changes taking place between man and environment. The life process is a becoming. Developmental events along life's axis express the growing complexity of pattern and organization evolving out of multiple previous man-environment interactions. Each repatterning is a revision of the immediately preceding pattern. At each point in space-time, man is what he has been becoming but he is not what he has been. Moreover, he cannot go back to what he has been. Life proceeds unidirectionally and is inextricably bound within the space-time dimension.

Numerous and varied events attend the process of human development and are incorporated into ongoing developmental patterning and repatterning. Earlier developmental patterns are replaced by later ones. The particular pattern that identifies the human field at any given point in space-time is unique. The same is true for the environmental field. It is out of the simultaneous interaction between these two patterns that change occurs.

This principle neither denies nor ignores the reality of past events. The life process is a constantly evolving series of changes in which the past has been incorporated and out of which new patterns have emerged. This principle does place the past in a context of nonrepeatability and postulates that the determinants of change are only what man is at any given moment coupled with the state of the environment at the same moment.

This principle is in contradiction to an all-too-common practice of interpreting various behavioral manifestations in adults as equivalent to developmental behaviors occurring in an earlier developmental stage. Under this latter view, adults may be subjected to handling deemed appropriate to an earlier period, to the detriment of the individual.

Pattern and organization are basic to this principle. It is pattern which is revised in the man-environment interaction. Pattern and organization take on greater complexity as life evolves. Change reflects this dynamic repatterning and growing complexity.

This principle predicts that change in human behavior will be determined by the simultaneous interaction of the actual state of the human field and the actual state of the environmental field at any given point in space-time. Probable outcomes of this interaction encompass a range of possibilities some of which may be deemed more likely than others. Predictions of probable outcomes take on greater accuracy as means for determining and specifying states of the human and environmental fields achieve greater precision and as relationships between these states and subsequent events are established.

This principle may be stated in symbolic form thus:

$$S = f\ S\text{-}T_1\ (M_1 \rightleftarrows E_1)$$

in which S stands for Synchrony
S-T stands for space-time

and can be read as: "Synchrony is a function of the state of the human field at a specified point in space-time interacting with the environmental field at the same specified point in space-time."

Principle of Helicy

The principle of helicy subsumes within it the principles of reciprocy and synchrony, and postulates further explanatory and predictive dimensions of nursing's theoretical system. The principle of helicy connotes that the life process evolves unidirectionally in sequential stages along a curve which has the same general shape all along but which does not lie in a plane. Encompassed within this principle are the concepts of rhythmicality, negentropic evolutionary emergence, and the unitary nature of the man-environment relationship.

The life process is characterized by probabilistic goal-directedness. Though the specific goal may not be known, increasing complexity of pattern and organization is a constant attendant of the developmental process. Man-environment interactions are directed toward achieving new dimensions of complexity. They are *not* directed toward achieving homeostasis or equilibrium (stable or unstable). The life process is continuously innovative and requires, for its understanding, a concept of man evolving.

Rhythmicalities portend probabilistic predictions. Life evolves along a spiralling longitudinal axis bound in the curvature of space-time. With each turn of the spiral along the axis, similarities appear. Spirals along the axis are further embedded within the spiralling of the axis itself [Figure 1]. Rhythmic phenomena are expressions of the reciprocal relationship between man and environment. The rhythms of life are inextricably woven into the rhythms of the universe. Man and environment constitute a unitary whole.

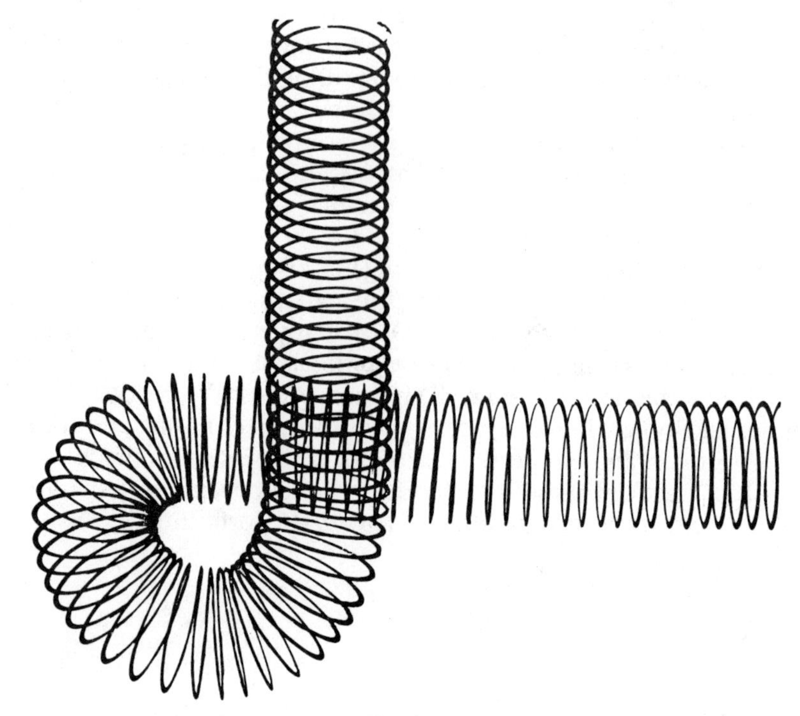

Figure 1.

The principle of helicy postulates an ordering of man's evolutionary emergence. The rise of cognition and feelings is encompassed. Predictive potential exists for a wide range of events in the real world. Cyclical similarities can be identified and probabilities determined. Earthbound man's advent into outer space and the bringing of extrasensory perception and other paranormal phenomena within the purview of recognized scientific endeavor are logical expressions of this principle.

This principle may be stated in symbolic form thus:

$$H = f\ S\text{-}T_1\ (M_1 \rightleftarrows E_1)\ \underset{\rightsquigarrow}{i}\ f\ S\text{-}T_2\ (M_2 \rightleftarrows E_2)\ \underset{\rightsquigarrow}{i} \text{—} f\ S\text{-}T_n\ (M_n \rightleftarrows E_n)$$

in which H stands for Helicy
$\rightsquigarrow$ stands for the spiral of life
i stands for innovation

and can be read as: "Helicy is a function of continuous innovative change growing out of the mutual interaction of man and environment along a spiralling longitudinal axis bound in space-time."

Principle of Resonancy

The principle of resonancy postulates that change in pattern and organization of the human field and the environmental field is propagated by waves. The life process in man is a symphony of rhythmical vibrations oscillating at various frequencies. Between man and environment there is a rhythmic flow of energy waves. An ordered arrangement of rhythms characterizes both the human field and the environmental field and undergoes continuous dynamic metamorphosis in the man-environment interaction process.

Man experiences his environment as a resonating wave of complex symmetry uniting him with the rest of the world. The life process may be likened to cadences—sometimes harmonic, sometimes cacophonous, sometimes dissonant; rising and falling; now fast, now slow—ever changing in a universal orchestration of dynamic wave patterns.

A multiplicity of waves characterizes the universe. Light waves, sound waves, thermal waves, atomic waves, gravity waves flow in rhythmic patterns—largely unseen, unheard, and unopen to man's capacity to see, hear, or perceive. The colorful auras of radiation waves surrounding radiating bodies are generally beyond the visible range of the human eye. These, and other waves, are integral facets of nature's rhythms.

The pattern of the human field is a wave phenomenon encompassing man in his entirety. The whole of man senses, feels, perceives, and reasons. Literary works speak of man swept by waves of grief or joy, loneliness, tenderness, and pain. The sick may "ache all over."

The resonance of change is a continuously propagating series of waves between man and environment, characterized by invariance under transformation. The predictive potentials of this principle arise out of a perception of the life process as an unending flow of wave patterns. The developmental process in growth of the individual is a good example of this principle.

Principles of Homeodynamics

The principles of homeodynamics postulate a way of perceiving unitary man. Changes in the life process in man are predicted to be inseparable from environmental changes and to reflect the mutual and simultaneous interaction between the two at any given point in space-time. Changes are irreversible, nonrepeatable. They are rhythmical in nature and evidence growing complexity of pattern and organization. Change proceeds by the continuous repatterning of both man and environment by resonating waves.

Evidence of conditions under which these principles hold arises out of examination of the real world. Investigations of a range of phenomena are necessary to provide the substantive data which can further the translation of these principles into practical application. Scientific research in nursing is beginning to underwrite the moving boundaries of nursing advances. Maintenance and promotion of health, disease prevention, diagnosis, intervention, and rehabilitation—nursing's goals—take on added dimensions as theoretical knowledge provides new direction to practice.

CHAPTER 39

The Theoretical Basis of Nursing

Martha E. Rogers

The theoretical base of nursing is an emergent—a new product. The inevitability of its unfolding is written in nursing's long commitment to human health and welfare. A hastening of developmental creativity, evident on all sides, insures nursing's quickening transition from pre-science to science. Concern for the human predicament is explicit in nursing's critical struggle "to know" that "people may benefit."

As new worldviews strain to emerge from the chrysalis of time-hardened traditions, probabilities for better achieving human health and welfare increase. Man's advent into outer space marks an era of accerelating evolution perhaps unequaled in the history of this planet. Science and technology, social complexification, and growing awareness of man's interrelatedness with nature, testify to a negentropic universe of escalating innovation and diversity. Humanitarian advocates vie with machine disciples while the horizon pimples with evolutionary emergents full of surprises for the future.

For many years nursing has been accumulating facts, observations, and ideas—building blocks for new ways of trying to understand man. The seeds for serious conceptual development, long dormant in the absence of an organized conceptual system, are now taking root in the fertile soil of a science of synergistic man—the phenomenon central to nursing's purpose. The science of nursing is identified by an organized conceptual system out of which to derive testable hypotheses and within which to lodge the findings of nursing research.

Nursing is humanitarian science which has as its central focus synergistic man—unitary man. The science of nursing is a science of man. Nursing's descriptive, explanatory, and predictive principles add new dimensions to the nature and direction of health services. Knowledgeable intervention is begin-

Rogers, M. E. (1971, March). *The theoretical basis of nursing.* Paper presented at the University of Illinois School of Nursing, Chicago, IL.

ning to replace experiential naiveté as nursing seeks to maintain and promote health, and care for and rehabilitate the sick and disabled.

Nursing's concern with man as a single, coherent, integrated system whose behavior cannot be predicted by the behavior of any of his component parts taken separately provides a foundation for theorizing a conceptual framework of high practical value. Synergistic man is more than and different from the sum of his parts. Nurses have long verbalized a generalized concern for "total" man expressed in the semantic ambiguity of "comprehensive care" which might be translated as a summation of acts dealing with various particulars of man if one had the time, and one's feet held out.

But unitary man is an entity in himself. He cannot be explained as an aggregate of cells, organs, and systems nor is he a summation of biological, physical, social, and psychological attributes.

The most detailed knowledge of hydrogen and oxygen does not describe water nor do the characteristics of sodium and chlorine predict the nature of harmless table salt. Neither does knowledge of psychology, biology, physics, et cetera provide a description of "MAN." Apparent similarities between human behavior and behaviors categorized as psychological, physiological, and social are as fallacious as would be a proposal that molecular or atomic behavior correctly described psychological or biological behavior. The characteristics of man are those of the whole and cannot be predicted from the characteristics of the parts.

An energy field has replaced the cell as the fundamental unit of living systems. Pattern and organization identify the field and give unity to a conceptual model of whole man. The human field comes into view only as the parts disappear. The field and the parts of the field cannot be seen simultaneously. When one perceives man, one cannot perceive psychological, or biological, or physical, or social phenomena (or systems, organs, and cells).

The human field is characterized by openness, unidirectionality, pattern and organization, sentience and thought. Man lives in a universe of open systems of which he is one. Mutual, simultaneous interaction between man and environment speaks to their complementary relationship in contradiction to a long-established and still pervasive dichotomous view made explicit by present-day fear mongerers who deal in the fallacies of adaptation, ecological negativism, and disease-oriented commitments to causation, whether single or multiple. The dire portenders of a dubious future are still caught in the demonstrable obsolescence of such concepts as homeostasis, adaptation, and steady-state.

A static view of man is implicit in the antiquated though nonetheless cherished concepts of homeostasis and equilibrium—dynamic or otherwise. These views are deeply rooted in an entropic view of the universe despite evidence of the negentropic nature of life and nonlife. They are coupled with a perception of man victimized by environmental and cosmic forces: clearly a dichotomous and false view of man and environment. Man continues to think he can perhaps control the environment, whereas at most he only rearranges it. In contradiction to this belief he expresses his submission to the environment by stating man must adapt to environmental vagaries whether of his own or nature's making. Man does *not* adapt. Man and environment evolve together.

Having misread the fourth dimension as spacialization of time rather than dynamization of space, man commonly fails to perceive the innovative and probabilistic imperatives inherent in the man/environment relationship. Static space is deemed to have slits through which man peers in sequential moments of linear time—except of course in the mobility afforded by the time machines of science fiction. Creative evolution on the other hand bespeaks dynamic space-time; continuous change. Nor is space-time to be perceived as linear.

Man is a multidimensional energy field whose boundaries extend beyond his visible mass. The human field occupies space-time, including the past and future as well as other dimensions. The human field varies continuously in density, intensity, and in size. Theoretically an energy field extends to infinity. Man and environment are contiguous, and together equal the universe. The life process evolves in rhythmic concert with a multidimensional environment. Change is omnipresent and continuous, nonrepeating and increasingly diverse. Life is transcendence. It does not seek some balance. The pleasure principle is out.

Human beings, the raison d'etre of nursing, are continuously manifesting new ways of behaving and new ways of becoming, whether they be deemed sick or well.

Broad principles and a range of knowledges must be constantly pulled together in novel ways in order to implement nursing's evaluative, habilitative, and rehabilitative services to people.

The study of unitary, or whole man if you like, is a necessary prelude to understanding and intervening in the multiple events which take place along the continuum of life. Normal and pathological processes must be treated with complete equality—the multiplicity of events that may take place along life's varied course. The unidirectional, innovative process is probabilistic and irreversible. Categorical diseases, so-called pathological states, and particulate phenomena are dangerously misleading bases for determining the health status of either individuals or populations. The intrusion of value systems into the evaluative process is a further source of distortion—all potentials for diminishing human safety.

Pattern and organization identify the human field and the environmental field. Indices of human functioning reflect the totality of the field. The patterning of indices (both human and environmental) provides descriptive data for potentially productive nursing intervention. The specific nature of the intervention will be individualized and creative thought rooted in probabilistic generalities.

Nursing is service to people, not to disease entities, to a range of pathological conditions, or to psychological aberrations. Moreover, the first line of defense in building a healthy society lies in maintenance and promotion of health, areas of concern initiated by nursing and integral to nursing's purposes. Nor should maintenance and promotion of health be confused with prevention of disease. Prevention of disease is a negative concept, demonstrably impossible of achievement (and fortunately so because if it were possible the magnificence of universal evolution would be denied). Resolution of health problems is directly related to the dynamic innovative potentialities of life to transcend itself.

Nursing's conceptual model provides the frame of reference from which the principles of homeodynamics are derived. The principles of homeodynamics provide a way of perceiving man and his environment. They predict the nature and direction of human development and underlie knowledgeable nursing practice. The principles of reciprocy, synchrony, and resonancy are subsumed within and extended in the principle of helicy. The fourth principle of homeodynamics, the principle of helicy, postulates the innovative, unidirectional evolution of life rhythmically along a spiral in mutual, simultaneous interaction with the environment. Human and environmental fields are multidimensional, contiguous with one another, and coextensive with the universe.

In this view the aging process is one of growing complexity, heterogeneity, and diversity. Traditional indices of aging lose their validity and new criteria for judging the aging process must be used. As life progresses, the human field takes on new dimensions of complexity, little recognized as forerunners of the transformation of energy inherent in the life-death cycle. The commonly perceived running down in aging is an artifact, the result of our own limited vision and particle views. Perceptions of the aged change. Nursing intervention becomes a positive process directed toward enabling the aged to achieve their own probabilistic goals as whole human beings sans obeisance to the sterility of human insults and physical routines currently practiced. Death is deemed a transformation of energy.

A theory of accelerated evolution derives from nursing's conceptual system. A lengthening of the waking state, a half century of vastly accelerated motion, radiation increments, major and rapid atmospheric changes, man's advent into outer space, and mixing of the planet's gene pools on a heretofore unheard of scale, among a multiplicity of other factors, combine to support such a proposal. Man's emergence from the sleeping state to lengthening awareness is evidenced both phylogenetically and ontogenetically. A swiftening [sic] of change in the sleep:wake ratio marks the space age.

The already dynamic system we know as man is being subjected to increased environmental motion in rapidly escalating amounts. From horse to train, to car to plane, to jet to supersonic transport, and to rocket—with the last but a clumsy precursor of the future's electrical field propulsion systems—further innovation proceeds. And soon there will be the space station shuttles. Nursing research directed toward investigating the relationship between added environmental motion and human development among premature infants, full-term newborns, 3- to 4-month-old infants, and 11- to 12-month-old infants provides consistent and significant evidence in support of a speeding up of development. A pilot study of adults has laid the groundwork for a full-scale investigation of this population, and a study of preschoolers is getting under way. The rocking cradle, the rocking bed, and the rocking chair should be added to nursing's armamentarium for intervention.

A theory of accelerated evolution postulates a range of questions concerning real world phenomena. Might one propose that the population explosion is nature's way of providing an adequate pool from which will come progenitors of an unknown future? Paranormal phenomena are not only a reality but in today's world they have become scientifically respectable. For many centuries man has deemed the five senses of seeing, hearing, tasting, smelling, and touching to be the avenues by which man learned to know his world. Is it not reasonable to postulate that so-called paranormal events constitute manifestations of an evolutionary emergent—a sixth sense destined to become a commonplace in life's near tomorrow? The threads are weaving into a rope.

With probabilistic certainty one may predict there will be many tendrils of distortion as the evolutionary rope is twined. Life forms transcend themselves. Universal rhythms are revised. Why is it that cancer cells fail to evidence rhythmic behavior? Might one propose that efforts to restore traditional rhythms to cancer cells are misdirected and futile? Can it be that cancer is a distortion of evolutionary emergence—one of life's many probings for new rhythms not yet determined? Can new directions in human field repatterning based on nursing's conceptual system lead to more credible intervention for synergistic man?

The gravitational "constant" is now noted to be "not constant." The universe is expanding. This planet is expanding in measurable increments. Volcanoes and earthquakes reflect more than chemical reactions. The shifting of the earth's land masses most recently explicit in the California quake are more than rearrangement. Density seems to be diminishing! Might one speculate a comparable phenomenon in living systems? Is a lessening of human field density a correlate of paranormal phenomena, of man's forward thrust into a new dimension of the universe–outer space?

The science of nursing is an optimistic science. A negentropic universe bespeaks a future of unequaled promise. The travails of the present—and there are many—must be re-examined in the light of life's and the environment's progressive development. Man's search for meaning brings new values and new visions. Universal dimensions beyond man's present comprehension lurk in the shadows and beckon the imaginative.

But not all is speculation. The knowledges nursing possesses, though in critical need for expansion, elaboration, alteration, and revision through theoretical research in nursing, are of high social significance. The way in which we perceive man and his world is the reality within which we act. Nursing's hypothetical generalizations and unifying principles are the guidelines of professional practice. Human service is nursing's goal. An organized body of theoretical knowledge arrived at by scientific research and logical analysis is indispensable to even minimally safe nursing services in today's rapidly changing milieu. Moreover, the knowledge nurses bring to bear upon the job to be done must be the best available. Nursing cannot afford to be guided by obsolete concepts.

CHAPTER 40

Nursing: A Science of Unitary Man

Martha E. Rogers

The explication of an organized body of abstract knowledge specific to nursing is indispensable to nursing's transition from pre-science to science. The need for such a body of knowledge can be identified in an escalation of science and technology coordinate with public demands for health services of a nature and in an amount scarcely envisioned by either the askers or the providers.

Traditionally nursing's goals have encompassed both the sick and the well, and the consideration of environmental factors has also been integral to nursing's efforts. Education and practice in nursing have been without interruption, directed toward maintenance and promotion of health, prevention of illness, and care and rehabilitation of the sick and disabled. Recognition that people are more than and different from their parts has characterized nursing from the time of Florence Nightingale to the present.

Nursing as a learned profession is both a science and an art. A science may be defined as an organized body of abstract knowledge arrived at by scientific research and logical analysis. The art of nursing is the utilization of the science of nursing for human betterment, and its fulfillment is a lifetime endeavor. Historically the term *nursing* has been used as a verb signifying "to do." Perceived as a science the term *nursing* becomes a noun signifying "to know." The education of nurses requires the transmission of nursing's body of theoretical knowledge. The practice of nursing is the use of this body of knowledge in service to people. Research in nursing is the study of the phenomenon central to nursing's concern.

The uniqueness of nursing, like that of other sciences, lies in the phenomenon by which nursing's focus is identified. The focus of the science of nursing, unitary man, is a logical outgrowth of nurses' long established pre-

---

Rogers, M. E. (1980). Nursing: A science of unitary man. In J. P. Riehl & C. Roy (Eds.), *Conceptual models for nursing practice* (2nd ed.) (pp. 329–331). New York: Appleton-Century-Crofts. Reprinted with permission.

scientific interest in people. Moreover in a universe of open systems (to be discussed later in this chapter) consideration of the environment must be deemed integral with the study of unitary man. Specifically then, the science of nursing seeks to study the nature and direction of unitary human development integral with the environment and to evolve the descriptive, explanatory, and predictive principles basic to knowledgeable practice in nursing. No other science or learned professional field deals with unitary man as a synergistic phenomenon whose behaviors cannot be predicted by knowledge of the parts.

A conceptual system constitutes the substantive base of a science of nursing. Such a system is arrived at by the creative synthesis of facts and ideas and is an emergent—a new product. Theories derive from the conceptual system and are tested in the real world. The findings of research are fed back into the system, and the system undergoes continuous alteration, revision, and change commensurate with the new knowledge. A science is open-ended. The elaboration of a science emerges out of scholarly research.

Developing a Conceptual System for Unitary Man and Environment

Four building blocks are essential in the development of the conceptual system presented in this paper, (1) energy fields, (2) universe of open systems, (3) pattern and organization, and (4) four dimensionality. A brief discussion of each of these areas follows.

Energy Fields

Energy fields have been noted in the literature for several decades as constituting the fundamental unit of both the living and the non-living. *Field* is a unifying concept. Energy signifies the dynamic nature of the field. Energy fields extend to infinity. They have no real boundaries. However for purposes of study of a given phenomenon one may specify imaginary boundaries according to arbitrary criteria. This conceptual system is concerned with two energy fields: (1) the human field and (2) the environmental field. More specifically, man and environment *are* energy fields. They *do not have* energy fields. A field has meaning only in its entirety. It is indivisible. The unitary human field is not a biologic field or a physical field or a social field or a psychologic field, each of which deal [sic] with only a part of unitary man. The human field is more than and different from the sum of its parts. Unitary man cannot be understood by knowledge of his parts anymore than ordinary table salt can be predicted by a knowledge of sodium and chlorine. Unitary man has his own integrity. One cannot generalize from parts to a whole. The characteristics and behaviors of unitary man are specific to unitary man. The science of unitary man is a new product. Moreover the phrase *matter and energy* is redundant. Matter is energy manifesting itself in dynamic wave patterns. An energy field is the fundamental unit of unitary man and of environment.

Openness

Energy fields extend to infinity. Consequently they are open—not a little bit open, not sometimes open, but continuously open. The long-established view of the universe as an entropic, closed system is rapidly losing ground. Proposals that living systems were open systems led Von Bertalanffy to postulate that living systems manifested negative entropy. Evidence has continued to accumulate in support of a universe of open systems. The closed-system model of the universe is contradicted and obsolescence of such concepts as steady-state, adaptation, equilibrium and the like is made explicit.

Pattern and Organization

Pattern and organization identify an energy field. These are continuously changing. Moreover in a universe of open systems change is always creative and innovative. Human and environmental fields are continuously characterized by wave pattern and organization but the nature of the pattern and organization is always novel, always emerging, always more diverse.

Four-Dimensionality

The human and environmental fields are postulated to be four-dimensional. When Einstein proposed that the three coordinates of space and the coordinate of time be synthesized to arrive at a new dimension—the fourth—and postulated the theory of relativity, the universe took on an entirely new look. Newtonian absolutism was contradicted. The concept of four-dimensionality postulated a world of neither space nor time. Unfortunately words are as yet inadequate to communicate the scope and depth of this concept. A useful analogy of this difficulty can be found in Edwin A. Abbott's book titled *Flatland* (1952). This four-dimensionality is not a spatial dimension nor is it to be confused with fourth dimensions being proposed by other disciplines such as mathematics and psychology. A four-dimensional world is clearly different from a three-dimensional world. Efforts to schematize four-dimensionality require substantial abstract thinking. In spite of the risk of oversimplification and potential error the following sketch [Figure 1] may be useful. Imagine unitary man as a four-dimensional energy field embedded in a four-dimensional environmental field.

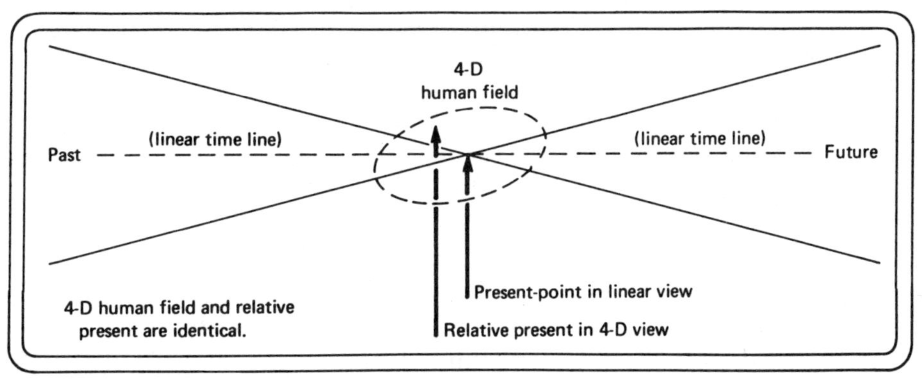

Figure 1.

The four-dimensional human field is characterized by continuously fluctuating imaginary boundaries. The present as a point in time is not relevant to a 4-D model. Rather the four-dimensional human field is the 'relative present' for any individual. Some implications for the explanation of paranormal events come into view. Four-dimensional reality is perceived as a synthesis of nonlinear coordinates from which innovative change continuously and evolutionally emerges.

The building blocks presented above are integral to the imaginative synthesis out of which a conceptual system emerges. Definitions of unitary man and environment give specificity to the conceptual system and are stated as follows:

Unitary Man: a four-dimensional, negentropic energy field identified by pattern and organization and manifesting characteristics and behaviors that are different from those of the parts and which cannot be predicted from knowledge of the parts.

Environment: a four-dimensional, negentropic energy field identified by pattern and organization and encompassing all that outside any given human field.

Each human field is unique, and so too is each person's environmental field. The human field and its environment field are coextensive with the universe. Unitary man and environment are integral with one another. Further, this system is postulated to be a humanistic model and not a mechanistic one. Human behavior manifests reason and feelings. Further it is postulated that man has the capacity to participate knowingly and probabilistically in the process of change.

Principles of Homeodynamics

Principles and theories derive from the organized conceptual system. First to be discussed are the principles of homeodynamics. These are broad generalizations that postulate the nature and direction of unitary human development. They are stated as follows:

Principle of helicy: The nature and direction of human and environmental change is continuously innovative, probabilistic, and characterized by increasing diversity of human field and environmental field pattern and organization emerging out of the continuous, mutual, simultaneous interaction between the human and environmental fields and manifesting non-repeating rhythmicities.

Principle of resonancy: The human field and the environmental field are identified by wave pattern and organization manifesting continuous change from lower-frequency, longer wave patterns to higher-frequency, shorter wave patterns.

Principle of complementarity: The interaction between human and environmental fields is continuous, mutual, simultaneous.

These principles have validity only within the context of this conceptual system of unitary man. Their meaning has specificity within their definitions and provides for unambiguous communication. The principle of complementarity is in actuality subsumed within the principle of helicy. However for purposes of clarity as well as to emphasize the significance of mutual simultaneity and its contradiction of highly cherished "causality," it seems important to identify it specifically.

Reality "is" according to one's perception of it. How one perceives it depends on the conceptual model one holds of the world. What we see, how they see it, and the questions they ask differ according to their conceptual models. Within the context of this conceptual system, then, unitary man and his environment are in continuous, mutual, simultaneous interaction, evolving toward increased differentiation and diversity of field pattern and organization. Change is always innovative. There is no going back, no repetition. Causality is contradicted. Living and Dying are developmental processes. This is an optimistic science but not a utopian one.

The illusion of causality is one that many persons, including scientists, have great difficulty relinquishing. J. T. Fraser (1975) notes that "since Aristotle, Western thought has held causality and its corollary, lawfulness, almost sacrosanct." Heisenberg's principle of uncertainty, Plancks' quantum theory, and Einstein's relativity, introduced early in this century shook the physical world. Later Bertrand Russell (1953) pointed out, "The reason physics has ceased to look for causes is that, in fact, there are no such things. The law of causality is a relic of a bygone age, surviving, like the monarchy, only because it is erroneously supposed to do no harm." The appearance of causality is an illusion, a mirage. History tells us of persons burned at the stake for declaring the earth revolved around the sun. Michael Polanyi's (1958) comment that "almost every major systematic error which has deluded men for thousands of years relied on practical experience" is worthy of note. The appearance of causality does not make it so. In a universe of open systems mutual simultaneity is explicit.

Theories deriving from the conceptual system provide a means of describing, explaining, and predicting . . . unitary man. Only a few such theories will be presented in this paper. Their implications for better understanding unitary man and for determining the nature and direction of nursing intervention will be discussed briefly.

Theory of Accelerating Evolution

Change is postulated to proceed in the direction of higher wave frequency field pattern and of organization characterized by growing diversity. Higher frequencies portend acceleration. Multiple references of the past decade or so, including the best seller *Future Shock* by Alvin Toffler, testify to a speeding up of change. Simple forms change less rapidly than complex ones. Developmental norms of 30 to 40 years are no longer valid. People are sleeping less and living longer. The nature of motion common in today's world changes and its speed increases by leaps and bounds. SSTs and rockets to the moon are only a beginning. The Rand Corporation is currently developing a very high speed transit "tubecraft" that will whisk people across the country by electromagnetic waves at approximately 14,000 miles per hour. Travel time from New York City to Los Angeles is expected to be 21 minutes. Homes are filled with electrical equipment. Increasingly higher frequency waves are identified in atmospheric changes and radiation increments as well as in the practicalities of ultraviolet rays and ultrasonics. Man and environment evolve and change together. The doom sayers who propose that man is destroying himself are in quicksand. On the contrary there is a population explosion, increased longevity, escalating levels of science and technology and multiple other evidences of man's development potentials in the process of actualization.

One would anticipate that new norms might very probably include higher blood pressure readings and increasingly active children. *Normal* means average and average means a majority of the population. What is "normal" for one person need not be "normal" for another. What was normal 40 years ago would not be normal today. Large numbers of the public at every age are, today, reported to manifest blood pressure readings higher than the norms established some years back. Blood pressure is itself a rhythmical phenomenon. Accelerating change characterized by higher wave frequency field pattern and organization might be expected to manifest itself in new norms for blood pressure readings plus a wider range of distribution of differences among individuals. Similarly one might anticipate a speeding up of evolutionary development currently noted in the large number of children who are being labeled hyperactive.

Explaining Paranormal Events

Consider the point made earlier that "human field" and "relative present" are identical. Moreover what is a relative present for one person is different from that for someone else. Examine the implications for explaining precognition, deja vu [sic], clairvoyance and the like. Clairvoyance, for example, is rational in a four-dimensional human field in continuous mutual, simultaneous interaction with a four-dimensional environmental field. So too are such events as psychometry, therapeutic touch, telepathy, and a wide range of other phenomena. Within this conceptual system such behaviors become "normal" rather than "paranormal."

Rhythmical Correlates of Change

Human field rhythms are not to be confused with biologic rhythms or psychologic rhythms or similar particulate phenomena. Human field rhythms are manifestations of the whole. Sleep/wake patterns when perceived as field behaviors point up both developmental emergence from sleeping to waking and signify evolutionary potentials of "beyond waking." Not only is there substantial evidence that man is sleeping less today (at all age levels) but that the sleep/wake pattern has changed.

In many studies in a range of disciplines increased physical motion has been noted to be associated with biologic, physical, and psychosocial development. But what about human field motion? Are the pragmatics of "taking a slow boat to China" or of comments such as "my motor is running too fast" (or too slow) or "stop the world I want to get off" suggestive of changing patterns of human field motion? What about the "multi-stimuli" classrooms in which many children seem to prosper? Validation of postulated indices of human field motion and developmental evolution is being sought in investigations currently in progress in the Division of Nursing at New York University.

When perceived as rhythmical developmental processes, living and dying take on different meanings. Perception of time's passing is clearly different from time estimation. Evolution from the pragmatic to the visionary bespeaks the fulfillment of new potentials and growing diversity.

Implications for Practice

The implications of such theories for human services must be examined if the goals of a learned profession are to be met. There is nothing in this conceptual model that predicts man will be freed from all "disease" and live happily ever after. So-called disease and pathology are value terms applied when the human field manifests behaviors that may be deemed undesirable. Values are continuously changing. Errors are often introduced. New knowledge revises old views. A few examples of changes in nursing practice based on the science of unitary man are presented below.

The Aging Process

Aging is a process that is continuous from conception thru [sic] dying. *Aged* is a term used to identify persons generally according to some established arbitrary chronologic decision. In this conceptual system aging is a developmental process. Moreover aging is a continuously creative process directed toward growing diversity of field pattern and organization. It is not a running down. The aged need less sleep and the patterned frequencies of sleep/wake are more diverse. A liking for sharp tastes among the aged bespeaks rather than deteriorating taste buds more likely an appreciation of the complexities of a range of taste phenomena. Cognitive skills are reported to increase with aging. Color preferences change in the direction of higher wave frequencies. Aging is not a disease. New life-styles are being promulgated by the aged themselves. Nursing's role in maintaining and promoting the health of the aged requires major changes in attitudes and nursing practice.

Hypertension and Hyperactivity

These behaviors are properly viewed as manifestations of evolutionary emergence. The mass marketing of iatrogenesis needs to cease. Why are third-graders being taught to use sphygmomanometers? What is the significance of mushrooming numbers of sphygmomanometers in multiple shopping centers? What is the meaning of a society of drug takers (and I am not referring to illegal use of hard drugs)? What is the relationship between labels and hypochondriasis and other forms of behavior? Change is developmental. Diversity is to be valued. True, parents whose indoctrination and wave patterns proclaim they need 8 hours of sleep in every 24 hours may have difficulty with their healthy three-year-old who refuses to sleep more than 4 hours in each 24-hour period. A nurse must demonstrate imagination and ingenuity in helping such parents to accept the "normality" of their child and to design ways of enabling both parents and child to fulfill their different rhythmic patterns without either's being condemned. New relative norms with marked flexibility and open-endedness must be initiated. A positive attitude toward changing diversity is imperative.

The use of this conceptual system as a basis for description, explanation, and prediction is far-reaching. Broad principles to guide practice must replace rule-of-thumb. The unitary human being is different from the sum of his parts. Principles drawn from the biologic, physical, and psychosocial sciences, no matter how excellent they may be in their own respective fields, cannot be used to describe, explain, or predict about unitary man. Calling nursing science a science of unitary man signifies nursing's potential for fulfillment of its social responsibility in human service.

References

Abbot E A: Flatland. New York, Dover, 1952

Fraser J T: Of Time, Passion, and Knowledge. New York, Braziller, 1975, p 40

Polanyi M: Personal Knowledge. Chicago, The University of Chicago Press, 1958, p 183

Russell B: On the notion of cause, with applications to the free-will problem. In Feigl H, Brodbeck M (eds): Readings in the Philosophy of Science. New York, Appleton, 1953, p 387; cited in Kerlinger, Fred, Foundations of Behavioral Research. New York: Holt, Rinehart, and Winston, Inc. 1964

Toffler A: Future Shock. New York, Random House, 1970

CHAPTER 41

Science of Unitary Human Beings

Martha E. Rogers

Some years ago Elizabeth Kemble* pointed out that ". . . much has been written and said concerning the spirit, art, and science of nursing. No one will deny the importance of all three in the effective practice of nursing. But the noble spirit alone is not enough. The art of nursing falls short even with a fine spirit. It is only when nursing practice is based on a theoretically sound foundation that the spirit and art can come into full being." The theoretically sound foundation that gives identity to nursing as a science and an art requires an organized abstract system from which to derive unifying principles and hypothetical generalizations. Through basic and applied research, principles and theories are tested. New understandings emerge. New questions arise. Description, explanation, and prediction take on new meanings. A substantive body of knowledge specific to nursing takes form.

The uniqueness of nursing, like that of any other science, lies in the phenomenon central to its purpose. Nursing's long-established concern with human beings and their world is a natural forerunner of an organized abstract system encompassing people and their environments. The irreducible nature of individuals as energy fields, different from the sum of their parts and integral with their respective environmental fields, differentiates nursing from other sciences and identifies nursing's focus.

A Science of Unitary Human Beings basic to nursing requires a new world view and a conceptual system specific to nursing phenomena of concern. The development of a science portends the emergence of abstract concepts and a corresponding language of specificity. Scientific language evolves out of the general language. Terms specific to the system are defined for clarity and precision. Uniformity of usage provides for communication. Rigorous research can

Rogers, M. E. (1986). Science of unitary human beings. In V. M. Malinski (Ed.), *Explorations on Martha Rogers' science of unitary human beings* (pp. 3–8). Norwalk, CT: Appleton-Century-Crofts. Reprinted with permission.

*Former Dean of the University of North Carolina School of Nursing at Chapel Hill, N.C.

be pursued and replicated. All terms, except those defined specific to the system, are interpreted in their general language meaning.

When nursing is perceived as a science, the term *nursing* becomes a noun signifying a body of knowledge. The education of nurses has identity in the transmission of nursing's body of theoretical knowledge. The practice of nursing is the creative use of this knowledge for human betterment. Research in nursing is the study of unitary human beings integral with their environment.

Science is open-ended. Change is continuous. New knowledge brings new insights. The development of a Science of Unitary Human Beings is a never-ending process. The conceptual system first presented some years ago has gained in substance. Concomitantly, errors have undergone correction, definitions have been revised for greater clarity and accuracy, and updating of content is continuous. Basic theoretical research is essential for ongoing development of this field of study.

The development of a conceptual system is a process of creative synthesis of facts and ideas out of which a new product emerges. Principles and theories derive from the system and are tested in the real world. The findings of research are fed back into the system, whereby the system undergoes continuous alteration, revision, and change. A conceptual system exists only in its entirety. It bespeaks wholeness and unity. It provides a way of perceiving people and their world.

The conceptual system that underwrites a Science of Unitary Human Beings does not derive from one or more of the basic sciences. Neither does it come out of a vacuum. A multiplicity of knowledges from many sources flows in novel ways to create a kaleidoscope of potentialities. Fundamental concepts are identified. Significant terms are defined congruent with the evolving system. A humane and optimistic view of life's potentials grows as a new reality appears. People's capacity to participate knowingly in the process of change is postulated.

Unitary human beings are specified to be irreducible wholes. A whole cannot be understood when it is reduced to its particulars. The use of the term *unitary* human beings is not to be confused with current popular usage of the term *holistic,* generally signifying a summation of parts, whether few or many. The unitary nature of environment is equally irreducible. The concept of *field* provides a means of perceiving people and their respective environments as irreducible wholes.

Four concepts are postulated to be basic to the proposed system, namely: energy fields, openness, pattern, and four-dimensionality. These concepts are defined consistent with the general language and are given specificity according to the conceptual system under discussion.

Energy fields are postulated to constitute the fundamental unit of both the living and the non-living. *Field* is a unifying concept. *Energy* signifies the dynamic nature of the field. *Energy fields* are infinite. Two energy fields are identified: the human field and the environmental field. Specifically, human beings and environment are energy fields. They do not have them. Moreover, human and environmental fields are not biological fields or physical fields, or social or psychological fields. Neither are human and environmental fields a summation of biological, physical, social, and psychological fields. This is not a denial of other fields. Rather, it is to make clear that human and environmental fields have their own identity and are not to be confused with parts.

A universe of open systems has been gaining support for three-quarters of a century. With introduction of relativity, quantum theory, and probability, the prevailing absolutism, already shaken by evolutionary theory, received a critical blow. By the 1920s Selye was proposing adaptation, and by the 1930s Bertalanffy introduced the idea of negative entropy. Soon Cannon advanced the idea of homeostasis. Space exploration began in the 1950s, and by the 1960s some physiologists suggested replacing the term *homeostasis* with the term *homeokinesis.* As new knowledge escalated, the traditional meanings of *homeostasis, steady-state, adaptation,* and *equilibrium* were no longer tenable. The closed-system, entropic model of the universe began to be questioned.

In a universe of open systems, causality is not an option. Acausality had come in with quantum theory. Bertrand Russell, some years later, noted, "The law of causality . . . is a relic of a bygone age, surviving, like the monarchy, only because it is erroneously supposed to do no harm."[1] Energy fields are open—not a little bit or sometimes, but continuously. The human and environmental fields are integral with one another. Causality is invalid. Change is continuously innovative.

Pattern is defined as the distinguishing characteristic of an energy field perceived as a single wave. Pattern is an abstraction. It gives identity to the field. The nature of the pattern changes continuously. Each human field pattern is unique and is integral with its own unique environmental field pattern. The term "pattern" is used only to refer to an energy field. Manifestations of field pattern emerge out of the human and environmental field mutual process and will be discussed later in this chapter.

Four-dimensionality characterizes the human and environmental fields. It is defined as a nonlinear domain without spatial or temporal attributes. All reality is postulated to be four-dimensional. The relative nature of change becomes explicit. Four-dimensionality is postulated to be a given of this system. It is not something one moves into or becomes. It is a way of perceiving human beings and their world.

Definitions increase in clarity and specificity as the conceptual system emerges. The unitary human being (human field) is defined as an irreducible, four-dimensional energy field identified by pattern and manifesting characteristics that are different from those of the parts and cannot be predicted from knowledge of the parts. The environmental field is defined as an irreducible, four-dimensional energy field identified by pattern and manifesting characteristics different from those of the parts. Each environmental field is specific to its given human field. Both change continuously, mutually, and creatively. The human and environmental fields are infinite and integral with one another.

Unifying principles and hypothetical generalizations derive from the conceptual system. The Principles of Homeodynamics are three in number and together postulate the nature and direction of change. These principles are set forth as follows:

Principles of Homeodynamics	
Principle of Resonancy	The continuous change from lower to higher frequency wave patterns in human and environmental fields.
Principle of Helicy	The continuous, innovative, probabilistic increasing diversity of human and environmental field patterns characterized by nonrepeating rhythmicities.
Principle of Integrality*	The continuous mutual human field and environmental field process.

*Formerly titled Principle of Complementarity.

Pattern is a key concept in these principles. The principles are stated so that they are mutually exclusive, to avoid the confusion that attended earlier definitions. The term *integrality* has replaced *complementarity* to gain greater accuracy and clarity of meaning.

Pattern was noted earlier to be an abstraction. Manifestations of field patterning are observable events in the real world. They are postulated to emerge out of the human-environmental field mutual process. Change is continuous, relative, and innovative. Increasing diversity of field patterning characterizes the process of change. Individual differences point up the significance of relative diversity. For example, changing rhythmicities possess individual uniqueness. Transition from longer sleeping to longer waking to beyond waking is highly variable between individuals. Moreover, further diversity is being manifest in so-called 'day people' and 'night people' as well as in other examples of rhythmical diversity.

Investigations testing the validity of the Principles of Homeodynamics and the postulated nature of change in field pattern manifestations appear in this text. Research in this area is ongoing.

A science has many theories. As these are tested, some will be supported; others may not. Replication of research may contribute to the level of confidence one may have in a given theory. Everyday events, when examined from a new world view, a different perspective, raise new questions and suggest new explanations.

A theory of accelerating evolution deriving from this conceptual system requires a fresh look at today's rapidly changing norms in blood pressure levels, children's behavior, longer waking periods, and other events. Higher frequency wave patterns of growing diversity portend new norms coordinate with accelerating change. Labels of pathology based on old norms generate hypochondriasis—not uncommonly iatrogenic in origin. "Normal" means "average." Normal (average) blood pressure readings in all age groups are notably higher today than they were a few decades ago. Evidence that these norms are jeopardizing the public's health is insubstantial. The relative nature of multiplying individual differences in a dynamic, continuously innovative system raises critical questions about the meaning of mass surveys and unrestrained encouragement of frequent blood pressure checks. Drugs are dispensed with largesse and not infrequently cause something less than healthy side effects. Health personnel have long deplored public failure to follow up on recommended "expert" treatment. Could it be that there is a folk wisdom that protects the unwary and the "doubting Thomases"?

Not only has the average waking period lengthened, but sleep-wake continuities are increasingly diverse. Developmental norms have changed significantly in recent years. Gifted children and the so-called hyperactive not uncommonly manifest similar behaviors. It would seem more reasonable to hypothesize hyperactivity as accelerating evolution than to denigrate rhythmicities that diverge from outdated norms and erroneous expectations.

Manifestations of a speeding up of human field rhythms are coordinate with higher frequency environmental field patterns. Radiation increments of widely diverse frequencies are common household accompaniments of everyday life. Atmospheric and cosmological complexity grows. Environmental motion has quickened. A very high-speed transit tube craft that can whisk people across the country by electromagnetic waves at approximately 14,000 miles per hour is already within man's capability. Moon villages and space towns are on the near horizon.

Human and environmental fields evolve together, integral with one another. The doomsayers who predict man's early self-destruction fail to recognize the innovative potentials that abound. Increased longevity, escalating science and technology, outer-space exploration, aroused concern for human rights, and multiple other evidences of man's evolutionary potentials in process of actualization bespeak a future people have scarcely envisioned.

With increased longevity, growing numbers of older persons are added to the population. Contrary to a static view engendered by a closed-system model of the universe, which postulates aging to be a running down, the Science of Unitary Human Beings postulates aging to be a developmental process. Aging is continuous from conception through the dying process. Field patterns are increasingly diverse and creative. The aged sleep less, and sleep-wake frequencies are more varied. Higher frequency patterns give meaning to multiple reports of time experienced as racing.

Aging is not a disease, nor is it analogous to the "one-hoss shay" of literary lore. Innovative developmental diversity manifests itself nonlinearly and in contradiction to the traditional emphasis on chronological age as a determinant in change. More diverse field patterns change more rapidly than the less diverse. Populations defy so-called normal curves as individual differences multiply. This conceptual system predicates a clearly different approach to the aged. Values are revised. A new sense of self-worth becomes evident among older people.

The emergence of paranormal phenomena as valid subjects for serious scientific research has nonetheless been handicapped by a paucity of viable theories to explain these events. The conceptual system presented here provides a framework for generating and testing viable theories. Some are reported in this volume. Alternative forms of healing, meditative modalities, and imagery are increasingly popular. The efficacy of Therapeutic Touch, developed by Dolores Krieger, has been documented. The implications for creative health services are notable. Noninvasive therapies and diminished use of drugs can be expected to replace the current mechanistic emphasis in treating human ills.

Nurses are concerned with the dying as well as with the living. Unitary human and environmental rhythms find expression in the rhythmicities of the living-dying process. Just as aging is deemed development, so too is dying hypothesized to be developmental. The nature of the dying process and after-death phenomena have gained considerable public and professional interest in recent years. Investigations into the nature and validity of a range of phenomena associated with dying are reported in the literature. Definitions of death are increasingly arguable. Questionable practices in securing organs for transplantation have led to legislative action. The right to die with dignity is being written into final testaments and debated in courts of law. Concomitantly, reports of near-death and after-death experiences are already listed among the best-sellers. A new approach to studying the dying process is provided by the conceptual system herein presented. The nature and continuity of field patterning subsequent to dying, while admittedly a difficult area to study, nonetheless is open to theoretical investigation.

Research findings support the nature of change postulated in the Principles of Homeodynamics. Some are reported in this book. Others have been completed or are nearing completion. New tools of measurement are necessary adjuncts to studying questions arising out of a world view that is different from the prevalent view. The research potentials of this system are infinite. It is logically and scientifically tenable. It is flexible and open-ended. Practical implications for human betterment are demonstrable.

Seeing the world from this viewpoint requires a new synthesis, a creative leap, and the inculcation of new attitudes and values. Guiding principles are broad generalizations that require imaginative and innovative modalities for their implementation. The Science of Unitary Human Beings identifies nursing's uniqueness and signifies the potential of nurses to fulfill their social responsibility in human service. Basic theoretical research in the Science of Unitary Human Beings is indispensable. Only then can the theoretically sound foundation continue to evolve.

References

1. Russell B: On the notion of cause, with applications to the free-will problem. In Feigl H, Brodbeck M (eds): *Readings in the Philosophy of Science.* New York, Appleton-Century-Crofts, 1953, p. 387.

CHAPTER 42

Nursing Science and Art: A Prospective

Martha E. Rogers

In little more than a decade the 21st century will arrive, accompanied by a plethora of manifestations of accelerating change. Futurists prophecy [sic] multiple scenarios, often in conflict with one another. Economics, education, health, lifestyles, robots, computers, environment, world affairs, and space travel are just a few of the areas undergoing scrutiny and subject to prediction. Social evolution from tribes to city-states to nations and now to "one world" foretell [sic] interplanetary and intergalactic communication with intelligent life beyond the present purview. Diversification and synthesis grow. New world views multiply and encompass the extraterrestrial.

Scientific and technological wonders escalate. A cashless society is well on its way. Low technology robots for home and workplace are in the making. Over a year ago, the U.S. Department of Transportation approved a Transrapid monorail for a proposed 8800-passenger-per-day line from Los Angeles to Las Vegas with a round trip cost of perhaps as little as $50.00 (half the current airfare) and travel time of 1 hour.

Moon mining and gravity-free manufacturing in space are anticipated within this century. Galactic grocery stores, educational centers, health services, recreational opportunities and the like are inevitable inclusions in a space-bound world society. A bill has been presented to Congress to establish space colleges with scholarships using a system similar to earlier agricultural colleges. A visionary design for a space station housing a think tank in orbit 23,000 miles from Earth provided the centerpiece last year of a Washington, DC, exhibit, the underlying idea being that weightlessness encourages creativity (Harger, 1986). The First National Conference on Nursing in Space met in April, 1988, at the University of Alabama School of Nursing (Huntsville, AL).

Ethical issues take on new dimensions. What is the significance of biotechnology leading to genetic erosion through predicted loss of genetic diver-

Rogers, M. E. (1988). Nursing science and art: A prospective. *Nursing Science Quarterly, 1,* 99–102. Reprinted with permission.

sity as farmers cultivate only selected high-yield strains? Will human cadavers be kept on life support systems to provide for organ harvesting, research, and education of various health personnel (*Outlook '87 and Beyond,* Bethesda, MD: World Future Society)? Is a new definition of death in the making? How does a new world view explain these events?

Old realities contradict present knowledge and fall short of providing viable explanations of observable incidents. New realities are coming forth postulating new directions and promises of a hopeful future. Humankind is on the threshold of a new cosmology transcending an earth-bound past.

Nursing is integral with the rapidly changing world noted above. Moreover, many nurses have been moving apace to assure that there will be a substantive body of theoretical knowledge specific to nursing to underwrite the practice of nursing. New job frontiers are already here, but too few nurses are prepared to move into them. The future will find fewer and fewer nurses employed in hospitals. Educational programs in nursing at all levels must prepare for the future or the unemployables in nursing will continue to accumulate.

Nursing is postulated to be a science. A science is identified by the phenomenon central to its concern. For example, physicists study the physical world, biologists study biological phenomena, psychologists study the mind, and astronomers study the cosmos. The central concern of nurses has long been human beings and their environments. Definitions of specificity become necessary to differentiate nursing's focus from that of other sciences. For the science of nursing, human beings as well as environments are identified as irreducible energy fields. The uniqueness of nursing is its central concern with unitary, irreducible human beings and their respective environments. The purpose of nursing is to promote human health and well being.

A science may be defined as an organized body of abstract knowledge arrived at by scientific research and logical analysis. This body of knowledge provides a means of describing, explaining, and predicting about the phenomenon central to its concern. The creative use of the body of abstract knowledge in human service constitutes the art of nursing.

When nursing is specified to be a science, the term *nursing* becomes a noun signifying a body of knowledge. The abstract system specific to nursing is a new product, a synthesis of facts and ideas. It is rooted in a new world view compatible with the most progressive knowledge available and is a necessary prelude to the study of people and their world and to the derivation of principles and theories. More specifically, nursing is postulated to be a basic science. The phenomenon of concern is unique to nursing and has well established roots going back to nursing's prescientific era.

The study of nursing is the study of human and environmental fields. It is not the study of the biological world any more than the study of biology is the study of the physical world. Further, the study of nursing is not the study of nurses and what they do any more than biology is the study of biologists and what they do.

The development of an abstract system specific to nursing is a process of synthesis. A scientific language adds clarity and precision and is derived from the general language. A specific definition has meaning only within the science or framework connected with it. Nursing's abstract system does not come out of a vacuum. Neither does it derive from other basic or applied sciences, nor is it a summation of knowledge drawn from other fields.

Building blocks fundamental to the science of unitary human beings are postulated to include energy fields, a universe of open systems, pattern, and four-dimensionality. Definitions of specificity for these and other terms relevant to this system are as follows:

Learned profession: a science and an art.

Science: an organized body of abstract knowledge arrived at by scientific research and logical analysis.

Art: the imaginative and creative use of knowledge.

Negentropy: increasing heterogeneity, differentiation, diversity, and complexity of pattern.

Energy field: the fundamental unit of the living and the nonliving. Field is a unifying concept, and energy signifies the dynamic nature of the field; energy fields are infinite.

Pattern: the distinguishing characteristic of an energy field perceived as a single wave.

Four-dimensionality: a nonlinear domain without spatial or temporal attributes.

Conceptual system: an abstraction, a representation of the universe or some portion thereof.

Unitary human being (*human field*): an irreducible, four-dimensional energy field identified by pattern and manifesting characteristics that are specific to the whole and that cannot be predicted from knowledge of the parts.

Environment (*Environmental field*): an irreducible, four-dimensional energy field identified by pattern and integral with the human field.

A few brief comments concerning the above definitions seem in order. Energy fields constitute dynamic unity. They are infinite and they are abstract. People and environments are noted to be energy fields. They do not *have* energy fields; they *are* energy fields. A universe of open systems a quarter of a century ago moved forward to replace the closed system model of the universe. By the 1960s the advent of space exploration confirmed the obsolescence of such ideas as homeostasis, adaptation, steady state, and equilibrium. Negentropy moved to replace entropy. The universe is not running down. Causality is a contradiction of open systems. Moreover, association does not mean causality. Pattern is an abstraction that gives identity to human and environmental fields. One perceives manifestations of field pattern, but one does not perceive field pattern itself. Field pattern changes continuously. Moreover, it is always new and always more diverse. Four-dimensionality is a nonlinear domain without spatial or temporal attributes. People are not becoming four-dimensional. Rather, in this world view, all reality is four-dimensional. All other dimensions are abstractions.

The postulates specified earlier are integral to nursing's abstract system but are by no means all that is incorporated into a synthesis of facts and ideas by which a new product is identified. The science of nursing is the science of unitary human beings. The abstract system is an irreducible whole that represents a new way of looking at the universe. Principles and theories derive from the totality of the system. To study nursing from this reality requires consistency with the totality of the system.

Characteristics and manifestations of unitary human beings are specific to the whole, namely, the human energy field and the environmental energy field. Testable hypotheses derive from the system. Principles are broad generalizations. They are statements of relationships. They help to describe, explain, and predict the nature of human and environmental change.

The following principles of homeodynamics derive from this abstract system:

Principle of resonancy: The continuous change from lower to higher frequency wave patterns in human and environmental fields.

Principle of helicy: The continuous, innovative, probabilistic, increasing diversity of human and environmental field patterns characterized by nonrepeating rhythmicities.

Principle of integrality: The continuous, mutual human field and environmental field process.

Many theories continue to derive from this system. Some have been tested, some are in the process of being tested, and others are being prepared for testing (see Malinski, 1986). Testable hypotheses continue to emerge.

Basic and applied research are both necessary to nursing's future. Basic research provides new knowledge. Applied research tests knowledge already available. Basic research in the science of nursing is an essential prelude to applied research in this field.

A new world view, in this instance nursing's abstract system, signifies a new reality, raises different questions, and suggests new answers. The goal of nurses is to participate in the process of change so that people may benefit. The future is one of growing diversity, of accelerating evolution, of nonrepeating rhythmicities. Change is inevitable. The nature of change is probabilistic.

A few examples of ways in which this system contradicts traditional views may help to clarify new directions. For example, the aging process has engaged the attention of people for centuries. In recent decades, it has assumed the proportions of a major disease. Even so, there is documented evidence that more and more people are living well beyond a 65-year retirement age and little evidence that longevity is associated with prevailing practices in health or medical fields. In the science of unitary human beings, aging is a normal developmental process. It is not a disease. Increasing longevity is an evolutionary process. Why shouldn't people sleep less as they grow older? What is wrong with increasingly enjoying sharp tastes? In a nonlinear reality without spatial or temporal attributes and manifesting accelerating change, might not one expect visions of note emerging regardless of chronological age? Human aging is not to be determined by physical or biological or social-psychological criteria. Human longevity is a developmental field process to be viewed positively and creatively and with cognizance of individual diversity.

So-called disease entities have less and less validity. Causality and cure are feeble claims. The good cholesterol and the bad cholesterol often sound more like television's fictional good guys and bad guys than a scientific verity. Ecological errors perpetrated by scientists can be as devastating as anything the general public does. A quick look at the latest disease entity to engage the attention of the western world, in particular, is AIDS. Interestingly enough, the AIDS virus is not a newcomer. Moreover, incidence statistics concerning this condition are open to many questions. Might one propose that AIDS is an example of man's ecological ignorance? Is it possible that the massive use, misuse, and abuse of antibiotics and various chemicals, with growing numbers of individuals allergic to such drugs, is a significant variable associated with the emergence of AIDS? History is replete with the going and coming of epidemics of many kinds. Such events often seem to have a beginning and ending of their own. People participate in the process of change but not necessarily with knowledge and wisdom. People do not control anything, as human and environmental fields are integral to each other; they are in mutual process. They are not at war with one another. A new world view is necessary for a more productive approach to studying AIDS. Cancer, cardiac conditions, and a multiplicity of less frequent conditions need to be reexamined from a new reality. Potentials for human betterment growing out of a new world view come into sight.

Noninvasive therapeutic modalities are emphasized in this new reality. The practice of therapeutic touch, developed by Krieger (1981), is already in use in many places around this planet. The use of humor, sound, color, and motion continue to undergo investigation. Findings of research in the science of nursing are being reported in the literature and are finding their way into the practice arena wherever people are. Imagery and meditative modalities have much to offer in this reality. Emphasis on human rights, client decision making, and noncompliance with traditional rules of thumb are necessary dimensions. Community-based health services must take precedence over shrinking hospital-based sick services. Although both provide meaningful services, it is the broad community-based health promotion services that provide the umbrella. Autonomous nursing practice directed by nurses holding valid baccalaureate and higher degrees with an upper division major in nursing science are [sic] central to the future. Moreover, the term *community-based* takes on enhanced meaning as it is defined to include multiple extraterrestrial centers.

The future demands new visions, flexibility, curiosity, imagination, courage, risk taking, compassion, and an excellent sense of humor.

References

Harger, J. (1986). Far out idea: Think tank in space. *Insight,* pp. 64–65.

Krieger, D. (1981). *Foundations for holistic health nursing practices: The renaissance nurse* (pp. 138–148). Philadelphia: Lippincott.

Malinski, V. (1986). *Explorations on Martha Rogers' science of unitary human beings.* Norwalk, CT: Appleton-Century-Crofts.

CHAPTER 43

Nursing: Science of Unitary, Irreducible, Human Beings: Update 1990

Martha E. Rogers

The countdown for the 21st century has begun. New facts and ideas continue to generate syntheses for new world views. Genetic engineering engenders a mechanistic explanation of life and spawns ethical issues that far exceed Aldous Huxley's (1932) *Brave New World.* Concomitantly, "caring" has become an "in" word as the public is told that the mother who cares gives her child Castoria and the wife who cares feeds her spouse Nutragrain. Major American contemporary health problems are iatrogenesis, nosocomial conditions, and nosophobia. Toxic terrorism is rampant with the health fields frequently providing the terrorists themselves.

Entrepreneurship marks one of the fundamental changes in today's economy. New careers coordinate with new world views and exacerbating innovative technology mount. Potentials for careers in outer space challenge even the most imaginative. Homo spacialis looms on the horizon as moon villages, space towns, and Martian communities foretell a new world.

Nursing's transition from pre-science to science must be explicit if nurses are to provide knowledgeable innovative services in a space-bound world society. A new world view compatible with the most progressive knowledge available (Lauden, 1977) is a necessary prelude to studying human health and to determining modalities for its promotion both on this planet and in outer space.

As a learned profession, nursing is both a science and art. The *uniqueness of nursing,* like that of any other science, lies in the phenomenon central to its

---

Rogers, M. E. (1990). Nursing: Science of unitary, irreducible, human beings: Update 1990. In E. A. M. Barrett (Ed.), *Visions of Rogers' science-based nursing* (pp. 5–11). New York: National League for Nursing. Reprinted with permission.

focus. Nurses' long-established concern with people and the world they live in is a natural forerunner of an organized abstract system encompassing people and their environments. The irreducible nature of individuals is different from the sum of the parts. The integralness of people and environment that coordinate with a multidimensional universe of open systems point [sic] to a new paradigm: the *identity of nursing as a science.* The purpose of nurses is to promote health and well being for all persons wherever they are. The art of nursing is the creative use of the science of nursing for human betterment.

A science is an organized abstract system. It is a synthesis of facts and ideas; a new product. Historically, the term "nursing" has been used as a verb signifying "to do." When nursing is identified as a science the term "nursing" becomes a noun signifying "a body of abstract knowledge." Theories derive from this organized body of abstract knowledge. Consequently, theories deriving from a Science of Unitary Human Beings are specific to nursing just as theories deriving from biology are specific to biological phenomena, theories deriving from sociology are specific to sociological phenomena, and theories of physics are specific to the physical world. Moreover, one must keep in mind that the study of biologists and what they do is not the study of biology. Similarly, the study of nurses and what they do is not the study of nursing.

A science has many theories. Nursing is the study of unitary, irreducible, indivisible human and environmental fields: people and their world. Complexity of investigatory methodology is not a substitute for substantive content in any field. Florence Downs (1988) noted recently ". . . our research efforts are replete with sophisticated methods applied to unsophisticated content" (p. 20). The education of nurses has identity in transmission of nursing's body of theoretical knowledge. The practice of nurses is the creative use of this knowledge in human service. Research methods are empty without substance to study. Research in nursing specifies a body of knowledge specific to nursing; research in other fields is not a substitute.

Developing nursing's abstract system demands a new world view. A language of specificity provides for precision, clarity, and communication. Replication of research becomes possible. Nursing, like other sciences, is a synthesis of facts and ideas—a new product. It is not a summation of principles and theories from other fields dealing with different phenomena and rooted in different paradigms. Nursing's focus on unitary human beings and their world as defined in this system is unique to nursing [Table 1].

Table 1. Key Definitions Specific to the Science of Nursing

Energy Field:	The fundamental unit of the living and the non-living. Field is a unifying concept. Energy signifies the dynamic nature of the field; a field is in continuous motion and is infinite.
Pattern:	The distinguishing characteristic of an energy field perceived as a single wave.
Multidimensional:	A nonlinear domain without spatial or temporal attributes.
Unitary Human Beings: (Human Field)	An irreducible, indivisible, multidimensional energy field identified by pattern and manifesting characteristics that are specific to the whole and which cannot be predicted from knowledge of the parts.
Environment: (Environmental Field)	An irreducible, indivisible, multidimensional energy field identified by pattern and integral with the human field.

A universe of open systems underwrites the growing diversity of people and their environments. Furthermore, it should be emphasized that people *are* energy fields. They do not *have* them. All reality is postulated to be multidimensional as defined herein. One does not become multidimensional. Rather, this is a way of perceiving reality. The use of the term "multidimensional" to replace the term "four-dimensional" does not represent any change in definition. Efforts to select words best suited to portray one's thought are difficult at best. Multidimensional provides for an infinite domain without limit.

The abstract system exists as an irreducible whole. Principles and theories derive from this irreducible whole. The nature of change finds expression in the principles of homeodynamics. New knowledge is contributing continuously to revisions of thinking. A significant change in one word in the principle of helicy occurs. Interestingly enough, the change is consistent with the abstract system and new knowledge supports it. Clarification is in order. The reader is familiar with the transition from absolutism to probability. The literature now points up that unpredictability transcends probability. Eugene Mallove (1989) writes, "To find in the late 20th century that unpredictability plays a significant role in the orderly celestial arena is not only a surprising development but a revolutionary one in the history of science" (p. 12). Peterson (1989) discusses further the unpredictability of self-organized critical systems.

The deletion of probability from the abstract system underlying the science of unitary human beings and the addition of unpredictability strengthens [sic] consistency and supports [sic] the nature of change proposed in the principles of homeodynamics. The principles are now stated below in Table 2 as revised.

These principles provide fundamental guides to the practice of nursing. They continue to undergo investigation and to generate both basic and applied research in the science of nursing.

Energy fields are in continuous motion. Field pattern has been a central concept in this system from its inception over 2½ decades ago. It is interesting to note that Ferguson (1980) wrote in her book *The Aquarian Conspiracy* that "Synthesis and pattern seeing are survival skills of the 21st century." Ferguson's comment is certainly apropos to the Science of Unitary Human Beings. Pattern within nursing's abstract system is itself an abstraction that reveals itself through its manifestations. Manifestations of patterning emerge out of the human/environmental field mutual process and are continuously innovative. The evolution of life and non-life is a dynamic, irreducible, nonlinear process characterized by increasing complexification of energy field patterning. The nature of change is unpredictable and increasingly diverse (see Table 3).

Table 2. Principles of Homeodynamics

Principle of Resonancy:	Continuous change from lower to higher frequency wave patterns in human and environmental fields.
Principle of Helicy:	Continuous, innovative, unpredictable increasing diversity of human and environmental field patterns.
Principle of Integrality:	Continuous mutual human field and environmental field process.

Table 3. Manifestations of Field Patterning in Unitary Human Beings

The evolution of unitary human beings is a dynamic, irreducible, nonlinear process characterized by increasing diversity of energy field patterning. Manifestations of patterning emerge out of the human/environmental field mutual process and are continuously innovative. Pattern is an abstraction that reveals itself through its manifestations.

The nature of unitary field patterning is unpredictable and creative. Change is relative and increasingly diverse. Some manifestations of relative diversity in field patterning are noted below.

lesser diversity		greater diversity
longer rhythms	shorter rhythms	seems continuous
slower motion	faster motion	seems continuous
time experienced as slower	time experienced as faster	timelessness
pragmatic	imaginative	visionary
longer sleeping	longer waking	beyond waking

The "seems continuous" noted in Table 3 refers to a wave frequency so rapid that the observer perceives it as a single, unbroken event. Not only is field pattern diversity relative for any given individual but there is also a marked increase in diversity between individuals. The implications of this for increased individualization of nursing services are explicit.

The Science of Unitary Human Beings is equally applicable to groups as to individuals. Groups are defined as two or more individuals. The group energy field to be considered is identified: It may be a family or a social group, a crowd or some other combination. Regardless of the group identified, the group field is irreducible and indivisible to itself and integral with its own environmental field. The environmental field is unique to any given group field. The principles of homeodynamics postulate the nature of group field change just as they postulate the nature of individual field change.

Questions concerning whether mother/fetus are one field or two often arise. It may be handled either way. The mother/fetus may be deemed a single indivisible field—a group field if you like. This field would be irreducible. If one determined to focus on the mother or on the fetus, these would be individual fields integral with their own unique environmental fields. Regardless of the field one chooses to study, it is essential to remember that one cannot generalize from parts to a whole. For example, studying the members of a group will not provide knowledge about the group.

The Science of Unitary Human Beings encompasses our advent into outer space. Today's astronauts are envoys to our outer space-directed future—a future that is already here. Planet Earth is integral with the larger world of human reality. The outer space future will not be how to use planetary knowledge and skills in space but rather the elaboration of a new world view in which new knowledge and new modalities raise new questions, provide new answers, and signify different evolutionary norms. Homo spacialis (Robinson & White, 1986) is proposed to transcend Homo sapiens in approximately two generations of space dwelling. Planet-bound physiological norms are already inadequate parameters for humankind in space. They are increasingly irrelevant for space travelers and to forthcoming Homo spacialis. So-called pathology on Earth today may signify health for the space bound.

Testable hypotheses derive from nursing's abstract system. Research enables one to understand the nature of human evolution and its multiple unpredictable potentialities. Description, explanation, and vision strengthen a nurse's ability to practice according to the level and scope of a given nurse's preparation and knowledge in the science of nursing. Holistic trends force new ways of thinking and spell new world views. Gould (1977) once wrote, "Facts do not speak for themselves. They are read in the light of theory" (p. 21). Unitary human health signifies an irreducible human field manifestation. It cannot be measured by the parameters of biology or physics or the social sciences and the like. The principles of homeodynamics postulate the nature of change with equal relevance for individuals and for groups, for Homo sapiens and Homo spacialis and beyond.

Education for all is undergoing considerable review. Davis (1989) has noted that "The shelf life of an education today doesn't last a working lifetime" and emphasizes "a shift to a life-time of learning rather than one of knowing" (p. 16). Basic and applied research in the science of nursing is a must.

The Science of Unitary Human Beings sparks new interventive modalities—that evolve as life evolves from earth to space and beyond. Spin-offs from space can lead to more effective services for Homo sapiens on planet Earth. Non-invasive modalities will prevail. A positive attitude toward change is generated. Vision and imagination grow. The purpose of nurses is to promote human betterment wherever people are—on planet Earth or in outer space.

Health services are properly community based. Satellite services such as hospitals provide an orientation to pathology—not to health. As health promotion takes over, fewer and fewer people will need sick services as they currently exist. Today's world is rapidly becoming an entrepreneurial society and nurses are already into the stream of the entrepreneurial world. There is critical need for mutual respect for differences between all health personnel, between nurses, between health fields, and between fields of science.

The practice of nursing will be characterized primarily by non-invasive modalities. Research in the science of nursing is already providing support for skills deemed unscientific in the past. An excellent example is Krieger's (1979) work in therapeutic touch—relate this to the art of evening care, of back-rubs, even that cool hand on a fevered brow. There are many more examples.

As diversity grows so too does individualization of services. How do nurses best participate in enabling people to fulfill their own rhythmicities? Meditation, imagery, relaxation have undreamed of potentials. Unconditional love is beginning to receive the attention it deserves. Attitudes of hope, humor, and upbeat moods are already documented to be often better therapy than drugs.

Basic research in the Science of Unitary Human Beings is increasing (Ludomirski-Kalmanson, 1985; Malinski, 1986). Concomitantly, Senator Clairborne Pell, in the February 1988 issue of *Omni,* points out that various methods are used to prevent research that is out of the mainstream from ever getting off the ground and deplores the gearing of all research monies toward traditional disciplines of science. Nurses would do well to recognize that biomedical research is not research in nursing.

Read the chapters in this book within the context of a new world view. Examine them carefully for contradictions. Envision a future not yet here.

Enjoy your forays into the unknown. Change is continuous, inevitable, and exciting.

References

Davis, S. (1989, April). Envisioning the future. *Futurific,* 16–18.

Downs, F. (1988). Nursing research: State-of-the-art. *Journal of the New York State Nurses' Association, 19*(3), 20.

Ferguson, M. (1980). *The aquarian conspiracy: Personal and social transformation in the 1980s.* Los Angeles, J. P. Tarcher.

Gould, S. J. (1977). This view of life. *Natural History, 52,* 20–24.

Huxley, A. (1932). *Brave new world.* New York: Modern Library.

Krieger, D. (1979). *The therapeutic touch: How to use your hands to help or to heal.* Englewood Cliffs, NJ: Prentice Hall.

Lauden, L. (1977). *Progress and its problems: Toward a theory of scientific growth.* Berkeley: University of California Press.

Ludomirski-Kalmanson, B. (1985). An empirical investigation in support of M. Rogers' principle of integrality. In *Proceedings of the 10th National Research Conference* (pp. 201–204). Toronto, Ontario, Canada: University of Toronto Faculty of Nursing.

Malinski, V. (Ed.) (1986). *Explorations on Martha Rogers' science of unitary human beings.* Norwalk, CT: Appleton-Century-Crofts.

Mallove, E. T. (1989, May-June). The solar system in chaos. *The Planetary Report,* pp. 12–13.

Pell, C. (1988, February). First Word. *Omni, 14,* 32–34.

Peterson, I. (1989, July). Digging into sand. *Science News. 138,* 42.

Robinson, G. S., & White, H. M. (1986). *Envoys of mankind.* Washington, DC: Smithsonian Institute Press.

CHAPTER 44

Space-Age Paradigm for New Frontiers in Nursing

Martha E. Rogers

In February 1957, Lee DeForest, father of modern electronics, stated: "To place a man in a multistage rocket and propel him into the controlling gravitational field of the moon . . . will never occur regardless of all future scientific endeavors" and compared such proposals to the wildest dreams of Jules Verne (Friedman, 1989). This was just 12 years before the Apollo moon landing.

Manned voyages to Mars now seem likely by the year 2000, with a projected round trip of as little as two months (*Futurific,* Feb. 1990). Currently, 125 students from 26 countries are enrolled in the International Space University—an international, non-profit, interdisciplinary institution designed to educate the world's future space professionals (Burke, 1989). Out of 2,500 applicants to the National Aeronautics and Space Administration (NASA) for admission to the Astronaut Corps in 1990, 106 made it to the interview stage—all expertly qualified in diverse scientific and technological fields. At the end of the process, 23 applicants were selected. Numbers of astronauts to be selected are increasing, but competition is sharp. Technical skill, enthusiasm, communication skills, and experience in areas outside one's own discipline are essential, but the sine qua non of being an astronaut is generally noted as the ability to be a team player (Triplett, 1990).

Increasing space travel capabilities are manifest in many countries. Establishment of moon villages, space towns, and Martian communities are near and presage a major emigration of "earth-kind" in the not too distant future. Interplanetary and intergalactic communication with intelligent life beyond our present purview portends new meanings to citizenship in a space-encompassing world society. Interestingly enough, each dollar NASA spends for re-

Rogers, M. E. (1990). Space-age paradigm for new frontiers in nursing. In M. E. Parker (Ed.), *Nursing Theories in Practice* (pp. 105–112). New York: National League for Nursing. Reprinted with permission.

search and development generates $9.00 in private spending (*Futurific,* Feb. 1990).

A new oneness attends planet Earth's integration into the space world: a new synthesis in which spin-off from space exploration marks planet Earth's future.

Astronauts—precursors of "spacekind"—portend outward emigration by Homo sapiens and their transcendence by "Homo spatialis." This transcendence will be an evolutionary process, not an adaptive one. According to Robinson and White (1986), this process could take place in two generations of space living (about 50 years). Life support systems in reverse will then be needed for the earth-bound traveler from space. (There are those who are already predicting a shortage of Homo sapiens on planet Earth as emigration expands). A cartoon in a recent issue of *Omni* depicts two Homo spatialis by the bedside of a very sick "Earthman." One "Spaceman" is saying to the other "If he lives he'll be nothing more than a Homo sapiens."

New world views abound. Synthesis and holism are predominant among these views. James Lovelock, in *The Ages of Gaia* (1988), proposes a scientific synthesis in harmony with the Greek conception of the Earth as a living whole, as Gaia. Buckminster Fuller (1981) argues firmly for Earth as a spaceship. Leslie Kenton, writing in the *Noetic Sciences Bulletin* (1990), emphasizes the fallacy of depending on well-meaning actions and good intentions while we continue to operate with a paradigm that views reality as fragmented. Holistic world views are being studied by such persons as David Bohm, Fritz Capra, Rupert Sheldrake, and Rene Weber—both as individuals and in groups. My own work focuses on developing a holistic world view by proposing a science of unitary, irreducible beings that is coordinate with a world view that includes outer space.

Noninvasive therapeutic modalities are increasingly emphasized by a range of health care workers. New modalities will emerge out of evolution toward spacekind, which will spark more effective modalities for earthkind. A holistically oriented space-age paradigm is the substance of nursing's science of unitary, irreducible human beings.

Traditional world views are increasingly untenable and fail to explain contemporary events. Today's health care system is dangerously deficient and cannot be cured simply by adding more dollars or by other simplistic proposals. Toxic terrorists abound. Remember the two grapes from Chile and the Alar apples from Washington state. Colman McCarthy in an Editorial in *The Washington Post* last year wrote, "Dairy cows are shot through with so many drugs that milk ought to be sold as a prescription-only product." *Science News* in its September 23, 1989, issue notes "Green House warming is being recognized as a terrorist threat—not a scientific reality." The *Baltimore Sun* recently headlined a wire-service story thus: "Cow gas blamed for global warming." Another report based on ten years of weather satellite data shows no evidence of global warming from the greenhouse effect (*Arizona Republic,* March 1990). The debate goes on.

AIDS doesn't kill everyone who gets the virus. Infectious diseases are not new to this planet. Hope, attitude, mood, and laughter are reported to be as effective in strengthening the autoimmune system as drugs and vaccines. Today's major health problem is nosophobia: a morbid dread of disease.

Denial of human freedom to select medical care other than allopathic has helped spawn the Coalition for Alternatives in Nutrition and Health Care, a group that is promoting a health care rights amendment which would prohibit Congress from making any law restricting individuals' rights to chose and practice the type of health care they want.

As nurses move in the mainstream of a growing entrepreneurial society, subtle harassment and euphemisms are not unknown deterrents to nurses and are further aggravated by nurses who support anti-educationism in nursing and dependency on others. Failure to value differences between nurses and other health care personnel adds to the problem.

Accelerating change, an unpredictable future, and mushrooming social and ethical issues threaten the status-quoers. James Madison, in a speech given June 16, 1788, made this statement:

> I believe there are more instances of the abridgement of the freedom of the people by gradual and silent encroachments of those in power than by violent and sudden usurpation.

A humorous note seems fitting here:

> What with the threat of nuclear war, acid rain, crime in the streets, and AIDS—sometimes it seems as if it hardly pays to give up smoking.

Nursing is inseparable from the new world view and the process of change. Holistic trends are on the way to becoming a massive torrent. A new vision of a world encompassing far more than planet Earth is in the making. The science of nursing emerges out of a space-age world view. The evidence of diversifying wholeness is substantial. For instance the pace of evolution from clans to tribes to city-states to nation-states to one planet is accelerating.

The Science of Nursing

My discussion of nursing begins with the premise that nursing is a learned profession: a science and an art. A science is an organized body of abstract knowledge. The art involved in nursing is the creative use of science for human betterment. As a science, nursing generates many theories.

The uniqueness of nursing, as in other sciences, is identified in the phenomena of concern. Nursing is the study of unitary, irreducible human beings and their respective environments. As a science, the term "nursing" is a noun signifying an organized body of abstract knowledge. Theories of nursing derive from this abstract system of knowledge. The science of unitary human beings is rooted in a new world view coordinate with today's knowledge. The science of nursing is a synthesis of facts and ideas; it is a new product.

Many fields emerge out of new world views, holistic in focus. Fields differ according to the phenomena of concern. The following attributes are some of those included in the holistic world view presented here.

- *Energy Fields:* The fundamental unit of the living and the non-living. Field is a unifying concept. Energy signifies the dynamic nature of the field. Fields are infinite and continuously open.
- *Pattern:* The distinguishing characteristic of an energy field perceived as a single wave.

- *Multidimensional:* A nonlinear domain without spatial or temporal attributes.

The above terms represent definitions of a specificity within the science of nursing. General language definitions are relevant unless a term is defined with specificity. Two further terms of significance in this world view are defined as follows:

- *Unitary Person:* An irreducible, multidimensional energy field identified by pattern and manifesting characteristics that are specific to the whole and cannot be predicted from knowledge of the parts.
- *Environment:* An irreducible, multidimensional energy field identified by pattern and integral with a given human field.

People *are* energy fields. They do not have them. Continuous change emerges out of nonequilibrium and exhibits punctualism not gradualism. Change is accelerating. Chaos theory is transforming the way we think the world is (Crum, 1989; Peterson, 1989; Percival, 1989; Stewart, 1989).

Principles of Homeodynamics

Principles of Homeodynamics derive from the abstract system and postulate the nature of change. The principles are listed as follows.

Principle of Resonancy: The continuous change from lower to higher frequency wave patterns in human and environmental fields.

Principles of Helicy: The continuous innovative, unpredictable, increasing diversity of human and environmental field patterns.

Principle of Integrality: The continuous mutual human field and environmental field process.

Manifestations of field pattern assist in relating the abstract to the everyday world.

Manifestations of Field Patterning in Unitary Human Beings

The evolution of unitary human beings is a dynamic, irreducible, nonlinear process characterized by increasing diversity of energy field patterning. Manifestations of patterning emerge out of the mutual human/environmental field process and are continuously changing. Pattern is an abstraction that reveals itself through its manifestations.

The nature of unitary field patterning is unpredictable and creative. Change is relative and increasingly diverse. Some manifestations of relative diversity in field patterning are noted below.

Individuals experience lesser diversity and greater diversity, longer rhythms, shorter rhythms, and rhythms that seem continuous. Individuals experience motion as slower, faster, and continuous. Individuals experience time as slower, faster, or unmoving. Individuals are sometimes pragmatic, sometimes imaginative, and sometimes visionary. Individuals experience periods of longer sleeping, longer waking, and periods of being beyond waking.

Nursing Education and Practice

The world view and abstract system I present encompass earthkind and spacekind. Manifestations of change are holistic, continuous, and manifestations of pattern emerging out of the human and environmental field process. Homo spatialis is a product of evolution—a new species transcending Homo sapiens. It should be noted that changes that occur in Homo sapiens in space need not be labeled pathology. In fact, one would properly perceive such changes as manifestations of the human and environmental field process. This world view and this abstract system represent a new reality. The new reality encompasses new ways of thinking, new questions, new interpretations—and requires consistency with the system if one is to study it. Stephen Jay Gould wrote in the *Natural History Journal* a comment of relevance here, "Facts do not speak for themselves. They are read in the light of theory." Research and investigation in the science of unitary human beings is on-going (Malinski, 1986; Barrett, 1990; Sarter, 1990 [Editors' Note: Reference should be Sarter, 1988]).

The study of nursing as a science is the study of the phenomena central to nursing; unitary, irreducible human beings and their environments. It is *not* the study of other fields or theories deriving from other fields. A sociological theory is just that, no matter who studies it. Such a theory may be very good and the investigator may make a significant contribution to sociology. The study of nurses and what they do is not the study of nursing anymore than the study of biologists and what they do is the study of biology.

The education of nurses, whether technical, professional, or advanced, is properly rooted in a sound general education appropriate to the level of preparation sought. Everyone needs to include extraterrestrial content in their learning.

Central to the education of nurses must be study of the science of unitary human beings. Further, we must commit ourselves to a lifetime of learning. The nature of the practice of nursing (the use of knowledge for human betterment) is rooted in what one knows and in the imagination, creativity, compassion, and skill one uses. Nurses focus on health promotion. In the educational process we do not need to teach students how to do everything. Rather we need to teach them how to figure out how to do everything.

Health services are community based. Services such as hospitals, nursing homes, and the like supplement the base. There is a great need among all health care workers to develop mutual respect for differences.

Noninvasive modalities mark the future of nursing practice on this planet and in outer space. Therapeutic touch, imagery, meditation, relaxation, and the like will increase. Diversifying wholeness emphasizes the growing need for more individualization of services. Nonrepeating rhythmicities in sound, color, taste, fragrance, and the like have undreamed of potentials. Caring is a practice modality getting much attention from nurses, but caring does not identify nurses any more than workers in any other field. Almost everyone is capable of caring. The nature of caring in a given field depends on the body of scientific knowledge specific to that field. Humor, laughter, mood, and attitude have been found to be significant in health promotion and maintenance.

As a holistic reality revolutionizes our thinking and as space exploration and space living provide spin-off from space that can be helpful on planet Earth, nursing will change, as will other fields. We are on the threshold of a fantastic and unimagined future. Our potential for human service is greater than it has ever been. On with it!

References

Barrett, E. (1990). *Visions of Rogers' science-based nursing.* New York: National League for Nursing.

Burke, J. T. (1989). ISU tunes in on voyager watch. *The planetary report, IX*(6), 4.

Cow gas blamed. (1990, March). *Arizona Republic,* p. A6.

Crum, R. (1989, fall). Why Johnny kills. *New York University Magazine, 4*(2), 34.

Each dollar NASA spends. (1990, February). *Futurific, 14*(2), 37.

Friedman, S. T. (1989, February). Who believes in UFO's? *International UFO Reporter, 14*(1), 6–10.

Fuller, R. B. (1981). Critical Path. New York: St. Martin's Press.

Gould, S. J. (1977, February). This view of life. *Natural History, 52,* 20–24.

Kenton, L. (1990, spring). Member forum. *Noetic Sciences Bulletin, V*(1), 6.

Lovelock, J. (1988). *The ages of Gaia.* New York: W. W. Norton & Co.

Malinski, V. (1986). *Explorations of Martha Rogers' science of unitary human beings.* Norwalk, CT: Appleton-Century-Crofts.

Manned voyages to Mars. (1990, February). *Futurific, 14*(2), 37.

Percival, I. (1989, October). Chaos: A science for the real world. *New Scientist, 123,* 42–47.

Peterson, I. (1989, July). Digging into sand. *Science News, 136,* 40.

Robinson, G., & White, H. (1986). *Envoys of mankind.* Washington: Smithsonian Institution Press.

Sarter, B. (1988). *The stream of becoming: A study of Martha Rogers' theory.* New York: National League for Nursing.

Stewart, I. (1989). *Does God play dice?: The mathematics of chaos.* Cambridge, MA: Brasil Blackwell, Inc.

Triplett, W. (1990, April/May). The class of 1990. *Air & Space, 5*(1), 73–77.

CHAPTER 45

Nursing Science and the Space Age

Martha E. Rogers

Humankind is on the threshold of a new cosmology transcending an earthbound past. In less than a decade the 21st century will arrive, accompanied by many manifestations of accelerating change. Futurists prophecy [sic] multiple scenarios, often in conflict with one another. Genetic engineering engenders a mechanistic explanation of life and spawns ethical issues that far exceed Huxley's (1932) *Brave New World.* Economics, education, health, world affairs, lifestyles, as well as robots, computers, environment, and space travel are just a few of the areas undergoing scrutiny. Interplanetary and intergalactic communication with intelligent life beyond the present purview portends new meanings for citizenship in a space-encompassing world society. These new world views also take into account the extraterrestrial.

The science of unitary human beings encompasses this human advent into outer space. Today's astronauts are envoys to the human space-directed future. Astronauts, the precursors of spacekind, portend an outward emigration by Homo sapiens and, what is more, their transcendence by Homo spatialis. This transcendence will be an evolutionary, not an adaptive process.

Planet earth is integral with the larger world of human reality. Thus, the space future will not consist of how to use planetary knowledge and skills in space, but an elaboration of a new worldview in which new knowledge and modalities raise new questions, provide new answers, and signify different evolutionary norms. According to Robinson and White (1986), Homo spatialis will transcend Homo sapiens in approximately two generations of space living (about 50 years). Particulate phenomena such as physiological norms are already inadequate for judging the parameters of humankind in space. Even more, the so-called pathology on earth today may signify health for the spacebound.

Rogers, M. E. (1992). Nursing science and the space age. *Nursing Science Quarterly, 5,* 27–34. Reprinted with permission.

Homo spatialis looms on the horizon as moon villages, space towns, and Martian communities foretell a new world. Moon-mining and gravity-free manufacturing in space are anticipated within this century. Galactic grocery stores, educational centers, health services and recreational opportunities are each inevitable inclusions in a space-bound world society.

Increasing space travel capabilities are already manifest in many countries; a new oneness attends planet earth's integration into the space world, a new synthesis in which spinoffs from space exploration mark planet earth's future.

Should all of this seem impossible, one need only recall that in February 1957, Lee DeForest, father of modern electronics, stated: "To place a man in a multistage rocket and propel him into the controlling gravitational field of the moon . . . will never occur regardless of all future scientific endeavors." He compared these proposals to the wildest dreams of Jules Verne (Friedman, 1989). DeForest made this statement just 12 years before the Apollo moon landing.

A New World View for Nursing

Nursing's transition from pre-science to science has also accelerated, but it must become explicit if nurses are to provide knowledgeable innovative services in a space-bound world society. The explication of an organized body of abstract knowledge specific to nursing is indispensable. The need for such a body of knowledge can be identified in an escalation of science and technology coordinate with public demands for health services of a nature, and in an amount, scarcely envisioned by either the consumers or providers.

A new worldview compatible with the most progressive knowledge available (Lauden, 1977) has become a necessary prelude to studying human health and to determining modaliites for its promotion both on this planet and in outer space. The science of nursing is rooted in this worldview, a pandimensional view of people and their world.

Traditionally nursing's goals have encompassed both the sick and the well, and the consideration of environmental factors has also been integral to nursing's efforts. Education and practice in nursing have been directed toward promotion of health without interruption. The recognition of people as distinct from their parts has characterized nursing from the time of Florence Nightingale to the present.

The introduction of systems theories several decades ago set in motion new ways of perceiving people and their world. Since then, science and technology have escalated. The exploration of space has revised old views, and thus new knowledge has merged with new ways of thinking. Nothing less than a second industrial revolution has been initiated, far more dramatic in its implications and potentials than the first. The pressing need to study people in ways that would enhance their humanness has coordinated with the accelerating technological advances and forced a search for new models. A major hindrance to the evolution of viable models, however, was noted by Capra (1982) when he wrote about the difficulty encountered while trying to apply the concepts of an outdated worldview to a reality that could no longer be understood in terms of these concepts.

The science of nursing was arrived at by the creative syntheses of facts and ideas and is an emergent, a new product. These principles and theories were derived from the abstract system and were tested in the ordinary world. The findings of this research have accumulated and changed commensurate with the new knowledge. A science is open-ended. The elaboration of a science emerges out of scholarly research. Thus, the findings of research are fed back into the system, whereby the system undergoes continuous alteration, revision, and change. A science then, exists only in its entirety, it bespeaks wholeness and unity, and it provides a way of perceiving people and their environment.

The science of unitary human beings has not derived from one or more of the basic sciences. Neither has it come out of a vacuum. It flows instead in novel ways from a multiplicity of knowledge, from many sources, to create a kaleidoscope of potentialities. In turn, fundamental concepts are identified and significant terms are defined congruent with the evolving system. A humane and optimistic view of life's potentials grows as a new reality appears. Then, people's capacity to participate knowingly in the process of change is postulated.

Since nursing is a learned profession, it is both a science and an art. The uniqueness of nursing, like that of other sciences, lies in the phenomenon central to its focus. For nurses, that focus consists of a long established concern with people and the world they live in. It is the natural forerunner of an organized, abstract system encompassing people and their environments. The irreducible, indivisible nature of individuals is different from the sum of their parts. Furthermore, the integrality of people and their environments coordinates with a pandimensional universe of open systems, points to a new paradigm, and initiates the identity of nursing as a science. The purpose of nurses is to promote health and well-being for all persons wherever they are. The art of nursing, then, is the creative use of the science of nursing for human betterment.

A theoretically sound foundation that gives identity to nursing as a science and an art requires an organized abstract system from which to derive unifying principles and hypothetical generalizations. Through basic and applied research, theories are tested, new understandings emerge, and new questions arise. As a result, description and explanation take on new meanings, and a substantive body of knowledge specific to nursing takes form.

A science may be defined as an organized body of abstract knowledge arrived at by scientific research and logical analysis. This knowledge provides a means of describing and explaining the phenomena of concern. A science can also have more than one paradigm or abstract system, but the phenomena of concern remain constant. A worldview is a paradigm from which one can derive principles and theories that may guide practice. More specifically, however, nursing is postulated to be a basic science. Surely, this science does not come out of a vacuum. Neither does it derive from other basic or applied sciences, nor is it a summation of knowledge drawn from other fields. Nursing, instead, consists of its own unique irreducible mix.

Since science is open-ended and change is continuous, new knowledge brings new insights. Thus, the development of a science of unitary human beings is a never-ending process. This abstract system first presented some years ago has continued to gain substance. Concomitantly, early errors have undergone correction, definitions have been revised for greater clarity and accuracy, and updating of content is ongoing. Basic theoretical research, then, continues to be essential for the ongoing development of this field of study.

Both basic and applied research are necessary to nursing's future; basic research provides new knowledge while applied research tests the new knowledge already available. Multiple methodologies that may be used in the pursuit of the new knowledge include quantitative and qualitative methods and encompass philosophic, descriptive, and other approaches. The application of the science of unitary human beings to nursing, from a holistic worldview, also demands new tools and new methods. Moreover, it is only through research that the theoretically sound foundation can continue to evolve.

Historically the term "nursing" has been used as a verb signifying "to do," rather than as a noun meaning "to know." When nursing is identified as a science the term "nursing" becomes a noun signifying a "body of abstract knowledge." Consequently, theories deriving from a science of unitary human beings are specific to nursing, just as theories deriving from biology are specific to biological phenomena, theories deriving from sociology are specific to sociological phenomena, and theories of physics are specific to the physical world.

The study of nursing is not the study of the biological world any more than the study of biology is the study of the physical world. Further, the study of nursing is not the study of nurses and what they do any more than biology is the study of biologists and what they do. Nursing instead, is the study of unitary, irreducible, indivisible human and environmental fields: people and their world. The complexity of investigatory methodology is not a substitute for substantive content in any field. Downs notes ". . . our research efforts are replete with sophisticated methods applied to unsophisticated content" (Downs, 1988, p. 20). The education of nurses gains its identity by the transmission of nursing's body of theoretical knowledge. The practice of nurses, therefore, is the creative use of this knowledge in human service. Research methods are empty without substance to study. Thus, research in nursing specifies a body of knowledge specific to nursing, and research in other fields is not a substitute.

The uniqueness of nursing, like that of any other science, lies in the phenomenon central to its purpose; people and their worlds in a pandimensional universe are nursing's phenomena of concern. The irreducible nature of individuals as energy fields, different from the sum of their parts and integral with their respective environmental fields, differentiates nursing from other sciences and identifies nursing's focus.

Unitary human beings are specified to be irreducible wholes. A whole cannot be understood when it is reduced to its particulars. The use of the term unitary human beings is not to be confused with the current popular usage of the term holistic, generally signifying a summation of parts, whether few or many. The unitary nature of environment is equally irreducible. The concept of field provides a means of perceiving people and their respective environments as irreducible wholes.

The Science of Unitary Human Beings

The significant postulates fundamental to the science of unitary human beings include energy fields, openness, pattern, and pandimensionality. The de-

Table 1. Key Definitions Specific to the Science of Nursing

Energy Field:	The fundamental unit of the living and the non-living. Field is a unifying concept. Energy signifies the dynamic nature of the field. A field is in continuous motion and is infinite.
Pattern:	The distinguishing characteristic of an energy field perceived as a single wave.
Pandimensional:*	A non-linear domain without spatial or temporal attributes.
Unitary Human Being: (Human field)	An irreducible, indivisible, pandimensional energy field identified by pattern and manifesting characteristics that are specific to the whole and which cannot be predicted from knowledge of the parts.
Environment: (Environmental field)	An irreducible, pandimensional energy field identified by pattern and integral with the human field.

*Formerly titled Four-Dimensional and Multidimensional.
Reprinted with permission from the National League for Nursing, *Visions of Rogers' science-based nursing,* 1990, p. 9. Update 1991.

velopment of a science portends the emergence of abstract concepts and a corresponding language of specificity. Scientific language evolves out of the general language. Additionally, terms specific to the system are defined for clarity, precision, and communication so that rigorous research can be pursued and replicated. Terminology, except that defined specifically to the system, is interpreted in its general language meaning (see Table 1).

Theory concerning a universe of open systems has been gaining support for three quarters of a century. Since the introduction of the theory of relativity, of quantum theory, and of probability, the prevailing absolutism, already shaken by evolutionary theory, has received a critical blow. By the 1920s Selye had proposed adaptation, and by the 1930s von Bertalanffy introduced the idea of negative entropy (Rogers, 1970). Soon after Cannon advanced the idea of homeostasis. Space exploration began in the 1950s, and by the 1960s some physiologists suggested replacing the term homeostasis with the term homeokinesis. As this new knowledge escalated, the traditional meanings of homeostasis, steady-state, adaptation, and equilibrium were no longer tenable. The closed-system, entropic model of the universe began to be questioned and evidence has continued to accumulate in support of a universe of open systems (see Table 2).

In a universe of open systems, causality is not an option. Energy fields are open, not a little bit or sometimes, but continuously. A universe of open systems explains the infinite nature of energy fields, how the human and environmental fields are integral with one another, and that causality is invalid. Change, then, is continuously innovative and creative. Moreover, association does not mean causality.

New worldviews abound. Synthesis and holism are predominant among these views. Lovelock (1988) proposed a scientific synthesis in harmony with the Greek conception of the earth as a living whole, as Gaia. Fuller (1981) had argued that earth is a spaceship, and Kenton (1990) emphasizes the fallacy of depending on well-meaning actions and good intentions while people continue to operate with a paradigm that views reality as fragmented. Holistic new worldviews are being proposed by such persons as Bohm (1980), Capra (1982), Sheldrake (Weber, Bohm, & Sheldrake, 1986), and Weber (1986). In addition, Rogers' work focuses on developing a pandimensional worldview by proposing

Table 2. Some Differences between Older and Newer Worldviews

Older Views	Newer Views
cell theory	field theory
entropic universe	negentropic universe
three-dimensional	pandimensional
homeostasis	homeodynamics
person/environment: dichotomous	person/environment: integral
causation: single and multiple	mutual process
adaptation	mutual process
closed systems	open systems
dynamic equilibrium	innovative growing diversity
waking: basic state	waking: an evolutionary emergent
being	becoming

Initial development 1968; update 1991.

a science of unitary, irreducible human beings that is coordinate with a worldview that includes outer space.

Within this pandimensional view, energy fields are postulated to constitute the fundamental unit of both the living and the nonliving. Field, then, is a unifying concept and energy signifies the dynamic nature of the field. Energy fields are infinite and pandimensional; they are in continuous motion. Two energy fields are identified: the human field and the environmental field. Specifically, human beings and the environment *are* energy fields; they do not *have* energy fields. Moreover, human and environmental fields are not biological fields, physical fields, social fields, or psychological fields. Nor are human and environmental fields a summation of biological, physical, social, and psychological fields. This is not a denial of the importance of knowledge from other fields. Rather, it is to make clear that human and environmental fields have their own identity and are not to be confused with parts. Human and environmental fields are irreducible and indivisible. What may be quite valid in describing biological phenomena does not describe unitary human beings, any more than describing a molecule tells you about laughter.

A science of unitary human beings is equally as applicable to groups as it is to individuals. The group energy field to be considered is identified. It may be a family, a social group, or a community, a crowd or some other combination. Regardless of the group identified, the group field is irreducible and indivisible. The group field is integral with its own environmental field. The environmental field is unique to any given group field. The principles of homeodynamics postulate the nature of group field change just as they postulate the nature of individual field change. They are equally relevant for Homo sapiens, Homo spatialis, and beyond. Furthermore, these principles have validity only within the context of the science of unitary human beings, their meaning has specificity within their definitions, and together they postulate the nature and direction of change.

Pattern is a key postulate in this system (see Table 3). It is defined as the distinguishing characteristic of an energy field perceived as a single wave. Pattern is an abstraction, its nature changes continuously, and it gives identity to the field. Moreover, each human field pattern is unique and is integral with its own unique environmental field pattern. In fact, the term "pattern" is used

Table 3. Principles of Homeodynamics

Principle of Resonancy:	Continuous change from lower to higher frequency wave patterns in human and environmental fields.
Principle of Helicy:	Continuous, innovative, unpredictable, increasing diversity of human and environmental field patterns.
Principle of Integrality:	Continuous mutual human field and environmental field process.

Reprinted with permission from the National League for Nursing, *Visions of Rogers' science-based nursing,* 1990, p. 8.

only to refer to an energy field. The characteristics of unitary human beings are specific to unitary human beings. Pattern is not directly observable. However, manifestations of field patterning are observable events in the real world. They are postulated to emerge out of the human/environment field mutual process (see Table 4).

Change is continuous, relative, and innovative. The increasing diversity of field patterning characterizes this process of change. Individual differences serve only to point up the significance of this relative diversity. For example, changing rhythmicities possess individual uniqueness. The transition from longer sleeping, to longer waking, to beyond waking is highly variable between individuals. Moreover, further diversity is manifested in so-called "day people" and "night people" as well as in other examples of rhythmical diversity.

Field pattern has been a central idea in this system from its inception over 25 years ago. It is interesting to note that Ferguson (1980) wrote in her book *The Aquarian Conspiracy* that "synthesis and pattern seeing are survival skills of the 21st Century." Ferguson's comment is certainly apropos to the science of unitary human beings. Pattern reveals itself through its manifestations. These manifestations are continuously innovative while the evolution of life and non-life is a dynamic, irreducible, non-linear process characterized by increasing complexification of energy field patterning. The nature of change is unpredictable and increasingly diverse. The rhythms and motion that "seem continuous" refer to a wave frequency so rapid that the observer perceives it as a single, unbroken event. Not only is field pattern diversity relative for any

Table 4. Manifestations of Field Patterning in Unitary Human Beings

The evolution of unitary human beings is a dynamic, irreducible, non-linear process characterized by increasing diversity of energy field patterning. Manifestations of patterning emerge out of the human/environment field mutual process and are continuously innovative. Pattern is an abstraction that reveals itself through its manifestations.

The nature of unitary field patterning is unpredictable and creative. Change is relative and increasingly diverse. Some manifestations of relative diversity in field patterning are noted below.

lesser diversity		greater diversity
longer rhythms	shorter rhythms	seems continuous
slower motion	faster motion	seems continuous
time experienced as slower	time experienced as faster	timelessness
pragmatic	imaginative	visionary
longer sleeping	longer waking	beyond waking

Reprinted with permission from The National League for Nursing, *Visions of Rogers' science-based nursing,* 1990, p. 9.

given individual, but there is also a marked increase in diversity between individuals. The implications of this for increased individualization of nursing services are explicit.

Pandimensionality

A universe of open systems underwrites the growing diversity of people and their environments. Pandimensionality characterizes these human and environmental fields and all reality is postulated to be pandimensional. Within this postulate the relative nature of change becomes explicit. The use of the term "pandimensional" to replace the terms "four dimensional" and "multidimensional" does not represent any change in definition. One does not move into or become pandimensional. Rather, this is a way of perceiving reality. Efforts to select words best suited to portray one's thoughts are at best difficult because words are often inadequate to fully communicate the meaning of a particular postulate. One useful analogy of pandimensionality, however, can be found in Abbott's (1952) *Flatland.* Here, the term pandimensional provides for an infinite domain without limit. It best expresses the idea of a unitary whole, and it is defined as a nonlinear domain without spatial or temporal attributes.

The abstract system exists as an irreducible whole; principles and theories derive from this irreducible whole. The nature of change finds expression in the principles of homeodynamics. New knowledge is contributing continuously to revisions of thinking. A significant change in one word in the principle of helicy occurred. Interestingly enough this change from probability to unpredictability is consistent with the abstract system, and new knowledge supports it. Some clarification is in order. The reader is familiar with the currently accepted transition from absolutism to probability. The literature now points up that unpredictability transcends probability. Mallove (1989) in the May/June 1989 issue of *The Planetary Report* writes, "To find in the late 20th Century that unpredictability plays a significant role in the orderly celestial arena is not only a surprising development but a revolutionary one in the history of science" (p. 12). Moreover, Peterson (1989) in the July 15, 1989, issue of *Science News* discussed further the unpredictability of self-organizing critical systems.

The deletion of probability from the abstract system underlying the science of unitary human beings and the addition of unpredictability strengthen consistency and support the nature of change proposed in the principles of homeodynamics. This continuous change emerges out of nonequilibrium and exhibits punctualism not gradualism. In addition, change is accelerating. Chaos theory, too, is transforming the way we think of the world (Crum, 1989; Peterson, 1989; Percival, 1989; Stewart, 1989).

Theories in the Science of Unitary Human Beings

A theory of accelerating evolution deriving from the science of unitary human beings puts in different perspective today's rapidly changing norms in blood pressure levels, children's behavior, longer waking periods, and other events. The higher frequency wave patterns manifesting growing diversity portend new norms to coordinate with this accelerating change. Labels of pathology that are based on old norms may generate hypochondriasis and iatrogenesis in patients. Normal means average. Normal (average) blood pressure readings in all age groups are notably higher today than they were a few decades ago. Not only has the average waking period lengthened, but sleep/wake continuities are increasingly diverse. Interestingly, gifted children and the so-called hyperactive not uncommonly manifest similar behaviors. It would seem more reasonable, then, to hypothesize that hyperactivity was accelerating evolution, rather than to denigrate rhythmicities that diverge from outdated norms and erroneous expectations.

Manifestations of the speeding up of human field rhythms are coordinate with higher frequency environmental field patterns. Humans and their environments evolve and change together. Therefore, radiating increments of widely diverse frequencies are common household accompaniments of everyday life. Environmental motion has quickened, while atmospheric and cosmological complexity continue to grow.

Accelerating change characterized by higher wave frequency field patterns might be expected to manifest itself in new norms with a wider range of distribution of difference among individuals. The doomsayers who claim that people are destroying themselves are in error. On the contrary, there is population explosion, increased longevity, escalating levels of science and technology, the development of space communities, and multiple other evidences of human potential in the process of actualization.

With increased longevity, there are growing numbers of older persons. And contrary to a static view engendered by a closed system model of the universe that postulates aging to be a decline, the science of unitary human beings postulates aging to be a continuously creative process. Aging evolves from conception through the dying process. The aging of a unitary human field is not a running down. Rather, field patterns become increasingly diverse as older people need less sleep, and sleep-wake frequencies become more varied. Higher frequency patterns give meaning to multiple reports of time perceived as racing.

The pandimensional nature of reality is of further relevance. A non-linear domain points up the invalidity of chronological age as a basis for differentiating human change. In fact, as evolutionary diversity continues to accelerate, the range and variety of differences between individuals also increase; the more diverse field patterns evolve more rapidly than the less diverse ones. Populations defy so-called normal curves as individual differences multiply.

In spite of this, the emergence of paranormal phenomena as valid subjects for serious scientific research has been handicapped by a paucity of viable theories to explain these events. The nature of the science of unitary human beings provides a framework to examine such theories. Pandimensional reality as conceptualized is a factor in deriving testable hypotheses.

The ability to explain precognition, deja vu, and clairvoyance becomes a rational process in pandimensional human and environmental fields. Within this science such occurrences become "normal" rather than "paranormal." The implications for creative health services under these conditions are notable. As a result, alternative forms of healing have become increasingly popular and some forms are surprisingly effective. Meditative modalities, for example, bespeak "beyond waking" manifestations, and the use of therapeutic touch has been documented as efficacious.

Theories continue to be derived from this science. As these theories are tested some will be supported; others will not. Replication and testing of theories by research methods will contribute to one's level of confidence in a given theory. Thus, everyday events, examined through this new worldview, will provide a fresh perspective, raise new questions, and allow new explanations.

Research results from studies concerned with unitary human beings and their environments support the nature of change postulated in the principles of homeodynamics (Barrett, 1990; Malinski, 1986; Sarter, 1988). New tools of measurement have become essential adjuncts to studying questions that arise out of a worldview quite different from the prevalent view. The research potentials of this new system are infinite. It is logically and scientifically tenable, flexible and open-ended. It is a new reality and encompasses new ways of thinking, new questions, and new interpretations. It also requires consistency with the system if one is to study it. The practical implications for human betterment are demonstrable.

The Science and Art of Nursing Practice

Seeing the world from this viewpoint requires a new synthesis, a creative leap, and the inculcation of new attitudes and values. The guiding principles of this science are broad generalizations that require imaginative and innovative modalities for their implementation. The science of unitary human beings identifies nursing's uniqueness and signifies the potential of nurses to fulfill their social responsibility in human service.

Nursing, therefore, is inseparable from the new worldview and the process of change. A new vision of a world encompassing far more than planet earth is in the making. The science of nursing emerges out of this space-age worldview. The evidence of diversifying wholeness is substantial. For instance, the pace of evolution from clans to tribes, to city-states, to nation-states, to one planet is accelerating.

The future, as well, is one of growing diversity, of accelerating evolution, and of nonrepeating rhythmicities. As such, it demands new visions, flexibility, curiosity, imagination, courage, risk taking, compassion, and above all, an excellent sense of humor.

The science of unitary human beings sparks new modalities that evolve as life evolves from earth to space and beyond. Spin-offs from space study and travel can lead to more effective services for Homo sapiens on planet earth. A positive attitude toward change will be generated while vision and imagination grow.

The purpose of nursing is to promote human betterment wherever people are, on planet earth or in outer space. As diversity increases, so too will individualization of services. How can nurses best demonstrate imagination and ingenuity in helping people design ways to fulfill their different rhythmic patterns? One method is to provide community-based health services. Community-based health services must take precedence over shrinking hospital-based sick services. Moreover, the term community-based takes on enhanced meaning as it is defined to include multiple extraterrestrial centers. Supportive services such as hospitals provide an orientation toward pathology, not toward health. Although both community agencies and hospitals provide meaningful services, it is the broad community-based health promotion services that provide the umbrella. As a defined orientation toward health takes place, fewer and fewer people will need the same type of sick services that currently exist. Nevertheless, nothing in this science suggests that humans will be freed from all "disease" and live happily ever after. Disease and pathology are value terms applied when the human field manifests characteristics that may be deemed undesirable. One of today's major health problems is nosophobia, a morbid dread of disease.

Autonomous nursing practice directed by nurses holding valid baccalaureate and higher degrees with an upper division major in nursing science is central to the future. Noninvasive therapeutic modalities are emphasized in this new reality (Barrett, 1990). The practice of therapeutic touch, developed by Krieger (1981), is already in use in many places around this planet. The use of humor, sound, color, and motion also continue to undergo investigation. Additionally, the concept of unconditional love is receiving attention. Attitudes of hope, humor, and upbeat moods have often been documented as better therapy than drugs. Imagery and meditative modalities have much to offer as well. Continued emphasis on human rights, client decision-making, and noncompliance with the traditional rules of thumb are also necessary dimensions of the new science and art of nursing. In addition to this, the noninvasive therapeutic modalities, increasingly emphasized by a range of health care workers, mark the future of nursing practice on this planet and in outer space.

The outcomes of the research in the science of nursing have been reported in the literature and are now finding their way into the practice arena wherever people are (Barrett, 1990; Malinski, 1986; Sarter, 1988). Such research enables one to understand better the nature of human evolution and its multiple, unpredictable potentialities. Description, explanation, and vision strengthen a nurse's ability to practice according to the level and scope of preparation and knowledge in the science of nursing. What is more, holistic trends open up new ways of thinking and spell new worldviews. Other new modalities will emerge out of this evolution toward spacekind that will spark more effective modalities for earthkind.

Caring is one practice modality getting much attention from nurses today. However, as such, caring does not identify nurses any more than it identifies workers from another field. Everyone needs to care; the nature of caring in a given field depends entirely on the body of scientific knowledge specific to the field. Caring is simply a way of using knowledge. Nurses care on the basis of ways they use the science of unitary, irreducible human beings.

Since today's world is rapidly becoming an entrepreneurial society, and nurses continue to move into its mainstream, a substantive knowledge base in a science of nursing has become indispensable. In addition, there is as well a critical need for mutual respect and valuing of differences between all health personnel: between nurses, between health fields, and between the fields of science.

Human beings are on the threshold of a fantastic and unimagined future. In light of this, the potential for human service is greater than it has ever been before. Many nurses have been moving apace to assure that there will be a substantive body of theoretical knowledge specific to nursing to underwrite the practice of nursing. The science of unitary human beings portends a new world in space, the next frontier.

References

Abbott, E. A. (1952). *Flatland,* New York: Dover.

Barrett, E. A. M. (Ed.) (1990). *Visions of Rogers' science-based nursing.* New York: National League for Nursing.

Bohm, D. (1980). *Wholeness and the implicate order.* Boston: Routledge & Kegan Paul.

Capra, F. (1982). *The turning point.* New York: Simon and Schuster.

Crum, R. (1989). Why Johnny kills. *New York University Magazine, 4*(2), 34.

Downs, F. (1988). Nursing research: State-of-the-art. *Journal of the New York State Nurses Association, 19*(3), 20.

Ferguson, M. (1980). *The aquarian conspiracy.* Los Angeles: Tarcher.

Friedman, S. T. (1989). Who believes in UFO's? *International UFO Reporter, 14*(1), 6–10.

Fuller, R. B. (1981). *Critical path.* New York: St. Martin's Press.

Huxley, A. (1932). *Brave new world.* New York: Modern Library.

Kenton, L. (1990). Member forum. *Noetic Sciences Bulletin, 5*(1), 6.

Krieger, D. (1981). *Foundations for holistic health nursing practices: The renaissance nurse.* Philadelphia: Lippincott.

Lauden, L. (1977). *Progress and its problems: Toward a theory of scientific growth.* Berkeley: University of California Press.

Lovelock, J. (1988). *The age of Gaia.* New York: Norton.

Malinski, V. M. (Ed.) (1986). *Exploration on Martha Rogers' science of unitary human beings.* Norwalk, CT: Appleton-Century-Crofts.

Mallove, E. T. (1989, May-June). The solar system in chaos. *The Planetary Report,* pp. 12–13.

Percival, I. (1989). Chaos: A science for the real world. *New Scientist, 123,* 42–47.

Peterson, I. (1989, July). Digging into sand. *Science News, 136,* 40.

Robinson, G. S. & White, H. M. (1986). *Envoys of mankind.* Washingon, D.C.: Smithsonian Institute Press.

Rogers, M. E. (1970). *An introduction to the theoretical basis of nursing.* Philadelphia: Davis.

Sarter, B. (1988). *The stream of becoming: A study of Martha Rogers' theory.* New York: National League for Nursing.

Stewart, I. (1989). *Does God play dice? The mathematics of chaos.* Cambridge, MA: Brasil Blackwell, Inc.

Weber, R. (Ed.). (1986). *Dialogue with scientists and sages: The search for unity.* New York: Routledge & Kegan Paul.

Weber, R., Bohm, D., & Sheldrake, R. (1986). Matter as a meaning field. In R. Weber (Ed.), *Dialogue with scientists and sages: The search for unity* (pp. 105–123). New York: Routledge & Kegan Paul.

SECTION FIVE

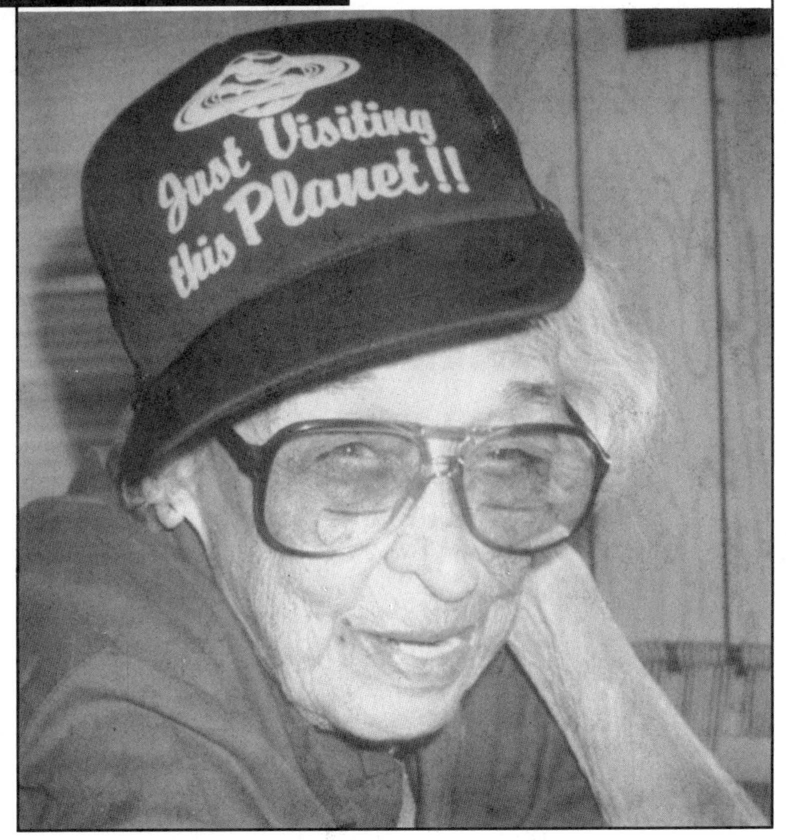

Just visiting. Martha E. Rogers at the 1991 summer meeting of Region 7 of the Society of Rogerian Scholars, Fernandina Beach, Florida. (Photograph by Martha H. Bramlett.)

Futuristic Visions

Section Editor
Elizabeth Ann Manhart Barrett

CHAPTER 46

On the Threshold of Tomorrow

Elizabeth Ann Manhart Barrett

If the future of nursing lies with the innovators, the rebels, the critical thinkers, Rogers as role model is unsurpassable. Her light has led the way. Quoting her role model, perhaps, Rogers noted that "Florence Nightingale said it rightly. No system can endure that does not march" (Rogers, 1983, p. 800). Nightingale and Rogers, sharing May 12 for entering the world 94 years apart, marched to their own unique yet similar drummers. They marched not alone but twirling the baton of leadership that freed a synergistic burst of power shared by all who participated in this nursing quest.

Rogers integrated zealous commitment for lighting candles to illuminate the darkness of ignorance in nursing and burning inspiration for lighting fires to accelerate the unrolling march of the profession. Beginning with an *n* of one, those who embrace the Rogerian paradigm have grown toward a critical mass with potential for not only transforming nursing but also provoking profound change in the health care system.

Convinced that "we are moving into a future filled with promise of the unexpected" (Rogers, 1986, p. 1), Rogers often told her students to "dream big." Her own view was continuously beyond the horizon. As she enthusiastically labored with love to achieve her ideals, no challenge was too great, no obstacle insurmountable.

Numerous futuristic themes representing her commitments concerning nursing permeated the entirety of her career. Some of these themes included:

1. Nursing as a learned profession
2. Nursing as a basic science whose phenomenon of concern is irreducible human beings in mutual process with their irreducible environments whether on earth or in space
3. Nursing as a noun meaning "to know" rather than a verb meaning "to do"
4. Baccalaureate education in nursing as preparation for beginning professional autonomous practice with a separate licensure

5. Collaboration between the baccalaureate-educated nurse and other peer professionals with a mutual respect for their differences and unique contributions to humans' search for health and well-being
6. Society's entitlement to nursing services of differing degrees of complexity delivered by nursing personnel prepared for various responsibilities
7. Optimism about people, the environment, and their mutual ongoing process of change

Nursing in Space

It is difficult to prioritize Rogers' contributions to nursing as a scientist, educator, politician, and futurist. Nor are these roles mutually exclusive. While one could argue that all of her work is futuristic, it is Rogers' contribution to nursing in space that is most uniquely futuristic. The science of unitary irreducible human and environmental energy fields provides direction for research that indeed will allow nursing to make a signal contribution to promotion of health and well-being for people—in space as well as on earth.

Rogers' interest in nursing in space as nursing of the future mushroomed in the late 1980s. This interest, however, was evident as early as the 1960s. For example, during the reign of Rogers' presidency, the sixth bienniel convention of the New York State League for Nursing (NYSLN) featured the theme of the "Nurse in the Space Age." This was 1962, seven years before a human walked on the moon (Rogers, 1962). Two years later in 1964 at the NYSLN convention Rogers remarked during her keynote address that "soon man will walk upon the moon" (Rogers, 1966).

Now who else in nursing was talking about space during the 1960s? Yet, this is not surprising since Rogers' work has been and continues to be consistent with current happenings in contemporary science. While not the same and unique to nursing, Rogers' paradigm is supported by similar, new worldview frameworks (Bohm, 1980; Gleick, 1987; Prigogine, 1980; Sheldrake, 1988).

Rogers' science and her dreams for humankind are science and dreams for spacekind as well. She maintained that the terrestrial and extraterrestrial cannot be separated and that the Science of Unitary Human Beings provided an explanatory system equally relevant for life and health on earth and in space (Doyle, Racolin, Rogers, and Walsh, 1990). She noted that space offers a new frontier, not the last frontier, where humans will experience in new ways the unimaginable and previously unknown. Knowing that the future is innovative and unpredictable, she has continually proclaimed that the future will not be a repetition of the past.

Autonomy Is Essential to Nursing's Survival

Evolutionary emergence, innovative complexification, and infinite potential bespeak Rogers' message for the future of humankind just as nursing science–based autonomous practice bespeaks the future of nursing's mandate for societal services. Concomitantly, another theme has concerned lines of demarcation and definitions of nursing, medicine, health care, and medical care. In this regard she quoted Nightingale, who admonished, "Experience teaches me

. . . that nursing and medicine must never be mixed up. It spoils both'' (Cope, 1958, p. 121). She was also clear that nursing care is not medical care. Rather, nursing care is an aspect of the overall umbrella of health care, which is more than medical care. As early as 1972 she prophesied that ''hospitals will become one of a wide range of satellite services'' (Rogers, 1972, p. 10). For many years she advocated nursing's role in health care reform.

Rogers spoke of differences among professions and the necessity for avoiding value judgments. Nevertheless, she was never hesitant to tell it as she saw it and challenged what she considered unethical behavior in nursing, medicine, health care institutions, and related industries. At the same time genuine interdisciplinary collaboration based on autonomous, distinct disciplinary purposes and distinct bodies of knowledge was an enduring goal with no room for compromise of values or scientific tenets.

Society of Rogerian Scholars

From 1982 to 1992 four international Rogerian conferences were held at New York University. They were sponsored by four New York University groups: Division of Nursing, Division of Nursing Alumni, Upsilon Chapter of Sigma Theta Tau International, and the Doctoral Students Organization. These conferences have presented state-of-the-science-and-art information regarding research, practice, and education based on Rogerian science. Opportunities for networking have been an important feature of these conferences. Future conferences are being planned.

Another avenue for future development of this science is the Society of Rogerian Scholars. The Society of Rogerian Scholars was chartered by the State of New York as a nonprofit corporation in 1988. All interested persons are invited to join this international organization. [For information, contact Society of Rogerian Scholars, Inc., telephone (800) 474-9793.] In addition to a newsletter published four times a year, a journal has been initiated with Violet M. Malinski and Sheila Cheema serving as co-editors of both the newsletter and journal. The history, mission statement, and purposes of the society will be quoted from the original 1988 bylaws and a brochure produced in 1992.

The idea for the Society of Rogerian Scholars was born in the living room of Martha Rogers' New York City apartment in November 1986. We were fortunate in having the opportunity to meet with Dr. Rogers twice a month for ongoing inquiry into the Science of Unitary Human Beings. Realizing that few people had this opportunity, we explored how to facilitate discussion and networking efforts among the widest possible audience. We decided that the best vehicle would be a formal organization that could provide services such as publishing a newsletter and sponsoring seminars. We called ourselves the Dreamers' Think Tank. The dream is reality—The Society of Rogerian Scholars, Inc. The founders and original Board of Directors were:

Elizabeth Ann Manhart Barrett, R.N., Ph.D., President
John R. Phillips, R.N., Ph.D., Vice-President
Thérése Connell Meehan, R.N., Ph.D., Secretary
Violet M. Malinski, R.N., Ph.D., Treasurer
Martha E. Rogers, R.N., Sc.D., F.A.A.N.

The mission of the Society of Rogerian Scholars, Inc., is to advance nursing science through an emphasis on the Science of Unitary Human Beings. The focus of the society is education, research, and practice in service to humankind.

The purposes are to:

1. Advance nursing as a basic science
2. Explore the meaning of a philosophy of wholeness for nursing
3. Foster the understanding and the use of the Science of Unitary Human Beings as a basis for theory development, research, education, and practice
4. Provide avenues for dissemination of information related to the Science of Unitary Human Beings
5. Foster a network for communicating the Science of Unitary Human Beings
6. Create forums for scholarly debate
7. Provide educational forums on the Science of Unitary Human Beings

Where Do We Go from Here?

Rogers has been known to many as a visionary, a prophet, a risk taker. Indeed, she is nursing's quintessential futurist. Hailing her as a futurist in no way conflicts with her endorsement of a future that is unpredictable. As she says, "one can speculate." Contrary to popular opinion, futurists do not predict the future; they are well aware that the future is unpredictable.

As a futurist, Rogers has suggested possibilities that might happen so that people could more fully participate in creating what they want to happen. Knowing the potentialities of the future, and even this does not frequently occur, facilitates free choice in actualizing possibles. Whether referring to individuals or members of various types of groups, including professions, organizations, and societies, Rogers emphasized that humans have many potentials, only some of which will be actualized. Her science was presented as an optimistic although not utopian view. Rogers exemplified this philosophy by being quick to differ sharply with discouraging doomsayers predicting disaster. Instead, she emphasized that humans change as the environment changes, and, therefore, predictions of disastrous human consequences of environmental changes may be off the mark.

Some believe the hundredth monkey phenomenon (Newman, 1979), with Rogers being the first monkey, is just beyond the horizon of the next millennium. Whether or not knowledge of the Science of Unitary Human Beings will reach the threshold of a critical mass beyond which it will become widely known and applied in nursing and beyond remains to be seen. Those who embrace Rogerian science–based nursing have grown in numbers throughout the continent and in numerous countries outside of North America.

Rogers charged nurses to go forward with further development of her legacy and proposed, "The future demands new visions, flexibility, curiosity, imagination, courage, risk-taking, compassion, and an excellent sense of humor" (Rogers, 1988, p. 102). Who among us will accept the challenge? Are we ready?

Only the future will reveal what changes in the science and art of nursing will flower from the seed she planted. Even now, one can hear the beat of her drum beckoning, "Press on, humankind and spacekind are waiting" (M. Madrid, personal communication, May 10, 1992).

References

The art of forecasting. (1986). Bethesda, MD: The World Future Society.
Bohm, D. (1980). *Wholeness and the implicate order.* London: Routledge and Kegan Paul.
Cope, Z. (1958). *Florence Nightingale and the doctors.* Philadelphia: Lippincott.
Doyle, M. B., Racolin, A., Rogers, M. E., & Walsh, P. C. (1990). A conversation with Martha Rogers on nursing in space. In E. A. M. Barrett (Ed.), *Visions of Rogers' science-based nursing* (pp. 375–386). New York: National League for Nursing.
Gleick, J. (1987). *Chaos.* New York: Penguin.
Newman, M. (1979). *Theory development in nursing.* Philadelphia: Davis.
Prigogine, I. (1980). *From being to becoming.* San Francisco: Freeman.
Rogers, M. E. (1962). Have you reserved your place in space? *League Lines, NYSLN, 8*(1), 7.
Rogers, M. E. (1966, June). *Quality nursing: Cliche or challenge?* Paper presented at the American Nurses Association Convention and Clinical Sessions, San Francisco, CA.
Rogers, M. E. (1972). Nursing's expanding role and other euphemisms. *Journal of the New York State Nurses Association, 3*(4), 5–10.
Rogers, M. E. (1983). Beyond the horizon. In N. L. Chaska (Ed.), *The nursing profession: A time to speak* (pp. 795–801). New York: McGraw-Hill.
Rogers, M. E. (1986, June). Commencement address. Presented at graduation, Mercy College, Dobbs Ferry, NY.
Rogers, M. E. (1988). Nursing science and art: A prospective. *Nursing Science Quarterly, 1,* 99–102.
Sheldrake, R. (1988). *The presence of the past.* New York: Times Books.

CHAPTER 47

The Future of Nursing

Martha E. Rogers

A century ago a group of the world's foremost mathematicians "proved" that a railroad train could not exceed 21 miles an hour because if it did, the air would be forced out of it and the passengers would die of suffocation.

Today researchers at the Rand Corporation in California are working on a very high speed transit "tube craft" system in which electromagnetic waves will shoot vehicles underground at 14,000 miles per hour to deliver passengers from New York City to Los Angeles in 21 minutes at a charge variously quoted from $6 to $50 a ticket. For outer space travel a starship engine is proposed that will make it possible to get from Earth to the Moon in 13 seconds and to the nearest star in 43 years—using already available technology. Distance is kaleidoscoping—soon the stars will be as close as next door.

Microelectronics are altering almost every aspect of human life. Instant information, home banking, self-guided planes and cars are coming off the drawing boards. Computerized records invade man's privacy. The drug industry furthers a mechanistic model of man. Ultra-sonic sewing machines make needle and thread out-dated. Flexible working hours have become so popular that the term "flex-time" is being considered for inclusion in the dictionary. 625 page books can now be microfilmed on one page, read with a viewer the size of a paperback book, sold for 25 cents, and thrown away at will.

Ecologists and environmentalists cry wolf. A multiplicity of drugs are avidly searching for some new disease to conquer. Human rights are abrogated faster than they are advocated. Bureaucratic imperatives grow. Iatrogenesis (medically induced disease), nosocomial diseases, and hypochondriasis are mass-marketed and constitute today's major health problems in the U.S.A.

Man is no longer planet bound. Space communities are on the threshold of reality. A human being has been reported to have been cloned. Genetic engineering has opened a Pandora's box and genetic counseling is rife with scientific invalidities deriving from outdated worldviews. The U.S. Supreme Court has approved patent rights for new life forms.

Rogers, M. E. (1980, March). *The future of nursing.* Paper presented at the University of Louisville, Louisville, KY.

Illness is the second largest business in the United States. Inflationary charges are rampant, with hospitals and medical doctors accounting for most of them—approximately double other areas. Profits are large and the quality of care is far from good. The January issue of *Nursing '77* reported a survey of 10,000 nurses in which approximately 40 percent stated they would not be hospitalized in the hospital in which they worked. Miller and Stokes in a paper titled "Health Status, Health Resources, and Consolidated Structural Parameters: Implications for Health Care Policy" which appeared in the September 1978 issue of the *Journal of Health and Social Behavior* reported that as the ratio of physicians and facilities to population increased, the death rate also increased. Concomitantly they also reported that as the ratio of nurses to population increased, the death rate decreased. Over half the prescription drugs in use are in the psychotropic, sedative, tranquilizer area. A litigious society is having a field day with a multitude of events proposed to be responsible for all manner of health problems—both real and imagined.

The public is demanding a nature and amount of health services not available and scarcely imagined. And let me make it clear—health services are *not* to be equated with medical services and hospital services. Medical doctors are only one of a range of health personnel—neither more nor less significant than any other health discipline. The public is asking for emphasis on community-based health services in contradiction to hospital-based sick services. Hospitals properly constitute one of a range of satellite services. An overabundance of medical doctors is a reality, and there are presently too many hospital beds. Many people are refusing to go to the hospital to avoid exposure to "extraordinary measures" to maintain vital signs. Hospitals are seeking to diversify their service and to advertise their wares not unlike the automobile, oil, and tobacco industries.

The stranglehold of the allopathic medical monopoly denies human rights to freedom of choice, informed consent, and a socially and economically viable national health plan (which I note has *not* yet been proposed). Efforts to control the practice of professionals in fields other than medicine, whether these be clinical psychologists, social workers, or dentists, or nurses, or some other discipline, ignore the reality that medical doctors have neither the knowledge nor competence to supervise or determine practice in any field except medicine. And let me be clear, nursing is not part of medicine. Medicine has stepped up its efforts to encroach on other fields—nursing and psychology in particular.

What does all this have to do with the future of nursing? Modern nursing's history encompasses many firsts in the nation's health services. Independence of action and the courage of their convictions characterized modern nursing's early leaders. They marched for woman suffrage—and went to jail for human rights. They believed that knowledge made a difference and that their responsibility was to the people they purported to serve. They knew what they were for, *not* just what they were against, and that is essential.

For more than a hundred years the scope of nursing has encompassed broad concern for the health of people. Nightingale's claim that the art of health nursing was as important as the art of sick nursing has been made explicit in nursing's century-old continuous and uninterrupted development of family health care, community-based health maintenance and promotion, and national and international leadership in designing and initiating public health measures—with care and rehabilitation of the sick and disabled a constant concomitant of nursing's efforts to maintain and promote health. Primary nursing care is as old as modern nursing. (And primary nursing care is not primary medical care). Direct accountability to the public is a legal fact.

Nursing's social and professional evolution has accelerated. The historical accident that initiated schools of nursing in hospitals delayed but did not stop nursing's entry into the nation's developing educational mainstream. Simultaneously power, profits, and politics rear pecking orders of seemingly growing strength. Escalating science and technology, feminism, new value systems, a massive corporate structure, and shifting power empires combine to threaten the status quo. Nurses are conned into leaving nursing with glittering euphemisms and promises that match the rainbows in the sky. Power, profits, politics, and propaganda are powerful.

Antieducationism, gullibility, dependency continue to plague nurses and nursing and to leave us vulnerable to the onslaught of vested interests. We must make an affirmative recommitment to nursing as a socially significant endeavor, assert our moral purposes, and regain the momentum of an earlier day. Concomitant with all other changes taking place, nursing is moving firmly and rapidly out of its prescientific era into a uniquely scientifically based field of endeavor.

Nursing's educational system prepares persons for three clearly different entry levels to practice. Licensure to practice is provided for only two of these levels: specifically, (1) the registered nurse level (for which associate degree programs and hospital schools prepare) and (2) the practical nurse level. No licensure is provided for the baccalaureate level of practice although human safety requires the knowledgeable judgments afforded by valid baccalaureate education in nursing.

That baccalaureate graduates currently take the same licensing examination as do hospital school and associate degree graduates is no more valid than if dentists were licensed according to their performance on a licensing examination for dental hygienists or medical doctors according to their scores on a physician's assistant examination or engineers according to how they achieved as engineering technicians. Moreover, a baccalaureate degree in a field other than nursing does *not* qualify a registered nurse to practice at a baccalaureate level in nursing.

Is the engineering technician who secures a baccalaureate degree in sociology qualified to practice as an engineer? Will a degree in psychology qualify the physician's assistant to practice as a medical doctor? Will a degree in biology for a dental hygienist create a dentist?

Failure to establish legal standards and to license at the baccalaureate level of practice in nursing leaves the public to be victimized by (1) persons granted baccalaureate degrees in the absence of a baccalaureate education in nursing, (2) unreasonable expectations of associate degree, hospital school, and practical nurse graduates, and (3) a health care system that endeavors to deny persons holding a valid baccalaureate degree in nursing their rights and responsibilities to use their knowledge for human betterment.

Concomitantly, there is continuing need for licensure of nurse graduates of associate degree and hospital schools (as long as the latter shall continue). These graduates are prepared for a career in nursing that society values and needs—a career worthy of honor and respect in itself. These graduates do not need to be "upgraded" in order to be socially significant. The words "registered nurse" and the letters "RN" identify this population. These nurses make decisions within the scope of their preparation and function with appropriate direction from nursing's baccalaureate and higher degree graduates.

Baccalaureate education in nursing prepares a general practitioner of nursing—a person who works directly with people, who gives direct nursing services, and who makes those intellectual judgments demanding substantive nursing knowledge. Do not confuse practitioners of nursing with nurse-practitioners.

Nursing's identity, its uniqueness, the sources of its scientific knowledge are imperative for socially responsible professional autonomy. If nurses are to be socially responsive participants and leaders in revolutionizing a health system that is in crisis, then there must be knowledgeable nursing commensurate with escalating science and technology and with human needs.

The identification of nursing as a learned profession demands that it be underwritten by an organized abstract system from which to derive hypothetical generalizations and unifying principles—the descriptive, explanatory, and predictive principles essential to knowledgeable nursing practice. Science is the study of relationships. A profession is a science and an art.

Nursing's leadership in designing and participating in the development and implementation of health services that spell mutual respect for the knowledge and skills of all is imperative. People are our business. They are why we exist. The future is something we create.

CHAPTER 48

A Scenario for Nursing in 2001 A.D.

Martha E. Rogers

In less than two decades the 21st century begins. Escalating science and technology have already foretold a changing pace. Communities in outer space have moved into reality. Alternatives in health services and in health personnel multiply. Nursing has emerged as a creative scientific endeavor attuned to accelerating diversity. Social responsibility has taken on new dimensions. Identifiable professional and technical careers magnify nursing's potential for human service. Anti-educationism has faded. Knowledgeable independence asserts itself. Nursing is a learned discipline.

Opportunities in nursing encompass planetary and cosmic settings. Humanitarian values burgeon. Vision expands. Interventive modalities are directed toward changing values in health. Independent professional practice, autonomous nursing centers, and interdisciplinary peer collaboration presage new avenues to well-being. The findings of research in nursing add novel perspectives in the evolution of life.

The pragmatics of "how we got there from here" are not so difficult as some imagine. Change is inevitable. The capacity of people to participate knowingly in the nature of change is supported. Within the context of rapidly changing times nurses too quicken their gaits. Licensure for baccalaureate level graduates as well as R.N. licensure for A.D.N. and hospital school graduates furthers public safety. Irreducible unitary human beings identify nursing's uniqueness. A knowledge base specific to nursing engenders interventive modalities commensurate with a new world view.

Nursing's paradigm generates unifying principles and hypothetical generalizations necessary to description, explanation, and prediction. Utilization of nursing knowledge for human betterment takes place wherever people are. Mutual respect for differences in knowledges and skills between levels of

---

Rogers, M. E. (1982, December). A scenario for nursing in 2001 A.D. *SAIN Newsletter,* pp. 1–2. Reprinted with permission.

nurses and between nursing and other fields emphasizes freedom of choice for alternatives in health personnel according to human need.

Autonomous nursing centers are well established on this planet and in outer space. Independent professionally educated (baccalaureate and higher degree) nurses are responsible for their own practice and for appropriate guidance of technical vocational nurses. Nursing is not dependent on any other discipline for either its knowledge or skills. Concomitantly interdisciplinary cooperation is demonstrable.

High speed transit systems on this planet enable nurses (as well as others) to work and study hundreds of miles from where they live should they wish to do so. Laser beams shoot people daily to space communities. Video technology provides multiple networks for uniting people toward probabilistic goals of self-fulfillment.

Designs for health utilize human potentials as a primary source of therapy. Hospitals, drugs, and scalpels are rare accouterments reserved for the esoteric and selected cases. Iatrogenesis, nosocomial conditions, and hypochondriasis are increasingly scarce as new designs replace an out-dated system.

Nursing in the year 2001 A.D. carries a major responsibility for determining the nature of services directed toward achieving human well-being. How nurses fulfill this responsibility is already in the making. Tomorrow's reality will far exceed our speculations.

CHAPTER 49

Beyond the Horizon

Martha E. Rogers

To peer into the future is to enlarge one's vision to glimpse a becoming, to see with that "third eye." It is to speculate upon a dream and to watch that dream unfold. It is to create a new reality.

Man's advent into outer space made explicit this new world. Escalating science and technology help to underwrite new paradigms and to hasten the ending of the industrial age. Noise, confusion, and insecurities mount as the speed of change reaches a crescendo. Old values lie moribund among the detritus of famous last words. Man moves to transcend himself. A new scenario comes into view.

The information explosion looks embryonic as man's emerging capacities to communicate in hitherto undreamed-of ways come into focus. Seemingly instant transportation outdistances the speed of light, illusory colors, shapes, sounds, smells, tastes diversify and proliferate in kaleidoscopic novelty. The impossible is possible.

Computers that can program themselves to produce a new race of "intelligence beings" superior to human life are serious subjects for workers in artificial intelligence. The United States Supreme Court has approved patent rights for new life forms. Civilian activities in outer space are not far off.

As the turmoil of change escalates, fanatic factions vie for supremacy. Violence is explosive. Prophets of doom clamor loudly, iatrogenic and nosocomial ailments go hand in hand with hypochondriasis. Holistic jargon and multiplying meditative modalities give vague intimations of new vistas in the making. Ethical issues and human rights stir the bureaucratic ashes of mass mediocrity and portend a concern for the individual.

In this not so mythical mosaic nurses whisk through airless tunnels in very high speed transit tubecraft with Los Angeles only 21 minutes from New York City (Rosen, 1976). They travel to the moon in 13 seconds and to the nearest star in 43 years (Heppenheimer, 1977). They live and work and play in

Rogers, M. E. (1983). Beyond the horizon. In N. L. Chaska (Ed.), *The nursing profession: A time to speak* (pp. 795–801). New York: McGraw-Hill. Reprinted with permission.

earth communities of incredible design. They are as diverse as the world they live in.

Individuality marks the people of the new world. Rhythmicities of extraordinary complexity weave pulsating patterns through threads of yesteryear and the "infinite now" expands. Alternatives in health care and health workers mushroom.

No utopia this. The search for meaning goes on. Beyond the horizon potentialities abound. J. B. S. Haldane's famous epigram comes to mind. "The universe is not queerer than we imagine, it is queerer than we can imagine."

Nursing changes coordinate with the larger world of man's perception. The confusion of nurses is the confusion of all people struggling to understand the contradictions, ambiguities, and uncertainties of a world caught up in a shifting panorama of infinite potentialities. Old securities have been shattered. Belief systems are threatened. Hierarchies are tumbling down. At the same time an optimistic view of man's future is beginning to permeate the current scene. Creative excitement is emerging out of the seeming chaos. New paradigms are taking hold.

To speculate upon the future can be an exciting game. To propose direction can be a dangerous one. To predict with any degree of certainty is to dare the impossible. The past presents no vistas of events to come. But people do have the capacity to participate in creation of this fabulous world of uncertainty. How little we know poses incredible hurdles. Errors in knowing magnify the problems. Nonetheless prediction gives direction to our gropings. Flexibility allows for fallibility. Vision promises the unexpected.

Let us peer beyond the horizon into a new world of nursing. A paradigm shift is explicit. People, long the center of nursing's purpose, appear as dynamic, irreducible wholes caught up in equally dynamic environmental wholes, together manifesting innovative patterns of growing complexity. And with Ferguson I would note that "synthesis and pattern-seeing are survival skills for the twenty-first century" (1980:300). An air of optimism is apparent.

The unfolding scene reveals a diversity of nursing personnel prepared for varying responsibilities of differing degrees of complexity in a multiplicity of settings on this planet and in outer space. All people fall within the scope of nursing. Principles and theories generated by nursing's new paradigm engage scholars and scientists in nursing as they seek to push back the frontiers of knowledge. Nursing educators incorporate the findings of nursing research into a rapidly growing body of substantive knowledge specific to nursing and transmit this knowledge to students seeking professional and technical careers in nursing. Practitioners of nursing translate this knowledge into novel and unexpected uses in their efforts to promote human health and welfare.

Nurses are not alone in this new world. A range of health workers participate in man's search for well-being. But the nature of health personnel and health services has changed dramatically. A new world view provides unity in diversity. Differences are held in high esteem. The public is oriented to health. People are active participants in the developmental process. Invasive therapies and drugs are rare. Health services issue from community centers as diverse as the life-styles of these variegated people. Facilities for sick services are notably diminished in number and are tangential to the primary purposes of a new design for health.

New perspectives reinterpret observable data. No longer is aging deemed a disease. Pregnancy is not a pathological event. Dying is a developmental process. Evolutionary emergence manifests individual differences that defy old norms. Innovation is viewed with enthusiasm. Problems are seen within a new context. Interventive modalities are directed toward promotion of health and well-being. Man and his world change together.

As nursing fulfills its social and professional responsibilities to people wherever they are, the dreams of tomorrow become today's reality. A clear, unambiguous commitment to nursing as a knowledgeable endeavor and a social necessity characterizes nursing personnel.

Education of nurses is firmly within the educational mainstream, but education itself manifests dramatic revisions. Man's past and future merge. Learning is broad, substantive, and exciting. Creativity is encouraged. Individual diversity and multiple career options abound. Theoretical knowledge specific to nursing provides a foundation on which to base practice. Career differences are valued and respected. A multiplicity of settings provides opportunity for testing theories. Imaginative concern for people is dominant.

Whatever the level of preparation or functional role or planetary or cosmic setting, a new sense of self and pride in nursing has taken hold. A new security embraces future uncertainties. The nature of nursing teems with innovations. Nursing is a major resource in its own right as people seek alternatives in health services.

These preliminary comments postulate a future for nursing as a basic science and public necessity. How realistic is this? Will there be nursing beyond the horizon? Multiple roads stretch into the future. Which ones lead to dead ends for nursing? What new alliances are in the making as fields encroach on one another's preserves in sometimes mighty territorial encounters? Will there be kaleidoscopic repatterning for new syntheses that can spell the disintegration of the traditional basic sciences and professional fields? What will people be like in this new world? These are heady questions.

In today's everyday world problems loom large, disagreements are common, and proposals for change are too often pedantic modifications of the past. Transition requires new perspectives. Practical realities demand imaginative resolution coordinate with accelerating change. Social responsibility is an indispensable adjunct in nursing's evolution. To realize nursing as an identifiable scientific field of endeavor dedicated to serving human kind requires creative action.

To establish nursing's identity as a science requires a phenomenon of concern unique to nursing, an organized conceptual system specific to the phenomenon, and unifying principles and hypothetical generalizations deriving from the system. The study of unitary man as an irreducible phenomenon is unique to nursing. It is not to be confused with the current ambiguities of holism, which is commonly associated with parts and sums of parts. A paradigm specific to nursing (and relevant to other fields concerned with man and environment) constitutes an organized abstract system. Principles and theories derive from the system. An aggregate of facts and theories drawn from various sciences do not provide a valid base for the practice of nursing. Neither do such aggregates contribute to knowledge of the unitary man. A firm belief in nursing as an organized body of abstract knowledge arrived at by scientific research and logical analysis is an essential prerequisite to nurses' ability to serve people knowledgeably. Nursing as a science and an art rings the death knell for nursing's antieducationists. It is no longer tenable to proclaim "a nurse is a nurse is a nurse," whether this is done through misleading statistics that clump baccalaureate graduates indiscriminately with associate degree and hospital school graduates; or through the subterfuge that attends the New York State Nurses Association 1985 Resolution with its grandfather clause that would mislead the public into thinking that all R.N.'s are qualified to practice at a baccalaureate level; or through certification procedures that ignore educational credentials; or through nurse-practitioner courses which provide medical skills for functioning as a physician's assistant to any R.N. in programs that range from 2 months to 2 years; or through other ways.

The uniqueness of nursing, like that of any other science, is found in the phenomenon of its concern. The practice of nursing derives from nursing's body of scientific knowledge specific to nursing. Justification for the education of nurses in institutions of higher learning, whether at the associate degree level or at the baccalaureate degree level, demands the transmission of substantive knowledge specific to nursing and appropriate to the student's level of study. Continued denial that education makes a difference leaves nursing vulnerable to proponents of trained subservience. Nor does the introduction of a professional doctorate in nursing change the issue or resolve the problem. The first undergraduate professional degree, whether it is labeled B.S. or M.N. or N.D., prepares for beginning professional practice. The confusion engendered by terminological differences only aggravates the situation. Antieducationists in nursing will not survive beyond the horizon.

Second, the battles over entry levels to practice will disappear as substantive knowledge in nursing is recognized. Nursing's educational system currently prepares persons for three different entry levels to practice. Licensure exists for the vocational (L.P.N.) and technical (R.N.) levels of preparation. Social responsibility demands that there be licensure for the professional (B.S.) level. Licensure exists to safeguard the public. It does not exist to serve the worker. Nor is certification to be confused with licensure. Moreover, as certification currently exists in nursing, there is little recognition of the need for a knowledge base specific to nursing or for the qualifications of those who certify (i.e., groups outside of nursing who claim to certify nurses to practice nursing). Proposals to place more control for certification with nurses continue to overlook a need for theoretical knowledge specific to nursing. Antieducationism in nursing denies safety to society and furthers the demise of nursing. "Beyond the horizon" demands a cohort of nurses firmly committed to "something to know in nursing" and ready and willing to assume the legal and personal responsibility it entails.

Next, nurses must get off the euphemistic merry-go-round. Nurse practitioners are not practitioners of nursing. Practitioners of nursing are not physicians' assistants. Primary nursing is not primary medicine. The "expanded role" might be better interpreted as a cover-up for medicine's encroachment on nursing's long established practices than as something new for nurses. Interestingly enough, many of those who have left nursing to become nurse-practitioner–physician assistants are destined to wake up in a dead-end avenue as an already documented oversupply of medical doctors becomes increasingly explicit. Of further significance it is reported that as the ratio of medical doctors and facilities to population increases, the death rate also increases, whereas as the ratio of nurses to population goes up, the death rate drops (Miller and Stokes, 1978). Such evidence suggests careful reexamination by those who have jumped on the bandwagon of medical skills as a way to save nursing and gain status.

The health care system is caught in a medical monopoly. Hospitals are big business (Goldsmith, 1980). Charges by hospitals and medical doctors have increased at a rate vastly in excess of the rest of the nation's economy. Too many hospital beds and frequent unnecessary hospitalizations are well documented. Hospitals are seeking to diversify their services and to advertise their wares, not unlike the products of the automobile, oil, and tobacco industries. A mammoth effort is ongoing to maintain a traditional power and profit structure replete with third-party payments. Meanwhile an awakening public is seeking alternatives in health services and personnel that they deem more effective as well as less costly.

Community-based health services developed under the aegis of nursing. A renewal of nursing leadership that will continue and enhance the broad scope of nursing's concerns and capabilities is essential. Nursing knowledge and nursing practice are the responsibility of nurses knowledgeable and competent to exercise such responsibility. Dependence on other fields denigrates professional autonomy, denies the identity of nursing, and leaves society without nursing services.

The *unification model* is a nurse-promulgated euphemism for earlier practices variously labeled as apprenticeships, joint appointments, and the like. The practitioner-teacher is magnified and substantive knowledge in nursing is minimized. Claims of economic and power pressures are used to excuse expediency. "A nurse is a nurse is a nurse" is avowed. Nurses are caught in a static web of their own shortsightedness. Some years ago Alfred North Whitehead stated that "when ideals sink to the level of practice, stagnation is the result" (McGlothlin, 1961). Those who seek to perpetuate the past, no matter how well-meaning they may be, are destined to fall by the wayside. They will not cross the horizon.

As nursing moves rapidly toward scientific identity and independent action, conflict with power and profit interests intensifies. Therapeutic modalities and health measures deriving from a science of unitary man can be expected to clash with practices directed toward treating part of man or the sum of his parts. Concomitantly the public is demanding freedom of choice, informed consent, and alternatives in health providers and health services. In the world of tomorrow autonomous nursing centers will augment independent professional practice in nursing. Referral systems within nursing and between nursing and other fields will expand. Emphasis on promotion of health will bring renewed optimism to a public too long deluged with threats of danger on every side.

The speed of change quickens. The horizon nears. Nursing in the twenty-first century has a new image. Problems of the twentieth century are no longer relevant. New concerns and new visions engage the nurses of tomorrow. Independence of thought and action, creative ideas, human compassion, and enthusiasm for the unknown abound. Diversity is a valued norm. Human health and welfare have new dimensions. Florence Nightingale said it rightly: "No system can endure that does not march."

References

Ferguson, Marilyn (1980). The Aquarian Conspiracy. Los Angeles. J. P. Tarcher, Inc.
Goldsmith, Jeff C. (1980). "The health care market: Can hospitals survive?" Harvard Business Review, September-October, 110–112.
Heppenheimer, T. A. (1977). Colonies in Space. New York: Warner Books, Inc.
McGlothlin, W. J. (1961). "The place of nursing in the professions." Nursing Outlook, 4:216.
Miller, Michael K. and C. Shannon Stokes (1978). "Health status, health resources, and consolidated structural parameters: Implications for public health care policy." Journal of Health and Social Behavior, September: 263–279.
Rosen, Stephen (1976). Future Facts. New York: Simon & Schuster.

CHAPTER 50

High Touch in a High-Tech Future

Martha E. Rogers

Adapting for my own use a statement made some years ago, I would say that it is not high technology that is causing our trouble, rather it is the people "whose feet tread the earth of a new world as their heads continue to dwell in the past."[1] Whether "those people" are scientists clinging to outdated world views, proponents of people as machines or collections of chemicals, nurses reluctant to exchange old technical resources for new tools of practice, or those fearful of unemployment generated by accelerating technological diversity—the argument prevails that high technology contradicts humane human services. In nursing, the debate too often sinks to this level of "high touch" versus "high tech," a view that overlooks the importance of both as tools in the knowledgeable practice of the science of nursing from which people may benefit.

'If This Is the Future . . .'

In December 1963 the Research Institute of America published a bulletin that began:

> The moment of truth on automation is coming . . . a lot sooner than most people realize. . . . The actions taken to cope with the coming crisis of automation will be more radical than business and government leaders publicly admit. . . . Automation has just begun to bite in. Up to now techniques have been in the process of development; today the major systems are complete. From this point on, they'll be spreading rapidly. The effect will be revolutionary on everything from office and plant to society itself.

Rogers, M. E. (1985). High touch in a high-tech future. In *Perspectives in nursing 1985–1987.* Based on presentations at the seventeenth NLN biennial convention (pp. 25–31). NLN Publication #41-1985. New York: National League for Nursing. Reprinted with permission.

The nearly 25 years since then have witnessed major developments in automation, rapid shifts in the state of the art in computers, thriving robots, and space travel, with moon villages and space towns soon to be realized.

Futurologists abound, although their predictions do not always match developments in real time. For instance, an article in *Science 84* was titled: "If this is the future—where's my 13 hour work week, personal helicopter, household robot, air-conditioned street, and auto pilot car?"[2] But do not despair. These and other wonders are in process.

When Thomas A. Edison invented the electric light, a demonstration for the public was installed in a New Jersey community. A committee of Englishmen came over to view this wonder and find out if it would really last. More specifically, they wanted to determine if the gas lighters would soon be out of jobs. The committee returned home confident that the electric light would never replace the gaslight. Today not only has the gas lighter passed into history, but it seems likely that the meter-reader may follow, as plans for a high-tech gas meter are implemented. Diversified Energies, parent company of the Minneapolis-based Minnegasco Gas Company, has applied for a patent on a radio-controlled gas meter that would transmit a signal to a central computer, which would automatically calculate the customer's bill.

A computer in every home is joining the chicken in every pot as the societal ideal. We are pressured to buy, buy, buy for home, school, and workplace on the high-tech market. Twenty years ago Secretary of Labor Willard Wirtz stated: "The machine now has a high school education in the sense that it can do most jobs that a high school graduate can do, so machines will get the job because they work for less than a living wage. A person needs 14 years of education to compete with a machine."[3] Today many fourth and fifth graders are computer literate. In less than another decade it can be expected that students entering college may be more comfortable with computers than the previous generation was with typewriters. College campuses are getting powerful new machines that can enhance education and research.

Not only are educational institutions rolling in computers, but the health care industry is alive with them. Nor is this a new event. In 1964, several departments at the Children's Hospital in Akron, Ohio, were linked to a central computer. It was predicted that nurses might have as much as 40 percent more time to spend with patients. Computer systems in hospitals and in a range of health care agencies look after patient records, record and analyze vital signs, collect patient histories, regulate medications, diagnose and treat, analyze test results, monitor vital signs and intravenous transfusions, and so forth, ad infinitum. Last year, *Omni* magazine carried an article about robot nurses.

Machines do *not* provide human services. Nor are machines a substitute for knowledgeable nursing services. Nonetheless, when used wisely and with judgment machines can be useful adjuncts as tools of practice. Their effectiveness and safety require nurses who are knowledgeable in the science of nursing, who are committed to people and their world as the focus of their concern, and who are socially responsible.

High technology is a manifestation of humankind's continuously innovative potential. Nostalgia for the "good old days" should not be allowed to obscure the "good old" outhouses, lack of central heating, and the other inconveniences that accompanied them.

The Job Frontier

High technology presages a new job frontier. Fear of unemployment as new machines are introduced is not new. That people are affected by accelerating technology is reflected in such phenomena as attrition without replacement of personnel, layoffs, and retraining programs. But these are by no means all attributable to high technology. Change is inevitable, and it is escalating on many fronts in many ways.

Moreover, one might reasonably propose that in the long term, as in the past, more jobs will be created than destroyed. Already there are mismatches between the nature of the labor supply and the demand for it. Preparing persons for jobs that are obsolete or no longer exist is tragic human waste. The past does not control the future.

"High tech" and "high touch" are not, in themselves, adversaries. Rather, the problem lies with nurses who perceive manual and machine skills as the substance of nursing rather than as tools that may be useful to implement the science of nursing. Many nurses have become enamored of machines. Pervasive anti-educationism, dependency, and naivete have exacerbated many problems. Concomitantly, the struggle for scientific identity and recognition as a learned profession continue to engage growing numbers of nurses.

"High touch" is a kind of shorthand for personal caring for people. It need not be physical touch, though it may include physical touch. It is a tool of practice. It has significance when it is rooted in a firm foundation in the science of nursing.

Some 25 years ago Elizabeth Kemble, then dean of the School of Nursing at the University of North Carolina at Chapel Hill, stated:

> Much has been written and said concerning the spirit, art, and science of nursing. No one will deny the importance of all three in the effective practice of nursing. But the noble spirit alone is not enough. The art of nursing falls far short even with a fine spirit. It is only when nursing practice is based on a theoretically sound foundation that the spirit and art can come into full being.[4]

Predicting the future can be dangerous. We live in a probabilistic world. We are also participants in creating the future. This future is by and large already here if we but open our eyes to see.

Nursing Today and Tomorrow

Nursing today is perceived by many to be in a state of crisis. The Chinese write the word *crisis* with two characters: the first signifies *danger* and the second *opportunity.* Nursing evolves within the larger world of people's experience. The health care system is in rapid change. It is up to us to seize the opportunities and to act with courage that people may benefit. Robert Browning's words, "A man's reach should exceed his grasp else what's a heaven for," are worth pondering.

Power, profits, and tradition vie with a "high tech/high touch" future. Cost containment has become a byword as diagnosis related groups (DRGs) seek to put a cap on rampaging overcharges by hospitals and physicians. But the situation is much larger and more complex than DRGs. Community-based health services are growing rapidly. A variety of health workers crowd the marketplace. Nearly 40 percent of nurses do not work in hospitals now. Before long this percentage can be expected to increase to the point where the larger percentage of nurses will work in community-based centers.

In Texas, 21 hospitals filed billions of dollars in false Medicare claims in a scandal that, according to the U.S. General Accounting Office, rivals defense contract overcharges.[5] And it seems unlikely that Texas hospitals are alone in massive Medicare overcharges. Hospitals are big business and big bucks. The second highest paid corporate executive in the United States last year according to *Forbes Magazine* is head of Humana, Inc., at nearly $18 million. Profit-making hospitals seem to be doing well.

The idea of people as machines and collections of spare parts wherewith to roboticize human beings enamors many. Human experimentation is not uncommon, and informed consent seems to have many meanings. A mechanist philosophy contradicts the unitary nature of humankind and our world and emerging world views.

Dislocations in the job market are already being felt in nursing. Blaming all of these on DRGs and other similar events will not solve the problems. We have too many nurses prepared for jobs that are not needed and too few to initiate and fill the jobs in nursing that are needed. Moreover, the practice of nursing focuses on people. Nursing does not exist to service the ends of any other field. The practice of nursing does not mean learning how to run a computer and how to nurse machines. . . .

Qualified faculty in nursing are indispensable. The fad of joint appointments only threatens to make us "jacks of all trades and masters of none."

Nursing practice will encompass independent nursing practice, autonomous nursing centers, and autonomous birthing centers, without the fallacy of so-called medical backup. However, standards of practice will be commensurate with educational preparation. Professional responsibility will rest with those holding valid and higher degrees in nursing.

There is critical need for mutual respect for differences among nurses and for differences between nurses and other personnel. Noninvasive modalities will predominate. All of us must undergo continual "retreading" for this new world. As we engage in the job that is before us there will be no time for burnout. We must *get out* of old ruts instead of *cop out* because of failure to envision the future.

An analogy to the situation of nursing today is that of an embryo in its eighth month in utero. It realizes things seem to be getting crowded. There is lots of waste floating around. The situation looks quite dismal. Then it begins to imagine what it might be like in the ninth month, the tenth, the eleventh month. The vision is truly frightening. What the embryo fails to realize is that in the ninth month there will be a major change—birth.

References

1. George S. Counts "The Impact of Technologic Change" in the Planning of Change, ed W.G. Bennis et al (New York Holt, Rinehart & Winston (1962) 21.
2. *Science 84* (January 1984): 34–43.
3. *Time*, March 5, 1965, 60.
4. Elizabeth Kemble, Unity of Nursing Care (Chapel Hill, N.C.: University of North Carolina, June, 1960).
5. Dallas Morning News, June 2, 1985; *USA Today*, June 3, 1985.

CHAPTER 51

Dimensions of Health: A View from Space

Martha E. Rogers

John Naisbitt concluded his book *Megatrends* with "My God. What a fantastic time to be alive!" These are truly exciting times. The future bodes well for risk takers and visionaries. Space exploration has a new reality. Space dwellers are already on the horizon.

Time magazine recently quoted Chairman Paine of the National Commission on Space as saying: "Somebody will be mining the moon by the year 2005. The only real question is what language they'll be speaking." Personally I am not sure it is that far off, but I tend to be impatient.

Scientific and technological wonders escalate. New worldviews multiply. Diversification marks the fields of business and industry. A cashless society is developing rapidly. Space towns, moon villages, and other extraterrestrial abodes are near. Galactic grocery stores, health services, educational centers, recreational opportunities, and the like are inevitable inclusions in a space-bound world society. Microwaving lunar soil to make bricks suggests implications beyond the building of houses and factories—possible clues relevant to the nature of evolutionary emergence in life forms. The liberal arts and sciences—essential bases in higher education for all students—properly include extraterrestrial matters.

Rapid and large-scale growth in the numbers of students at the University of North Dakota identifying majors in aeronautics and astrospace this fall points up significant interest in this broad area. One of the speakers yesterday emphasized the importance of interdisciplinary space studies. Moreover, I propose that the terrestrial and extraterrestrial cannot be separated. Peoples' advent into outer space is an expansion of frontiers—the capacity to experience in new ways the previously unknown.

Rogers, M. E. (1986, September). *Dimensions of health: A view from space.* Paper presented at the University of North Dakota Center for Aerospace Studies Conference on "Law and Life in Space," Grand Forks, N.D.

Change continues to accelerate. Developmental norms of even thirty to forty years ago are no longer valid. People are sleeping less and living longer. The paranormal is becoming normal.

People struggle to extricate themselves from no longer tenable worldviews. Utopian dreams of disease control flounder amidst outdated concepts of homeostasis, adaptation, and causality. Today's major health problems in the United States are iatrogenesis, nosocomial conditions, and hypochondriasis. Accelerating evolutionary diversity can be identified in so-called hyperactive children, rapidly changing lifestyles, astronauts who roam beyond this planet, and a host of other manifestations.

Cancer and cardiac conditions may be hypothesized to illustrate life's many probings for innovative expressions of emergent evolution which may or may not be deemed "good" in contemporary value systems. Dwellers in outer space may someday have to have support systems in reverse to visit this planet.

Capra in his book *The Turning Point* writes:

> We are trying to apply concepts of an out-dated world view to a reality that can no longer be understood in terms of these concepts.

Rupert Sheldrake has stirred the biological world with *A New Science of Life.* David Bohm has proposed *Wholeness and the Implicate Order.* Thomas Kuhn's paradigm shift is now up for second, third, fourth, et al. opinions.

Stephen Jay Gould, writing in *National History* (1977), noted:

> New facts collected in old ways under the guidance of old theories, rarely lead to any substantial revision of thought. Facts do not speak for themselves; they are read in the light of theory.

A new worldview compatible with the most progressive knowledge available is a necessary prelude to studying human health and to determining modalities for its promotion whether on this planet or in the outer reaches of space. Such a view focuses on people and their environments. Space exploration has opened new avenues. Communication technology provides new means.

An abstract system identifying a new reality evolves out of a synthesis of facts and ideas. Definitions of specificity contribute clarity and precision.

Energy fields are postulated to be the fundamental units of the living and the nonliving. Field is a unifying concept. Energy signifies the dynamic nature of the field. Energy fields are infinite. Human and environmental fields are specified to be irreducible, four-dimensional (defined as a nonlinear domain without spatial or temporal attributes), and identified by pattern (defined as the distinguishing characteristic of an energy field perceived as a single wave—an abstraction). These fields manifest characteristics specific to the whole and not predicted by knowledge of the parts.

People *are* energy fields. They do not have energy fields. Fields are infinite. A closed system model of the universe is contradicted. Such concepts as equilibrium, homeostasis, adaptation, steady state are outdated. Causality is invalid.

Principles and theories derive from this new worldview. The principles of homeodynamics postulate the nature of change. These principles are three in number and stated as follows:

Principles of Homeodynamics

Principle of Resonancy: the continuous change from lower to higher frequency wave patterns in human and environmental fields

Principle of Helicy: the continuous innovative, probabilistic, increasing diversity of human and environmental field patterns characterized by nonrepeating rhythmicities

Principle of Integrality: the continuous mutual human field and environmental field process

A theory of accelerating evolution deriving from this abstract system puts in different perspective today's rapidly changing norms in blood pressure levels, children's behavior, longer waking periods, and other events. Higher frequency wave patterns of growing diversity portend new norms coordinate with accelerating change. Labels of pathology based on old norms generate hypochondriasis and iatrogenesis. Normal means average. Normal (average) blood pressure readings in all age groups are notably higher today than they were a few decades ago. Evidence that these norms are jeopardizing the public health are [sic] insubstantial. In fact, astronauts and Olympic champions are reported to manifest blood pressure levels above the so-called norms.

Not only has the average waking period lengthened but sleep/wake continuities are increasingly diverse. Developmental norms have changed significantly in recent years. Gifted children and so-called hyperactive ones not uncommonly manifest similar behaviors. It should seem more reasonable to hypothesize hyperactive as accelerating evolution than to denigrate rhythmicities that diverge from outdated norms and erroneous expectations.

Manifestations of a speeding up of human field rhythms are coordinate with higher frequency environmental field patterns. Radiation increments of widely diverse frequencies are common household accompaniments in everyday life. Atmospheric and cosmological complexity grows. Environmental motion has quickened. Very high speed transit tube crafts on this planet are here and speeds are increasing. Yet only a century ago the world's finest mathematicians "proved" a train could never exceed 21 miles per hour because if it did, the air would be sucked out and the passengers suffocated.

Human-environmental fields evolve together in mutual process. The doomsayers who would have it that people are destroying themselves are in error. The prestigious club of Rome had to back up on its dire predictions of man's demise. On the contrary, there is a population explosion, increased longevity, escalating levels of science and technology, the development of outer space communities, and multiple other evidence of men's developmental potentials in process of actualization.

With increased longevity, growing numbers of older persons move into the picture. Contrary to a static view engendered by a closed system model of the universe which postulates aging to be a running down, the science of unitary human beings postulates aging to be a developmental process. Aging is continuous from conception through the dying process. Field patterns become increasingly diverse and creative. The aged need less sleep and sleep/wake frequencies become more varied. Higher frequency patterns give meaning to multiple reports of time experienced as racing. Aging is not a disease nor is it analogous to the "one hoss shay" of literary lore.

As developmental diversity continues to accelerate, the range and variety of differences between individuals also increase. More diverse field patterns evolve more rapidly than less diverse ones. Populations defy so-called normal curves and individual differences multiply.

The emergence of paranormal phenomena as valid subjects for serious scientific research has nonetheless been handicapped by a paucity of viable theories to explain these events. The nature of the paradigm presented here provides a framework for such theories. Four-dimensional reality as defined in this system is a signal factor in deriving testable hypotheses. The implications for creative health services are notable. Alternative forms of healing are increasingly popular—and some surprisingly effective. Meditative modalities bespeak "beyond waking" manifestations. Therapeutic Touch developed by Dolores Krieger, Ph.D., R.N., is documentedly efficacious. Proposals for think tanks in space to promote a person's creative potential need careful consideration and implementation.

Concern with the dying as well as with the living must be included. Unitary human rhythms find expression in the rhythmicity of the living/dying process. And just as aging is deemed developmental, so, too, is dying hypothesized to be developmental. The nature of the dying process and after-death phenomena have gained considerable public and professional interest in recent years. Yet rejection of the dying person continues to be all too common. Questionable practices in securing organs for transplantation have led to legislative action. The right to die with dignity is being written into final testaments. Concomitantly, reports of near death and after death experiences are already listing among the best-sellers. The dying process can be studied effectively within this system. The continuity of field patterning after death would seem to be a much more difficult area to investigate although by no means impossible.

Seeing the world from this viewpoint requires a new synthesis, a creative leap, and the inculcation of new attitudes and values. The goal of health workers and of the public focuses properly on the promotion of health. In a dynamic, continuously innovative world, one does not, for example, prevent disease. Rather in the process of change there are many potentialities, only some of which will be actualized. Therapeutic modalities will increasingly emphasize the noninvasive. Diversity will be accorded high value. Human health will not be measured by adding up parameters of biological, social, psychological, and like phenomena.

There are incongruities and contradictions between holistic directions and the forms of inquiry common today. New tools of measurement, new ways of thinking cannot be achieved by digging the same holes deeper. A view from space not only demands new ideas but makes explicit new holes to dig.

Will or should criteria for health on planet Earth be different from criteria for residents of space towns, moon villages, other planets, other solar systems, other galaxies? Are there implications for selecting space travelers and space dwellers for a healthy, happy life among the stars? What kind of health personnel and health resources should be provided? What should be our goals in relation to human and environmental field attributes? Questions will continue to arise as we probe new worlds.

And with John Naisbitt I repeat, "My God. What a fantastic time to be alive!"

CHAPTER 52

A Conversation with Martha E. Rogers on Nursing in Space

Martha E. Rogers, Maureen B. Doyle, Angela Racolin, and Patricia C. Walsh

Dr. Martha E. Rogers conversed with doctoral students on June 27, 1989 at New York University to explore her ideas on nursing in space, as well as her projections for the art and science of nursing within a new world view of transcendent unity and continuously escalating evolutionary change, and for the next evolutionary phase of human diversity—homo spatialis. The authors are grateful for this opportunity and for Dr. Rogers' willingness to let us explore with her.

Transcendent Unity

MER The main thing I want to get across is that we are talking about nursing in a whole new world of transcendent unity. We are not talking about planet bound anything, but rather, nursing in a universe where space encompasses the planet Earth. The spinoff in space is going to spell nursing on planet Earth as well as in space.

MBD You have said very clearly that we are integral with space. We cannot impose our view of Earth into space, rather Earth is integral with the larger view.

MER We are changing our vision. It won't be one of causality. (You know me and causality.) One will not affect the other, rather we will be integral with this enlarged universe.

AR Could you elaborate more on the idea of transcendent unity?

Rogers, M. E., Doyle, M. B., Racolin, A., & Walsh, P. C. (1990). *A conversation with Martha E. Rogers on nursing in space.* In E. A. M. Barrett (Ed.), *Visions of Rogers' science-based nursing* (pp. 375–386). New York: National League for Nursing. Reprinted with permission.

MER It's a nice phrase. Actually, I think what this is getting at is perhaps how people's advent into space will happen. It's really a transition from humankind to spacekind and it's really about how a space-directed people change, how the world changes, and how our view of the world changes. Because it does. Actually this is not different from the Science of Unitary Human Beings. It gives it more generality, and it extends it further.

When we talk about environment, man is not the only species on this planet and we are talking about an enlarged transcendent universe in which planet Earth is integral with outer space. After being space dwellers for a couple of generations, and generations are generally considered to be 25 years, one may propose that in approximately 50 years homo spatialis may transcend homo sapiens. There will evolve a new kind of species. What will this mean? I don't know.

AR In your presentation at the Third Rogerian Conference, you made a statement that today's realities would transcend traditional averages. When talking about space and space environment, you talked about the realities transcending traditional averages. I was wondering if that is talking about a similar kind of thing.

MER Oh yes. You are really asking, "What will tomorrow's norms be like?"

AR Yes. What will the norms and realities be like, what would you envision? Will there by any?

MER You see we are moving into living in space and we will have homo spatialis. How necessary is it to try to transfer Earth's atmosphere to outer space? How soon will people need support systems in reverse to visit planet Earth? Just as we have to have support systems in reverse if people play around under the ocean, there are people who will have to have support systems for space living. However, the norms will be in the enlarged universe, not planetary. It's going to be a whole different thing. Today the astronauts are the precursors of homo spatialis.

AR When you say the norms will be the norms of the enlarged universe, would that be synonymous with saying they would be universal or interplanetary?

Evolutionary Change

MER No, actually what I'm talking about is norms for continuously escalating evolutionary change and innovative, growing diversity. The speed of change has not only accelerated, it has gone up exponentially. There is a lot of evidence, of course, that the more change, the faster it speeds up itself; it's a normal thing. It is a fantastic time to be alive because we are on the edge of a new world, just as when life moved out of the waters onto dry land. We are at a major change. Perhaps it happened before, I don't know. The point is that right now I have no doubt that out in the cosmos there is something. I don't know what to call it, call it intelligent life, it is not like us.

Things we frequently hear about are proposed to be abnormal or pathological, for example, when they talk about the astronauts and the loss of calcium. Well, why is that considered bad? Maybe it is very normal in space. If it is normal and healthy, maybe if you're out there you don't need all that calcium. I consider physical bodies to be manifestations of field. This is a whole different way of looking. But if you take just our ability to see, we see within a very narrow range of the spectrum. Who's to say that there are not all sorts of intelligent fields out there outside our visible light spectrum. Just because our eyes don't see something doesn't mean it's not there.

The thing I'm saying is that change just is. For example, back in the 1950s Lee DeForest, the father of modern electronics, just 12 years before the Apollo landed on the moon, asserted that this could never possibly happen. Now that's also particularly interesting because early on when he first got into electronics, he was the one who proposed a cable across the ocean. He was sued and brought to court for lying to the public, for saying that such a thing could be done. Well, fortunately the courts said it was alright. Now here is a man who dared himself and then could not face up to a thing like man on the moon. So don't think for a minute that the status quo is going to hang around or that this isn't going to happen. It's already happening.

Now we are talking about a whole new breed. When I talk about homo spatialis I'm serious and so are others. Robinson and White, the authors of *Envoys of Mankind,* use the term frequently. I think it's a marvelous term. I didn't know what to call it, now I know.

PW How would you define homo spatialis?

MER It's the great big question in the sky. It's the next evolutionary phase of human diversity.

MBD Do you think homo spatialis will require food as we normally eat currently?

MER I don't know, and to me, it really doesn't matter. The point is, what is food? You see it's not input/output, but rather we're talking about the integralness of fields and how it might be manifest in some small way. Who's to know.

MBD We were wondering what they might sell in a galactic grocery store?

MER Right off they will sell potatoes and whatever (laughing). Maybe they won't need food, maybe they'll get food from the environment somehow.

PW How do you see our expansion into space taking place?

MER The first space islands are being built and they will be inhabited by the year 2000. It is projected that they will only hold about 20 people. But the day will come very quickly that things will change. When emigration to space begins, the demand here and on the moon and on whatever, is going to happen very fast. There are thousands of people longing to get up there already.

Initially, in a space island, the designs are such that they set up motions that will involve gravitational ties similar to those on Earth, however, they are set up in such a way that the heavier gravitational ties will be towards the center. As you move out, there will be less and less gravitational pull in the island. Now this can be great if you are talking about people with cardiac conditions, or emphysema, or the like because they will not have to battle against gravity. Now take the average person, who is an astronaut on a space island and spends his life on the outer edges. Pretty soon he may be in trouble if he moves to the middle of the island. And let's say he takes his wife and children, and they begin to have children. These children won't know what it's like to weigh a ton. You see all our patterns about what things weigh, a ton of lead or a ton of feathers, all depends on how you're looking at it. So it means the whole set of categories that we've grown up with are going to be gone. Think of the excitement!

Role of Nurse in Space and the Body of Nursing Knowledge

PW What do you think the role or function of the nurse will be on a space island?

MER I think the real purpose will be to promote human/space-kind well-being, whatever that may be. Well-being is a value, it is not an absolute. I think ways in which this will be done will be non-invasive in general, but I think it will involve modalities of which we have not yet even dreamed.

If one looks at allopathic medicine as we know it right now, it's going down the drain and going very rapidly, the reason being it is based on old world views. It is a historical absolute that somehow got the money and the prestige. There are many other medical areas equally important with allopathic medicine, for example, there are homeopathic, east oriental medicine, American Indian medicine, as well as herbalism. Various modalities other than medicine are under way—such as, non-invasive modalities, wholistic trends, unconditional love, etc. These are being tried in all sorts of ways, and we're finding that they have potential in relation to health and well-being. We don't know what will be involved in spacekind health promotion or what these new modalities will be. They are unpredictable.

PW Would nurse astronauts be actual mission specialists or would they be Earth support systems?

MER I think that they will not be astronauts or mission specialists at all, unless nurses decide that there is a body of scientific knowledge specific to nursing. The Science of Unitary Human Beings is the only proposal that has been made of that sort. Now people who are mission scientists have been very blunt about this issue when asked directly. If a nurse writes them to say she is interested, she will quickly be informed that they are looking for scientists basically and they do not perceive nurses as scientists. I think they see a nurse as someone who can monitor machines, that all nurses do is a technical, quasi-technical job and they have plenty of those sorts of people. They ask for engineers for their pilots, and there is no end to the support personnel for their pilot/engineers. These are people who essentially have graduate degrees. The pilots mostly have degrees in engineering, and the scientists particularly in mathematics, physiology, philosophy, and aeronautics. They have a broad based vision. To be included in this nurses have to be committed to having a body of knowledge specific to nursing that they will be willing to transmit and for which they will be responsible.

MBD If science is open-ended and constantly changing, how do you think our experience in space will influence the body of knowledge in nursing?

MER I don't think it will influence it at all. I think the Science of Unitary Human Beings provides the overall world view for an enlarged transcendent universe. Science tries to understand and describe reality.

AR We talk about a body of knowledge that is a science and which by definition is an organized abstract system. Something that I'm picking up on makes me question whether or not there is a contradiction in the whole idea of saying that we can have a science and a body of knowledge, which translates into the idea of research and theories, which ideally predict. But you are saying there is no predictability. So how does any of this fit?

MER When you say that, you see science is changing. But this is not going to throw out the physical world and biological world and all of that, just because things are unpredictable. There is no causality either, but there are relationships. Yes, I think a lot of these things are going to go, but I don't think it is important to be concerned with struggling with it. A science is identified by the phenomena of its concern. No other science has been concerned with people as irreducible energy fields. The Science of Unitary Human Beings is a new way of looking at people. Now this view of humans is neither more, nor less, nor bigger, nor greater, nor anything. It is a different phenomenon.

The thing that is true about science is that it is an organized abstract system, from which to derive theories. Now when nurses derive theories from sociology, those are not nursing theories, they are sociological theories. And a nurse might do excellent research in sociology, but it doesn't make it nursing just because a nurse does it, any more than if a physicist derived a theory from sociology, it would not be a physical theory, it would be sociological. Now here we have nursing as a basic science dealing with a phenomenon that is clearly unique to nursing; it is an organized system from which to derive multiple theories. A science generates many theories. There is no such thing as the theory of nursing any more than there is a theory of biology. For example, we have gotten caught up in this, and we have a lot of unlearning to do, since we confused research in other fields and thought if a nurse did it, that made it nursing. When we begin to look at nursing with this enlarged rapidly changing world view, the foundations and the principles of the Science of Unitary Human Beings are even more useful than before—they fit.

But science is never finished. It's always open ended. Physics which is so long established can be offered as an example. It is undergoing stresses that are as severe as science has experienced. Probability replaced absolutism and now there is unpredictability. A whole world of cards is falling apart. But we have lived through absolutism, we have survived probability and even Einstein didn't accept probability for a long time. He said, "I don't think God plays dice with the universe." And then there was quantum theory. Now we find that probability is no longer in. In addition, it is now known that the black holes don't just swallow everything. It seems that they also spit things back. And the idea of worm holes is fascinating; there are now some scientists who have come up with the recognition that there are ways that can be developed, practical ways of shooting through the universe instead of having to go around the long way. In other words, you may go off to another galaxy in almost no time flat. All we are dealing with here is time within our capacity to perceive it, and homo spatialis will not be caught in that kind of thing. It's all relative. Whatever we're seeing all around us are all sorts of manifestations of change; they are part of the evolutionary process.

Complexifying Wholeness

PW You have spoken of complexification. Could you explain what you are referring to?

MER You know I think back to the 1940s when Wendell Wilkie was running for president. One day he gave a talk and he talked about "one world." I think he was referring to peace, I don't know. The point is people got all excited, nobody wanted one world. And yet look at the changes from clans and tribes, to cities and states, to nations and now to one world—it's going to happen. And with this there is growing simplicity in the complexification.

PW I presume nursing has to follow along with this to keep up with it.

MER We don't follow along. We are integral with it. It's a matter of "Do we want to be around or not and, if so, how?" I think if we are going to claim that nurses have something important to contribute to people, then we are going to have to deal with complexification. Now sometimes I think that we are ahead of the game. And the more I get into it, the more I know we are. And certainly we are by no means the only ones who are trying to look at this sort of thing. There are David Bohm, Renee Weber, Rupert Sheldrake, and Fritz Capra among many others. In other words, we're moving to different concepts but with the same basic philosophical approach.

MBD When you talk about complexifying wholeness, via a new world view, and that evolves out of non-equilibrium, is that like saying that order emerges out of chaos?

MER No, I don't think so. I think we get caught up in what we mean by chaos. Now I think in one sense, yes, for example, the whole idea of unpredictability really emerged out of some of the work that was going on in mathematics in the new field called chaos. We grew up in absolutism, and that's part of the trouble now. People haven't even moved to a probabilistic universe. The thing is no matter what one may believe, the status quo is gone, it won't stay. Whatever one believes now in terms of evolution and change, there is no going back. You know we've had pulsating universes and all different things. Of course, the "big bang" is the "in" thing now and has been for a while. I think that too will pass, when it's going to pass, I don't know. At this point I'm willing to let anybody have it that wants it.

I do not think that whether or not the universe began as a "big bang" or some other way is going to make any difference in terms of how we try to explain the way things are. And it's going to change very rapidly. By the time we have large numbers of people emigrating into space and evolving into homo spatialis, we are going to find many things we could never even have imagined.

I think what is important is to keep an open mind and to be able to come to grips with how things seem to be moving now. This is where the Science of Unitary Human Beings has much to recommend it, since the principles of homeodynamics apply to the new world as well as today's. I agree that helicy needs a little bit of rewording, it's somewhat verbose, but I'm working on that. The principles represent a complete departure from old world views, but are consistent with the universe as we begin to know it now. The Science of Unitary Human Beings postulates unpredictability; it does allow for all these other things.

Nosophobia: Implications for Nursing Education

MBD You use the word "nosophobia." Do you think that perhaps we are going to take some of our problems into outer space?

MER You see, the thing about nosophobia, the morbid dread of disease, is that it is generated by greed. MDs and hospitals and multiple health professionals plus drug houses and the like are generating most of it and we are helping. The news media is very active in this also. For example, with AIDS everyone got all excited. Of course, it's a horrible thing, but so was cholera. AIDS has not begun to be as massive as cholera was. Cholera decimated three quarters of the European population in the thirteenth century. There is also very good evidence that part of this is directly traceable to the destruction of the immune system through the use of antibiotics and immunizations.

MBD What would you recommend that nurse eductors can do to prepare nurses for nursing in space? Would this be an integral part of a nursing curriculum, or would you see it as a specialization?

MER I think that if you are talking about right this minute, then we need doctorally prepared nurses who are qualified in nursing as a science. There may well be nurses with doctorates in other fields who are interested in space. Now many of those are not scientists in the sense of a mission specialist. I would also note that within one generation or less, the parameters of physiology, psychology, sociology, physics, etc. will not be appropriate or acceptable for determining human health and well being, or describing humans. They are simply not going to work. There is going to be a rapid change that we are going to see. It's going to happen. I don't think it is negative; I think it is exciting. The person who is flexible and who goes with the flow will have an advantage. There are people in other fields, and some in medicine, who are interested in this sort of thing. There is a growing move towards synthesis, towards unity and towards transcendence. I suggest you read Robinson and White's *Envoys of Mankind.* It's quite a readable book.

MBD I came across a statement in *Omni* by a woman who is a NASA research physician who claimed that they are developing criteria to measure an astronaut's sensitivity to self and others. Among other things, they feel this is important so that people will be able to function in tight quarters, for long periods of time, performing routine demanding tasks. Is it possible that studies being done by nursing doctoral students would be relevant to NASA and nursing in space?

MER If these studies are derived from the Science of Unitary Human Beings, then I think there would be some justification. There is no question NASA has already indicated that they need more studies about people and their relationships.

I would caution any researcher to be careful, that when you begin to split humans into pieces you are not studying people. There is all sorts of evidence that these things don't work, even when superficially they look like they are working. Many tests have been tried to predict who is going to be successful in space. They even get into something as pragmatic as motion sickness, which has no physiological parameters. No matter what has been tried, it cannot be predicted. Also, when someone goes up and has motion sickness, you can't predict if they will or will not have it again.

The Science of Unitary Human Beings is a new world view that more and more is being recognized. It does have a frame of reference that no other discipline has, and that also has a potential of encompassing space. It's not a question for space, but it is a question for human life. The whole idea of where we are within the overall picture has had to be changed, and I think the same thing is happening now.

PW What then would you recommend that we could do to start to participate in creating the future?

MER The first thing I would like to do is to commit ourselves to a world view that is consistent with the most up to date knowledge available. We have to commit ourselves to nursing as a science, a peer of other sciences. We are in desperate need of basic research, and we also need applied research. If we really teach nursing as a science to undergraduate students, students themselves would use it that way. Now there is a great deal of interest in using this science in employment. We have done a lot of talking about theory-based practice. What people don't realize is that it's nursing science–based practice. This is where our focus has to be.

PW Do you feel this commitment to nursing as a science and working within this framework will ensure having nursing as a major health presence in space?

MER Well, certainly everybody needs to be an educated person and needs a broad general education, including astronomy. The science of nursing should be taught to encompass the whole, starting at the undergraduate level. Now if you are talking about the immediate, one of the things that I am hoping is that the United States Air Force might invite me to go to NASA and do concentrated workshops with doctorally prepared nurses, and begin to see what we can do about building a scientific base. They might not buy it, I don't know, but I'm available. The point is that we will not go into Space unless we do something like that. And there is no other field equipped to provide the broad base of health promotion than yourselves from the Science of Unitary Human Beings. We are going to have to devise and define new modalities, because the business of the old procedure book just will not work.

MBD Do you think having a baby in outer space would be feasible?

MER Nobody really knows what it would be like. Now there is research going on, but it is limited to the primary mission objective. Research in the life sciences has not been the primary mission of any space program so far. The NASA technical memorandum #58,280 is a compilation of the Detailed Supplemental Objectives conducted by the space shuttle from 1981 through 1986. They can do no research in space of this sort on the life sciences or anything else, except as it is consistent with the primary mission objective.

PW How do you feel people knowledgeable in the Science of Unitary Human Beings, specifically nurses, can add to this?

MER I think it is essential that people who are involved in space travel and space immigration, and serving as mission specialists are people who are concerned with irreducible human beings. This is going to happen, whether it is nurses or somebody else. Right now we are ahead of the game and we have a responsibility to do something about it and to participate and share with others. One of the things the whole astronaut effort is strongly about is team work, in which there is mutual respect for differences. There is no one who runs the show. These teams are literally sharing, nobody thinks they have all the answers, or that they are going to tell everybody else what to do. They all have wide experience and vision and, of course, they are all committed.

We need more risk takers in nursing. If the doctoral student is going to go up into space, she or he needs to be thoroughly knowledgable and articulate in nursing as a science. The student needs to know the cosmos, to be widely read, to have a pilot's license, and to dream big. In research we are still trying to use deductive and inductive thinking without recognizing that the pressures and trends of wholistic thinking demand new ways of thinking. The chances to be creative are unlimited, you can shoot the works.

The Impossibility of "Going Home Again"

MBD I've heard you speak about when astronauts reenter Earth's atmosphere that they are never the same. It's like you can't really go home again because you have been so changed.

MER It is quite true, you know we never go back. You can't walk in the same river twice. I think what we are dealing with here is something where what happens is very dramatic. I may fly to another city and I will never be the same again no matter what, but it does not have the same impact as going into space would have. It's funny, there are people that think that if you go up in your own capsule, and take your own atmosphere with you that it should not make any difference. But we know that's not true. Everybody who has gone up has had all sorts of experiences. They are never the same. Some of them had startling experiences, certainly beyond normal.

MBD What I seem to hear from you is not only that you can't walk in the same river twice, or that you can't go home again, but why would you want to?

MER I wouldn't, but look at all the people who are trying so desperately to maintain the status quo. While some of it may be tied to greed, overriding that is a fear of change. It isn't just space. The whole idea of one world is very threatening to people. Look back on the interrelationships of tribes to cities to states. There are all sorts of things making it clear that we live in one world. The European economic community is already around and growing, a United States of Europe has been talked about for years, and there are reports that within three years a partial United States of Europe is expected to exist. If you look at how things are shaping up in different continents and different countries, it is clear that it is all moving toward this growing complexification. It looks like the wall in Germany might fall and the one in China is already cracked in a lot of places. Now if we have some of these strange little green men coming around here, it might unite people faster than you might think.

We have all these sorts of things going on that represent the continuous moving mass of interrelationships. I think it was Marilyn Ferguson who spoke of synthesis in pattern-seeing being essential for the twenty-first century. The whole concept of complexifying wholeness is where we are.

PW I have a question specifically for you. How did you evolve from the Slinky to space?

MER That's a goody. You see the Slinky was just an aid to thinking. It was one way of dealing with ideas. The Slinky signified open-endedness and non-repeating rhythmicities. But the Slinky had no meaning, except as a way to stimulate ideas. Once you get stimulated, then you no longer need the Slinky, you just keep on thinking and keep on going. It is extremely exciting!

References

Bohm, D. (1980). *Wholeness and the implicate order.* Boston: Routledge & Kegan Paul.

Boslough, J. (1985). *Stephen Hawking's universe.* New York: William Morrow.

Capra, F. (1975). *The tao of physics.* New York: Bantam Books.

Capra, F (1982). *The turning point.* New York: Bantam Books.

Capra, F. (1989). *Uncommon wisdom.* New York: Bantam Books.

DeForest, L. (1950). *Father of radio: The autobiography of Lee DeForest.* Chicago: Wilcox & Follett.

Ferguson, M. (1980). *The aquarian conspiracy.* Los Angeles: J. P. Tarcher.

Hawking, S. (1988). *A brief history of time.* New York: Bantam Books.

National Aeronautics and Space Administration. (1987, March). *Results of the life sciences detailed supplemental objectives conducted by the space shuttle: 1981–1986.* Technical memorandum (No. 58280). Houston, Texas: Lyndon B. Johnson Space Center.

Oberg, A. R. (1989, April). N.A.S.A.'s next generation. *Omni,* pp. 28, 80.

Robinson, G., & White, H. (1986). *Envoys of mankind.* Washington, D.C.: Smithsonian Institute Press.

Rogers, M. (1988, June). *Health in space.* Paper presented at the Third Rogerian Conference, New York City.

Sheldrake, R. (1988). *The presence of the past.* New York: Times Books.

Weber, R. (1986). *Dialogues with scientists and sages: The search for unity in science and mysticism.* London: Routledge, Chapman, & Hall.

SECTION SIX

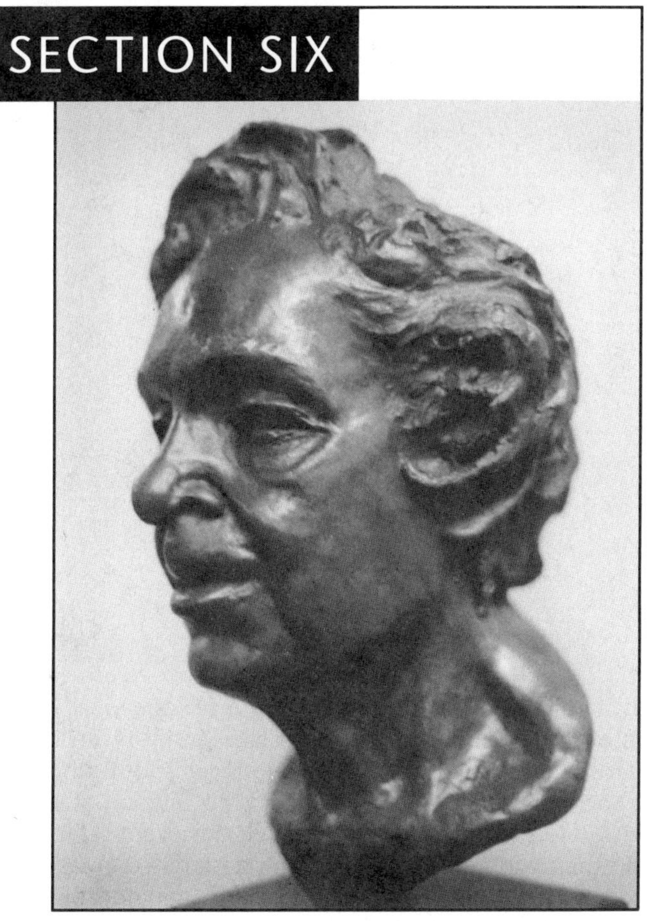

Portrait sculpture of Martha E. Rogers 1989.
(Portrait by Hamil.)

A Historical Salute to Martha E. Rogers on the Occasion of Her 75th Birthday

Section Editors
Violet M. Malinski and
Elizabeth Ann Manhart Barrett

On June 24, 1989, friends, family, and colleagues of Martha E. Rogers gathered for a celebration of a special birthday. Held at New York University, "A Historical Salute to Martha E. Rogers on the Occasion of Her 75th Birthday" was co-sponsored by the Society of Rogerian Scholars and the Division of Nursing, New York University. The committee that planned this event selected topics for presentation and then contacted experts in the designated areas to prepare and present papers addressing them. The speakers illuminated the social, nursing, and philosophical contexts within which Rogers developed her ideas, as well as her contributions to nursing science and to science at large. The papers appear here for the first time in print.

CHAPTER 53

The Social Context Within Which Martha E. Rogers Developed Her Ideas

Patricia Moccia

The ideas for this chapter originally flowed in the most linear fashion. If Martha Rogers was born in 1914, then there were certain social events in each of the decades since that must have shaped her ideas: the first and second world wars, Korea, Vietnam; the McCarthy hearings; the civil rights movement; economic conditions such as the Depression of the 1930s and apparent prosperity of the 1950s; cultural phenomena such as the big bands of the 1940s, Barbara Stanwyck, Joan Crawford, Clark Gable, Gary Cooper, and Disney animation; as well as intellectual arguments over existentialism and postmodernism surely had an influence. As the time line developed on the computer screen, echoes of her oft-repeated comments reverberated in the air: linear time, cause and effect, and three-dimensionality.

After recovering from the initial shock, I realized that I could release myself from the artificial constraints of linear time. From which social interactions with which people did Rogers' ideas emerge? Perhaps even, through which interactions with Rogers did famous women and men develop their perspectives on the world around them? Let us suspend linear time and explore a pandimensional history of the social context within which Rogers developed her ideas.

In preparation for her battles with organized medicine, for instance, I think Rogers must have been there in the 1880s when the Fabian Society was formed by writers such as Bernard Shaw (1898/1948), who was to write the following in the preface to his tragic play *The Doctor's Dilemma.* Is this Shaw or Rogers speaking?

> That any sane nation, having observed that you could provide for a supply of bread by giving bakers a pecuniary interest in baking for you, should go on to give a surgeon a pecuniary interest in cutting off your leg, is enough to make one despair of political humanity. But that is precisely what we have done. And the more appalling, the more the mutilator is paid. He who corrects the ingrowing toe-nail receives a few

shillings: he who cuts your insides out receives hundreds of guineas, except when he does it to a poor person for practice (p. 1).

Somewhere, sometime, Rogers might have said to Shaw, who then wrote it down:

> Doctoring is not even the art of keeping people in health (no doctor seems able to advise you to eat any better than his grandmother or the nearest quack). . . . The distinction between a quack doctor and a qualified one is mainly that only the qualified one is authorized to sign death certificates, for which both sorts seem to have equal occasion (p. 18).

Rogers not only did battle *against* organized medicine, she fought *for* nursing. In salute to her contributions to the nursing profession, consider how she led the fight for nursing's autonomy in New York State and across the nation. Did she do so within the Greek tragedy *Antigone?* As Rogers argued with other nurses about correct political strategy, was the following exchange between Antigone and her sister, Ismene, or between Ismene and Martha? Ismene pleads:

> . . . and what will be the end of us,
> If we transgress the law and defy our king?
> O think, Antigone; we are women; it is not for us
> to fight against men: our rulers are stronger than we,
> And we must obey in this, or in worse than this. . . .

Antigone responds:

> No; then I will not ask you for your help.
> Nor would I thank you for it, if you gave it.

Ismene:

> I do not defy them: but I cannot act
> against the state. I am not strong enough.

Antigone:

> Let that be your excuse then. I will go.

Ismene:

> I fear for you Antigone; I fear.

And Antigone spits back:

> You need not fear for me. Fear for yourself
> (Sophocles, 1957, p. 128).

Was it Antigone or Rogers that the Chorus referred to when they said: "She shows her father's stubborn spirit: foolish not to give way when everything's against her" (Sophocles, 1957, p. 139).

Thinking about Rogers' work as a nurse-educator and administrator, I have often wondered where M. Adelaide Nutting ever got the audacious courage to approach the Board of Trustees at Teachers College and argue so successfully that nurses be allowed to attend classes at Columbia University. I have often wondered from where such wisdom, leadership, and administrative talent emerged. If we suspend linear time, the question emerges of whether these two women had a conversation that spanned 80 years. Was Nutting watching in the wings as Rogers worked with the various deans of the School of Education and New York University to establish the Division of Nursing and expand its offerings to the thousands of nurses who have studied there?

Were Rogers' ideas for a nursing department formed by the experience of those who lived among the Chumash for at least a century before they were first discovered in Southern California by the Europeans in the 1500s? Living in tribes that were often headed by women, the Chumash were artists and astronomers who organized their society on the fundamental belief that a balance of supernatural forces existed in the world and that humans could enlist their aid through various ways such as dreams and public ceremonies. Central to their complex, competitive way of life was their belief that the role of individuals in the universe was to affect these forces for the social good.

There is little doubt in my mind that Rogers developed her ideas in societies led by women. Maybe she was at the Paris Commune in 1871 or in England for the 30 years that Elizabeth I ruled with, in the queen's own words, the "body of a weak and feeble woman, but the heart and stomach of a king" (Fraser, 1989, p. 224). Is it possible that Rogers was on the barge when Cleopatra distracted her enemies with her beauty as she ruled independent Egypt for 20 years in the 1st century B.C.?

Perhaps the teenage Rogers was interacting with the people of India who, from 1966 to 1986, lived in a society shaped by the commanding presence of Indira Gandhi, a woman described as tough, ruthless, and autocratic but also spiritual, courageous, and wise. Did Rogers sit as a student in her college lecture halls and hear what the prime minister of India said, long before she said it: "I am in no sense a feminist, but I believe that a woman is able to do anything." As Rogers continues her work today, perhaps she hears Indira Gandhi say: "I have often said that women today have a special role to play. The world's rhythm is changing, and women can influence and give it the right beat" (Fraser, 1989, p. 309).

Now for some perspectives on the social context within which Rogers developed her ideas about nursing science and the nature of reality. Consider—Rogers was undoubtedly there when the first man walked on the moon. The view from the moon's surface of earth rising must have been in her dreams as she developed her perspectives on reality. Richard Nixon greeted the returning astronauts with the words "the world was infinitely bigger" after the first man walked there. Somehow, Rogers knew that before either the astronauts or the former president did.

Perhaps Rogers' aura somehow extended to Zurich, where Lenin, Rosa Luxembourg, James Joyce, and Albert Einstein all lived and wrote at the turn of the century. Somehow she engaged the ideas of Einstein, who reportedly wrote (although I have never been able to find the exact citation):

> A human being is a part of the whole . . . he experiences himself, his thoughts and his feelings as something separated from the rest—a kind of optical delusion of his consciousness. This delusion is a kind of prison for us, restricting us to our personal desires and to affection for a few persons nearest us. Our task is to free ourselves from this prison by widening our circle of compassion to embrace all living creatures, and the whole of nature in its beauty.

Finally, when you consider the social context within which Rogers developed her ideas as an independent nurse, an educator, an administrator, and a scientist, I call the story of Ishtar to your attention. In northern and central Mesopotamia about 5000 B.C., Ishtar was worshipped as the queen of heaven and the goddess of the universe who ". . . out of chaos brought us harmony and from the chaos she has led us by the hand" (Stone, 1979, p. 107).

Most recently Ishtar has been written about in fiction by Rhoda Lerman (1973) in a novel entitled *Call Me Ishtar.* In the novel Ishtar is reincarnated as a suburban Jewish housewife in Syracuse, New York. While this might seem as far away from Rogers' life as one can get, the description is as close to her contributions as any I've ever read:

To whom it may concern:

What am i doing here? It's very simple. Your world is a mess. A mess!!!

Your laws are inhuman. Your religion without love. Your love without religion, and both, undirected are useless. Your pastrami is stringy and I am bored by your degeneracy.

But what's a mother do do? I am here to bring it all back together again. I have always been the connection between heaven and earth, between man and woman, between thought and act, between everything.

If your philosophers insist the world is a dichotomy, tell them that two plus two doesn't make four unless something brings them together. The connection has been lost.

But, I'm back. Cordially yours, I remain,
your Mother/Harlot/Maiden/Wife
The queen of Heaven

P.S. Call me Ishtar (pp. xi–xii).

Finally I would like to suggest that the social context within which Rogers developed her ideas can best be directed as the "thirteenth" or "other hour." According to Daly and Caputi's (1987) *Websters' First New Intergalactic Wickedary of the English Language,* such experience is defined as

—"the Time/Space when/where auras of plants, planets, stars, animals and all truly animate beings connect" (p. 282)

—"events that are not yet measurable, controllable, predictable—the Call of the Wild, the ever-recurring Spring of New Creation" (p. 283)

—"the possibilities of Metamorphosis, inspiring those who will shift the shapes of words, of worlds; and

—the Space/Times of New Beginnings, of whirring whirls." (p. 284).

References

Daly, M., & Caputi, J. (1987). *Websters' first new intergalactic wickedary of the English language.* Boston: Beacon.

Fraser, A. (1989). *The warrior queens.* New York: Knopf.

Lerman, R. (1973). *Call me Ishtar.* New York: Holt, Rinehart & Winston.

Shaw, B. (1898/1948). The doctor's dilemma. *Selected plays of Bernard Shaw, Vol. 1.* New York: Dodd, Mead.

Sophocles. (1957). Antigone. (Translated by E. F. Watling). New York: Penguin.

Stone, M. (1979). *Ancient mirror of womanhood.* Boston: Beacon.

CHAPTER 54

The Nursing Context Within Which Martha E. Rogers Developed Her Ideas

J. Mae Pepper

Although we know that Martha Rogers started to develop her ideas 75 years ago, I would like to limit my focus to the nursing context within which she grew in the past 35 years, beginning with the 1950s. In 1954, the same year that Dr. Rogers came to New York University, I entered a hospital diploma program, the dominant method used to prepare registered nurses at that time.

The employment pattern for registered nurses had dramatically shifted from what it had been throughout most of the first half of the 20th century.

Whereas "educated" nurses (commonly called "trained") had practiced primarily in the home, in the direct employ of the client (called "patient"), in the early 1900s, by the 1950s the registered nurse practiced primarily in the hospital setting. Although the early "educated" nurse practiced in the home setting, the moral context of that practice was not one of independence and autonomy. Reverby (1987) noted the contextual differences that existed between physicians and nurses:

> The medical student completing training went into private practice; the nursing student, however, went into private duty . . . nurses, even without the control of the hospital and medical hierarchy, were still supposed to be submissive to higher authority and morally committed to their work (p. 95).

Thirty-five years ago it was commonly accepted that only those registered nurses who had baccalaureate education should practice in the autonomous setting of the home. It is not surprising that Martha Rogers belonged to that elite minority in public health nursing. It is obvious to me that Dr. Rogers clearly understood nursing's primary mission, *maximizing the health of the public,* throughout her years of practice from 1937 to 1951, serving first as a rural public health nurse and then in leadership positions with Visiting Nurse Services. Health, people, and the universe in which we live were central themes for Martha Rogers even in the 1930s. That infinite vision remained with her when she changed her primary responsibility to nursing education, coming to New York University in 1954. That vision remains today. Let me focus on those times.

What was new and different in nursing in the 1950s? First, let's look at the opportunities that existed for any professional nurse who wanted to take on the mantle of leadership for the profession. In the editorial introduction to one of the most significant nursing books of the early 1950s, *Interpersonal Relations in Nursing* (Peplau, 1952), Bixler wrote, "There is something new in nursing . . . the concept of interrelationships among nurses, doctors, patients and others . . . nursing is conceived as psychodynamic in character. It is essentially organismic, nursing being presented in its wholeness rather than being compartmentalized" (p. vii). Bixler further noted that this organismic and interpersonal view should ". . . bring a new concept of their value as persons to many nurses and nursing students, and a new dignity because of the role they may play in aiding their patients to become resourceful even as they improve themselves" (p. viii). Nurses were asked to consider the idea that the quality of the nurse-patient relationship makes a substantial difference in the outcomes for both the nurse's and the patient's growth.

In explaining nursing as the dynamic process she called "psychodynamic nursing," Peplau (1952) noted that this represented a new trend. "Recognizing, clarifying, and building an understanding of what happens when a nurse relates herself helpfully to a patient are important steps . . . nursing is helpful when both the patient and the nurse grow as a result of the learning that occurs in the nursing situation" (Peplau, 1952, p. xii).

I believe Rogers integrated the new "dynamic" trend in nursing and was influenced by the interpersonal propositions developed by Peplau. Rogers' earliest and latest works present the human being as a sentient one, a feeling and thinking being. I believe that Rogers considered the notion of wholeness and explicated that concept far beyond what Bixler described when she spoke of Peplau's work.

To get a further picture of what nursing was like when Rogers went to New York University, one must recall some of the constraints on professional development that had to be reframed into opportunities. Recall that "between the Goldmark report of 1923 and the Ginsberg report of 1949, a number of studies and surveys indicated that the root of most difficulties was nursing schools' dual purposes of service and education. However, the studies resulted in limited reform" (Leddy & Pepper, 1989, p. 27). Diploma schools remained the dominant educational force for registered nurses until the early 1970s. Three more studies that were published around 1950 show how leaders were attempting to reframe the educational problem:

1. In 1948 Esther Lucille Brown recommended placing the preparation of professional nurses in the mainstream of higher education.
2. In 1949 Ginsberg recommended the preparation of professional nurses in baccalaureate programs, the preparation of technical nurses in community colleges, and the eventual discontinuation of practical nurse education (cited in Abdellah et al., 1973).

3. In 1953 Bridgman argued that nursing should have an upper division major like other academic disciplines and warned that superimposing a liberal education on a diploma base was not the solution (cited in Leddy & Pepper, 1989).

A sign of the times in the early 1950s is indicated in the professional identification of the leaders noted in these studies as well as others already mentioned. Many of these spokespersons for nursing were not nurses; good friends of nursing, but not nurses. I believe it is clear that Dr. Rogers was determined from her earliest days at New York University to reverse that situation—to specifically delineate that the business of nursing belonged to nurses and she and other nurse leaders would become the spokespersons for nursing.

What was new and different in nursing in the 1960s? For me, personally, one of the significant people who was new and different was Martha Rogers. I went to New York University in 1962. In addition to meeting Martha, one of the first things I did was purchase her first book, *Educational Revolution in Nursing,* published in 1961. I reread the book in an attempt to recreate what nursing was like in those days when Dr. Rogers was developing the science of nursing that has revolutionized nursing education, practice, and research.

Freeman, who wrote the foreword to the book, noted that Dr. Rogers' influence on nursing appeared in many guises, "in her work as director of one of the largest nursing education programs in the country, in her too infrequent publications" and "in her many contributions to organization activity" (Rogers, 1961, p. v). Freeman went on to state that perhaps the greatest impact Martha E. Rogers had was related to her "uninhibited thinking" (Rogers, 1961, p. v). Describing Rogers' book, Freeman wrote, "Dr. Rogers explores the meaning and nature of nursing and its relation to the broad sweep of human values and knowledge. From this she evolves a conceptualization of the kind of education needed to realize the potential of nursing for human betterment (Rogers, 1961, p. v). She continues, "This is a provocative book. There will be many who disagree with its basic premises; others will take exception to some of the specific concepts it includes. But with its purpose there can be no quarrel" (Rogers, 1961, p. vi). Noting the changing world at the beginning of the 1960s, Freeman advised readers, "It behooves everyone who is concerned with nursing to look deeply at the convictions, the reasons, and the values that determine what nursing and nursing education should be" (Rogers, 1961, p. vi). She further stated, "This book should help stimulate such thinking" (Rogers, 1961, p. vi). Note that she said "stimulate," not "contribute" to such thinking. Clearly the vision articulated by Rogers in 1961 represented a critical juncture for nursing and was pivotal to nursing's turning the corner, moving away from a dependent career focus to independent and interdependent professional accountability.

Rogers herself (1961) offered a word picture of some of the challenges facing nursing in the early 1960s:

> Out of the current indiscriminate lumping of nurses must arise a coherent conception of levels of nursing, consistent with the needs of society. Vocational, technical, and professional members of the nursing profession are significant contributors to the health and welfare of mankind, but continued use of the term "professional" to designate the broad range of knowledges and abilities among persons traveling under the umbrella of "Registered Nurse" is indefensible (p. vii).

In the same year as the first manned space flights, Rogers noted that "Atoms, missiles, and space travel foretell an era of unknown dimension" (p. vii). In addition to visualizing space travel as becoming commonplace, Rogers also immediately identified the opportunities and responsibilities for nurses to (1) consider the dimension of space as a significant factor in understanding the person/environment relationship and health and (2) assume the responsibility for remaining the number one health care provider both on earth and beyond.

Prior to and during the 1960s, conceptualizations of nursing were essentially descriptions of what the purpose and functions of nurses were—what the nurse does for/with people to achieve the stated purpose. Through these conceptualizations, the art of nursing flourished. Rogers recognized the limitations of approaching nursing in this singular way. Rather, given these early works on structuring nursing knowledge primarily by way of nurses' functions, she proposed to structure nursing knowledge using the approach of science, that is, set forth propositions that describe, explain, and predict human beings, environment, and health according to the purpose of nursing. Indeed, I believe that Dr. Rogers really was the first leader to articulate a truly scientific basis for nursing practice. The eleven nurses who formed the Nursing Development Conference Group (1973) and wrote the book, *Concept Formalization in Nursing* in 1973, noted that Rogers placed "nursing in a social context, viewing nursing as a service to society and as having a body of scientific knowledge" (p. 52).

Rogers also understood the power of knowledge and the significant changes that would occur in society, ending the industrial era. She knew long before "Megatrends" that our society would move into the "information era." She was visionary in her leadership, getting many nurses to join her in pursuit of the scientific basis for nursing. She convinced us that nurses must shift gears to emphasize health, expanding our horizon beyond illness in order to remain professionally responsible and competent to provide a critically needed service to society.

There is no greater legacy that can be left by a nursing scholar than to provide others in the discipline with a sense of personal importance and professional worth; to engage them in a lifetime of thinking, feeling, and acting like complete professionals—particularly when that scholar grew up professionally in a time when scholarship, autonomy, independence, and interdependence were not dominant values in nursing. We are indebted to Rogers for her contributions to nursing's professional development.

References

Abdellah, F. G., Beland, I. L., Martin, A., et al. (1973). *New directions in patient centered nursing.* New York: Macmillan.

Leddy, S., & Pepper, J. M. (1989). *Conceptual bases of professional nursing* (2nd ed.). Philadelphia: Lippincott.

Nursing Development Conference Group. (1973). *Concept formalization in nursing: Process and product.* Boston: Little, Brown.

Peplau, H. E. (1952). *Interpersonal relations in nursing.* New York: Putnam's.

Reverby, S. M. (1987). *Ordered to care: The dilemma of American nursing 1850–1945.* New York: Cambridge University Press.

Rogers, M. E. (1961). *Educational revolution in nursing.* New York: Macmillan.

CHAPTER 55

The Philosophical Context Within Which Martha E. Rogers Developed Her Ideas

Francelyn Reeder

Plato once said, "There are two worlds, the world of appearances and the world of ideas; souls are 'born remembering'—experiences are always strivings toward the world of ideas" (Plato, 1974, p. 200). Martha Rogers is probably a soul "born remembering." She once told me, "No one philosopher or philosophies could be singled out as having influenced my writing" (M. E. Rogers, personal communication, 1989). As her relative present encompasses roughly 20,000 to 30,000 years, it is clear that a presentation on the philosophical context of Rogers' works could not and would not be described in terms of the chronological years of her life, 1914 to the present, nor in terms of the prevailing views of this period. Unlike Kant's categories of space, time, and causality, Rogers would have begun life with categories of infinity, dynamic change, and comedy in the life span. This chapter is a reflection on "enduring ideas" within the life and work of Rogers and a playful as well as serious revisit to the context of her life of learning.

Rogers entered the life of loving, concerned parents who nurtured her in a context of great freedom to learn and grow. In a family that loved ideas, language itself was her primary teacher. In the context of freedom, Rogers' sense of her own little person (patterning) as an infant and a toddler evolved within the rhymes of the Oxford tradition (Opie & Opie, 1955). Walter de la Mare once remarked that "rhymes such as these free the fancy, charm tongue and ear, delight the inward eye and can lead the way to poetry itself" (cited in Opie & Opie, 1955, p. viii). At the age of 3, Rogers' father introduced her to the public library, where she loved the children's story hour. The rich world of oral tradition began to push back the frontiers of knowledge even then. The listening to and telling of stories was fun, she recalled (M. E. Rogers, personal communication, 1989). Her father would sit with her and ask her to tell him what she had learned.

The influence of family cannot be taken lightly in the story of Rogers' learning and creative scholarly works. Research on eminent personalities has disclosed that "a high degree of parental involvement in the learning experience of children is the one thing most strongly associated with becoming a creative person as an adult" (Goertzel, 1978, p. 301).

Autobiographical stories about school-age ways of learning provide another access to the origin of Rogers' expansive, evolving worldview. Picture her at the age of 5, standing on a chair reading the large family dictionary on a stand in the living room. Her parents were concerned that she was spending too much time reading instead of playing in the usual way of children her age. Recalling those experiences, Rogers said she learned concepts and ideas first by definition before she learned them in the world context. Life experiences, thereafter, only confirmed what she already knew (M. E. Rogers, personal communication, 1989). Again, the world of ideas has always been larger than life for Rogers and portends a future of infinite potentials. Learning was for her a process of "tying things together or synthesizing ideas rather than analyzing facts" (M. E. Rogers, personal communication, 1989). "A storing up and pondering of ideas" gave rise to more knowledge and new questions.

At the age of 7 years, Rogers' scope of world knowledge was enhanced through Greek and Egyptian mythology. Myths stir the heart of humans and have an appeal that is everlasting. The nature of myth itself provides a context for generating a broad sense of space and time and the evolution of ideas.

Rogers' works reflect a worldview similar to those she loved in mythology. Does the following description of Greek mythology evoke or resonate with Rogerian thought?

> The statements of myth have a direct reference to the past or to the universal present: only so far as the universal present implies the probable continuity of a condition have they any reference to the future. That Hephaistis limped and Hermes flew were, to the Greeks, facts true for all time. Why the simple present was excluded from the temporal reference of the myths, was clear from the nature of their subject matter (Rose, 1958, p. 67).

They were evolving!

Is the seed planted here for an eventual pandimensional human and environmental field without temporal-spatial attributes? In part, a worldview is both the process and the never-ending product of the imagination.

> Since the function of the imagination is to create, it is not to be expected that all its creations must conform to the attested experience of (human) kind or to what we may estimate as probable . . . therefore, most of the details of myths relate the improbable, but the probable and improbable alike were held to be true by the people at that time (Rose, 1958, p. 68).

Myths are still a source of inspiration and human values, fostering the growth of people toward the highest interests. Rogers remarked that her home and family were a source of many of her values and sense of social responsibility. From these sources, together with world literature and world religions, her own patterning was again confirmed. The values of human freedom and social responsibilities were taking form as she lived them.

At the age of 11 years, the nature of Rogers' ideas had been further enlarged by reading all 20 volumes of *The Children's Book of Knowledge.* Next, she delved into the *Encyclopaedia Britannica.* While this expansion of worldview was occurring, her knowledge and love of mathematics and algebra were expanding exponentially. It is not surprising that she would choose and love a mode of reasoning, use of symbols, and the method of combining them so as to convey to the mind at a single glance a long process of reasoning. It was her tendency to link potentials and actual scientific progress in a meaningful, evolving way.

Natural and physical sciences represent only one field of inquiry in the *Encyclopaedia Britannica.* Human nature and human life are the great objects of inquiry also present in literature, history, and philosophy. At an early age, the breadth and depth of Rogers' vision were nourished further by readings in anthropology, archaeology, cosmology, ethnography, astronomy, ethics, psychology, and aesthetics. In high school, eastern philosophy became a preoccupation and enjoyment. She loved to read because it made her stop and think. So it is today.

A broad education for a learned profession is staunchly upheld throughout Rogers' works. At the same time and with equal emphasis, she advocates research and logical analysis for the ultimate development of nursing science. To the critics who say that Rogerian nursing science is based on physics, she is quick to say, "Physics is only one source."

More can be said about the philosophical context attributed to Rogers' early life of learning. As a teenager, she recalls that she wanted to help people but did not clearly know how. Classes at the University of Tennessee in the science-med course did not provide the answer. Knoxville General Hospital had a School of Nursing, and Rogers decided to enroll in her 19th year of learning.

The hourglass of knowledge began to narrow. Militarized routines and a library limited to medical books constrained her human freedom and sensibilities. Opportunity was curtailed drastically in an impoverished classroom. Rogers left, with no intention of returning. However, something unexpected happened. She was brought face to face with a reality that would become a central concern of her life. Having left school, she took a ride on the local Knoxville bus that turned out to be opportunity for diversity. Rogers saw poor, tired, working-class people caught in the immediacy of everyday life. People without zest for life. She asked herself why. She resolved to return to nursing school. In spite of the learning conditions, nursing had promise as the opportunity to help people.

This early insight is expressed in later works. The purpose of nursing was a social mandate "to provide knowledgeable, compassionate service," where every individual has a creative potential to see patterns in life and human freedom to maximize this potential (M. E. Rogers, personal communication, 1989). Rogers loved her early nursing experience of caring for people in spite of doing so in a hospital setting. Next, knowledge of public health was music to her ears. The hourglass began to expand again. "Health" nursing in the environment was a possibility, like the nursing of Florence Nightingale, whom she admired greatly.

Even as a young woman in her twenties, Rogers thought that the world of nursing had not kept pace with either the progress of science or the march of civilization known to her through recorded history. She recoiled from the notion of learning by experience in nursing for several reasons, one being the true sense of learning.

For example, a shift in interpretation of experience in medical science was a strategic move away from a very broad range of human experience in learning described by Plato as "man and nature united" and by St. Thomas Aquinas as "passion and reason as wisdom." It represented a move in the scope of awareness allowable to the learner or inquiring person toward a very narrow, constricted view of experience. An example in 20th century philosophy of science is proscribed by Rudolf Carnap as "experience limited to five-sense perceptible immediate experience" (cited in Reeder, 1984, p. 15). Bacon's tenets for inductive method did not confirm Rogers' ideas. Limited to sensory observation, this view screened out the rich perspectives possible through conceptual thinking and imagination. In contrast Kant's (1980) notion of the active learner and advocacy of "a prior synthetic judgment" was a theory of knowledge that confirmed her ideas about creative learning. Again, Rogers' ideas were always larger than life, and imaginative thinking and synthesizing in historical events in her own life gave rise to original insights and meaning.

Rogers is passionate about what she has seen as she watched raids into what we could call "the vast fields of our ignorance," that is, ignorance and despair created in people by arrogant or unwarranted knowledge claims. Poincaré's voice echoed her conviction as she read his words: "One should be fearful only of an incomplete science which deceives itself and the people!" (cited in Whyte, 1944, p. 24).

Nihilism was a prevailing attitude at the turn of the century, spoken through the voice of Nietzsche. After 300 years of positivistic science the Western world still lacked a unity of science. In spite of this, scientific discoveries were often exaggerated by their authors. Without honesty and humility about knowledge claims, Rogers knew, as confirmed by Lancelot Whyte's works, incomplete and partial science could mislead the people at large.

Voices heard by Rogers included Descartes, who advocated "the method of doubt" in pursuit of certainty (cited in Rogers, 1970, p. 19) and Alfred North Whitehead (1925, p. 17) saying, "Seek simplicity and distrust it." Most recently, the voice of Paul Feyerabend (1981) warned society of scientific dogma and said, "take the responsibility to criticize its premises and its promises" (p. 156). These voices, in concert with Rogers (1961), warned nursing of its uncritical acceptance of knowledge received from other disciplines, particularly medical science and its claims about the human condition and its successful cures.

Rogers found the voice of a kindred spirit in the works of Lancelot Law Whyte (1944), an English theorist, in *The Next Development in Man.* Whyte used his experiences in observing philosophy and science to identify convergent paths in all realms of knowing that the intellect must take if a "unified" view of humankind in history was to be achieved. His major theme was designed to dispel the power of "antiman," a hopeless relativism in the West. In its place Whyte announced "unitary man." This term, although different from Rogers' conception of unitary human beings, was optimistic. It stood for a new type of human able to be more harmonious because of an awareness of the ordering of processes at all levels in nature, without and within. It could be said to be a forerunner of the reality described by Bohm (1980) in terms of the "implicate and explicate order of the universe," and it acknowledged the view first expressed in *The Phenomenon of Man* by Teilhard de Chardin (1965) of a synthesis of matter and spirit. Whyte's (1944) work traces everything to their common source: "the human *imagination* and its *organic roots*" (p. 3).

Whyte's voice was daring, born out of necessity, as was Rogers' voice. Her writings alerted the profession to the dangers it faced if, as a profession, it did not recognize the need for autonomy. Her first book, *Educational Revolution in Nursing* (1961), was informed by democratic ideals of human freedom and social responsibility. These voices, plus the ideals of liberal education voiced by Dewey (1929) and Whitehead (1925), among others, confirmed Rogers' ideals and challenged her to speak her own truth. The next work, *Reveille in Nursing* (Rogers, 1964), expressed the ideals of education. The third and major work gave birth to a unique science of nursing conceived through a life of learning and living. *An Introduction to the Theoretical Basis of Nursing* (Rogers, 1970) represents an original synthesis and organization of knowledge which is optimistic while evoking critical imaginative thinking. Rogers' ideas are indeed enduring ones.

References

Bohm, D. (1980). *Wholeness and the implicate order.* London: Routledge and Kegan Paul.

Dewey, J. (1929). *The sources of a science of education.* The Kappa Delta Pi lecture series. New York: Horance Liveright.

Encyclopaedia Britannica, 15th ed. (1982). Chicago: Encyclopaedia Britannica.

Feyerabend, P. (1981). How to defend society against science. In Hacking, I. (Ed.), *Scientific revolutions* (pp. 156–167). New York: Oxford University Press.

Goertzel, M. (1978). *Three hundred eminent personalities.* San Francisco: Jossey-Bass.

Kant, I. (1980). The limits of knowledge. In Rader, M. (Ed.) *The enduring questions* (4th ed.) (pp. 266–281). New York: Holt, Rinehart & Winston. Excerpts taken from *The critique of pure reason* (1780).

Opie, I., & Opie, P. (1955). Preface, *The Oxford nursery rhyme book* (pp. v–xi). Oxford: Oxford at the Clarendon Press.

Plato (1974). A theory of ideas. In *Republic,* Books V–VII (p. 361) (Trans. G. M. A. Grube). Indianapolis: Hacket.

Reeder, F. (1984). Philosophical issues in the science of unitary human beings. *Advances in Nursing Science, 6*(2), 14–23.

Rogers, M. E. (1961). *Educational revolution in nursing.* New York: Macmillan.

Rogers, M. E. (1964). *Reveille in nursing.* Philadelphia: Davis.

Rogers, M. E. (1970). *An introduction to the theoretical basis of nursing.* Philadelphia: Davis.

Rogers, M. E. (1976). Chapter 1. In Malinski, V. (Ed.), *Explorations on the science of unitary human beings.* Philadelphia: Davis

Rose, H. J. (1958a). *Handbook of Greek and Roman mythology.* London: Methuen.

Rose, H. J. (1958b). *Handbook of Greek mythology* (6th ed.). London: Methuen.

Teilhard de Chardin, P. (1965). *The phenomenon of man.* New York: Harper & Row.

Thompson, H., and Mee, A. (1928). *The new (children's) book of knowledge.* New York or London: Grolier Society, The Educational Book Company.

Whitehead, A. N. (1925). *Science and the modern world.* New York: Free Press.

Whyte, L. L. (1944). *The next development in man.* New York: Mentor.

CHAPTER 56

Rogers' Contribution to the Development of Nursing as a Science

Joyce J. Fitzpatrick

Within the latter half of the 20th century we have witnessed growth and change in nursing science in two important dimensions. First, the *content* of our science has been developed. Second, the *process* through which we shape our science has blossomed. Martha E. Rogers has been at the forefront of this scientific development within nursing, most often leading the revolution. Rogers is the 20th-century Nightingale. Born on the same day, May 12, ninety-four years after Nightingale, Rogers shares the same determination and motivation to change the world in which she lives. Her charisma has captivated nurses everywhere, urging all of us to expand our consciousness and awaken to our societal obligations to achieve maximum health potential for humankind.

In this chapter, I will explore Rogers' contributions to the content of nursing science, with particular attention to the basic components of Rogers' conceptual system, including the principles of resonancy, helicy, and integrality. Second, Rogers' science will be examined from the perspective of the characteristics of science. Lastly, Rogers' contributions to the process of scientific development will be addressed. The early writings of Rogers (1961, 1964) regarding educational reform for nursing are particularly relevant here, for Rogers' consistent efforts to design and advance our learned profession have led many nurse-educators and -scientists to their own contributions.

According to Rogers, the Science of Unitary Human Beings requires a new worldview and a conceptual system specific to nursing phenomena of concern. Creative synthesis of knowledge developed through the years has led to four basic concepts and three principles characterizing Rogerian nursing science (Rogers, 1970, 1980, 1986, 1987). Each of these is examined in relation to scientific developments advanced by Rogers. The brief review of content contributions is meant to be illustrative rather than exhaustive.

Energy Fields

Energy fields characterize person and environment; there are infinite, dynamic human and environmental fields unitary in their mutual process. In the early period of development of Rogers' conceptualizations, research focused on the electrical nature of the human field (Monck, 1968; Ramey, 1968). Contributions from these early studies assisted in refinement of definitions and further elaboration of the human and environmental field concepts. There continues to be considerable effort directed toward clarification of the concept of energy fields. Ference's (1979) classic research on human field motion is an important contribution to this area of study. Research related to Therapeutic Touch, most notably the work of Krieger and Quinn, demonstrates the translation to clinical phenomena (Heidt, 1981; Keller, 1983; Krieger, 1973, 1974, 1975; Krieger, Peper, & Ancoli, 1979; Quinn, 1982, 1984).

Openness

Openness characterizes the human and environmental fields. Continuous change and mutual process are manifest by these fields. In early explorations of boundary interactions nurse-scholars addressed the concept of openness. These nurse-researchers questioned field boundaries and energy exchange. These studies included those focused on perceived body space and boundaries such as those by Chodil (1978), Collett (1973), Hanchett (1979), Fawcett (1976), and Whall (1981).

Pattern

Pattern is defined as the distinguishing characteristic of an energy field perceived as a single wave; it gives identity to the field. The most noteworthy contributions to scholarly pursuits in this area include those of J. A. Smith (1981) and Newman (1983, 1986). Both have explored patterns of health, searching for new definitions of health that reflect new worldviews and a positive orientation to human potential. Additional noteworthy efforts to clarify and define health from Rogers' perspective include the research of Engle (1984, 1986), Reed (1983, 1986a, 1986b, 1987), Laffrey (1985, 1986), and Schorr (1983). Also, Rogers has directly influenced the theoretical work of Parse (1981, 1987), Newman (1972, 1976, 1982, 1983, 1986), and Fitzpatrick (1983, 1989), whose conceptualizations reflect an important pattern component. As part of this research area, Rogerian scholars such as Cowling (1983), Newman (1986), and Crawford (1982) have proposed the development of pattern profiles for clinical nursing assessments.

Pandimensionality

Pandimensionality characterizes the human and environmental fields and is defined as a nonlinear domain. It is without spatial or temporal attributes. Efforts to explore space and time within Rogerian nursing science have been extensive. In fact, perhaps the largest body of research has been in this area. While Rogers has cautioned us that pandimensionality goes beyond linear dimensions, the conceptual struggles inherent in the proposed understandings have led researchers to continue raising related theoretical and empirical questions. Research has been undertaken by such scholars as Newman (1972, 1976, 1982), M. J. Smith (1974, 1985), Rawnsley (1977), Fitzpatrick (1983), Engle (1984, 1986), and others.

Principle of Resonancy

The principle of resonancy postulates that change in pattern of the human and environmental field is propagated by waves. Programmatic research in this area has been extensive, particularly related to the manifestations of field patterning identified by Rogers. Spatial and temporal rhythms have been explored, as have light and sound waves and human field motion. Certainly, the rhythmic patterning essential to Rogers' conceptualizations has been a key area for scientific explorations. Of course, there is the classic research by Neal (1967) on infants' rocking. Examples are prominent in the research literature. Malinski (1980) and McDonald (1981) have investigated light waves; Fitzpatrick (1980, 1983), Reed (1983, 1986a, 1986b, 1987), Floyd (1983, 1984), and Newman (1982, 1986) have studied temporal and motion rhythms.

Principle of Helicy

The principle of helicy indicates that the process of change is one of increasing diversity. Raile (1983) explored creativity, actualization, and empathy as proposed measures of helicy in human development. Barrett's (1984) classic research on power has been directly related to the elaboration of the principle of helicy. Efforts to extend Barrett's research in various programmatic phases have been launched.

Principle of Integrality

The principle of integrality replaced that of complementarity; it describes the continuous mutual human and environmental field process. Rogers' thinking on the subject of wholism has influenced all of nursing. Pre-Rogers discussions of wholism were almost exclusively based on an understanding of addition of parts, the familiar biopsychosocial, cultural, spiritual conception of persons. Rogers' proposition that the whole is different from the sum of its parts is now often used in the rationale for our nursing actions. In fact, this component of Rogerian nursing science has made its way into everyday nursing language.

Characteristics of Science

Currently, much research is under way concerning not only the basic concepts and principles but more importantly the related theories (eg, the theory of accelerating change). Clearly the challenge for the 1990s is to more fully explicate and test the middle-range theories derived from Rogerian nursing science. This challenge is an important one, for without specificity and the rigorous application of scientific development, our progress cannot be rapidly advanced and widely accepted. Science has frequently been characterized as progressing from problems to problems of ever-increasing depth (Popper, 1968). Taken on this criterion alone, Rogers' science has propelled us to increasing depths. Traditionally held beliefs about patients and their health have been questioned and often discarded. We have been stretched by Rogers to consider maximum health potential in lieu of disease prevention. Individuals have been encouraged to knowingly participate in their future, thus enhancing their power and actualizing potentials for change (Barrett, 1983).

Science is first and foremost an intellectual discipline (Parsons, 1968). Science involves theory development, research, and constant intellectual activity to synthesize new knowledge as it is discovered and refined. Rogers' own writings and scholarly publications attest to the intellectual activity that has been prominent. Soon after completing her own doctoral studies, Rogers, through her academic leadership at New York University, began publishing her Science of Man as nursing science, providing a keen example for faculty and professional colleagues and, importantly, creating the new generation of nurse leaders, the graduate students whom she taught in courses and seminars.

Sciences are further characterized by a domain, a phenomenon of concern specific to that discipline. Far more than any other, Rogers had not only specified the domain of nursing's concern but also given it exact language. In fact, often in their misunderstanding of this requirement as a dimension of science, nurses have expressed concern with the new language and terminology introduced by Rogers. This distinct terminology has been introduced by Rogers as the specific language for nursing's phenomenon of concern. Novice Rogerians who are beginning study of the Science of Unitary Human Beings learn the building blocks of the conceptual system and are guided in their study by Rogers' precise definitions.

A number of other characteristics have been proposed for evaluation of conceptual or theoretical structures. In its very nature Rogers' scientific model has *explicit boundaries.* This very exclusion of other knowledge systems which established its scientific credibility also increases the concern within nursing knowledge circles. For somehow it is easier to cling to an eclectic *all-inclusive* view of persons. Often, the approach to science development in nursing, aside from Rogers' model, has been largely additive. As mentioned, Rogers has proposed that we shed our additive view of the ingredients of the psychological, sociological, physiological, biological, and spiritual perspective *and* rather than wait for the magic synthesis that leads one to nursing knowledge, that we create new knowledge. Rogers advocated studying the whole. She argued against reductionism and encouraged the development of new scientific approaches to basic nursing questions. Just as new scientific perspectives are being developed, so are new scientific methods.

Second, a conceptual or theoretical system should be *congruent with empirical evidence.* We should not assume that paradigms and theories are either true or false. We are often in search of the ideal truth. Rogers encourages us to ask ourselves to what extent conceptual systems are adequate in explaining the world or the phenomena of concern. Science is an approximation of reality, a search for truth, yes, but a search cognizant of the unreachable goal.

Such a discussion again brings one to the basic question, what is the phenomenon of concern to nursing? If one defines nursing science as practice theory, then this places boundary limits which could exclude the Science of Unitary Human Beings. If one defines nursing science as focused on practice theory with some allowance (inclusion) of theories and facts relevant to nursing practice, then the key factor becomes the definition of "relevant." Additional arguments regarding relevance of a scientific perspective have centered around the generality, usefulness, and significance of conceptual or theoretical systems. What if these three additional criteria are applied to the Science of Unitary Human Beings?

Does this conceptualization possess generality? Again, here the generality is the strength of the conceptualization. It is the abstract nature of conceptualizations of energy fields, pandimensionality, and wave patterns that lead pragmatists to become skeptical and ask, "How can I nurse an energy field?"

Is this conceptual system significant? Judging from the number of related theoretical developments and the applications in both research and in professional practice, one must conclude that this scientific development has had a marked impact on the further development of nursing science.

A fifth criterion to judge the adequacy of a conceptual or theoretical model is its capability of generating hypotheses. Rogers' conceptualization has consistently generated hypotheses for testing. A sixth criterion is that of internal consistency. All analyses of Rogerian nursing science support the basic inherent logic and consistency. Rogers does not waver. Systems are not a little bit closed, and persons are not sometimes whole.

The last criterion to be addressed is that of simplicity or parsimony. Science is the search for simplicity. William of Occam, a 14th-century philosopher, is credited with saying that entities should not be multiplied beyond necessity. This principle of parsimony means that no more forces should be postulated than are necessary to account for the phenomenon observed. In practice, this means that the simplest explanation is the best. Rogers' conceptualization, even in its complexity in terminology and essence, has a simplicity in form and structure.

Process of Science Development

Gortner (1980, 1983) has aptly described the development of a scientific ethos in nursing based on four principles of scientific work: confirmation, communality, competition and colleagueship, and continuity. Rogers has fostered these principles in her scientific pursuits and those of her colleagues and students. She has been responsible for thousands of graduate students' initial introduction to the Science of Unitary Human Beings. She has fostered dialogue and communication to develop a community of scholars. She has colleagues everywhere across the globe. Rogers has encouraged both competition and colleagueship as evidenced by graduates of educational programs she developed, and she has advocated programmatic research efforts related to the Science of Unitary Human Beings. Rogers has encouraged all of us to reach beyond what we ever expected was within our grasp. She has challenged, searched with us, and advocated that we re-search for new understandings.

Various examples could be used to describe Rogers' stature in the scholarly community of nursing. In the opening of the 1989 Forum on Doctoral Education, Rogers' statements were used as an introduction to a debate on scholarly content for the discipline of nursing. Rogers suggested that unless we develop an organized body of abstract knowledge specific to nursing, there is no purpose for doctoral programs in nursing and that we have often applied sophisticated methodologies to unsophisticated concepts.

Rogers and her nursing science are classics. One can hardly conceive of mention of the metaparadigm concepts, conceptual models, and nursing theories without front billing being given to Rogers. She has influenced the evolution of nursing and, at times, has plotted the scientific revolution.

Rogers' contributions to scientific developments within nursing have been coupled with her contributions to professional issues. She has consistently addressed our educational systems and the status of the profession, urging us to hold to our beliefs and societal commitments. Rogers has recognized and articulated the responsibility that the profession has to itself and ultimately to society, responsibility that dictates design of educational programs, areas and levels of practice, and scholarly, scientific, and professional behaviors. Our scientific debt to her is as compelling as our initial professional debt to Nightingale. Rogers is truly the 20th-century leader.

References

Barrett, E. A. M. (1984). *An empirical investigation of Rogers' principle of helicy: The relationship of human field motion and power.* Unpublished doctoral dissertation, New York University, New York.

Chodil, J. J. (1978). *An investigation of the relation between perceived body space, actual body space, body image boundary, and self-esteem.* Unpublished doctoral dissertation, New York University, New York.

Collett, B. (1973). *A study of the relationship between variation in body temperature, perceived duration and perceived personal space.* Unpublished doctoral dissertation, New York University, New York.

Cowling, W. R., III. (1983). *The relationship of mystical experience, differentiation, and creativity in college students.* Unpublished doctoral dissertation, New York University, New York.

Crawford, G. (1982). The concept of pattern in nursing: Conceptual development and measurement. *Advances in Nursing Science, 5,* 1–6.

Engle, V. (1984). Newman's conceptual framework and the measurement of older adults' functional health. *Advances in Nursing Science, 7,* 24–36.

Engle, V. F. (1986). The relationship of movement and time to older adults' functional health. *Research in Nursing & Health, 9,* 123–130.

Fawcett, J. (1976). *The relationship between spouses' strength of identification and their patterns of change in perceived body space and articulation of body concept during and after pregnancy.* Unpublished doctoral dissertation, New York University, New York.

Ference, H. M. (1979). *The relationship of time experience, creativity traits, differentiation, and human field motion: An investigation of Rogers' correlates of synergistic human development.* Unpublished doctoral dissertation, New York University, New York.

Fitzpatrick, J. J. (1980). Patients' perceptions of time: Current research. *International Nursing Review, 27,* 148–153, 160.

Fitzpatrick, J. J. (1983). A life perspective rhythm model. In J. J. Fitzpatrick & A. L. Whall (Eds.), *Conceptual models of nursing: Analysis and application* (pp. 295–302). Bowie, MD: Brady.

Fitzpatrick, J. J. (1989). A life perspective rhythm model. In J. J. Fitzpatrick & A. L. Whall (Eds.), *Conceptual models of nursing.* East Norwalk, CT: Appleton-Lange.

Floyd, J. A. (1983). Research using Rogers' conceptual system: Development of a testable theorem. *Advances in Nursing Science, 5*(2), 37–48.

Floyd, J. A. (1984). Interaction between personal sleep-wake rhythms and psychiatric hospital rest-activity schedule. *Nursing Research, 33,* 255–259.

Gortner, S. R. (1980). Nursing science in transition. *Nursing Research, 29,* 180–183.

Gortner, S. R. (1983). The history and philosophy of nursing science and research. *Advances in Nursing Science, 5,* 1–8.

Hanchett, E. S. (1979). *Community health assessment: A conceptual tool kit.* New York: Wiley.

Heidt, P. (1981). Effect of therapeutic touch on the anxiety level of hospitalized patients. *Nursing Research, 30,* 33–37.

Keller, E. (1983). *The effects of therapeutic touch on tension headache pain.* Unpublished master's thesis, University of Missouri, Columbia, MO.

Krieger, D. (1973). The relationship of touch with intent to help or to heal to subject's in-vivo hemoglobin values: A study in personalized interaction. *Proceedings of the Ninth American Nurses' Association Research Conference* (pp. 39–58). New York: American Nurses' Association.

Krieger, D. (1974). Healing by the laying-on of hands as a facilitator of bioenergetic change: The response of in-vivo human hemoglobin. *Psychoenergetic Systems, 1,* 121–129.

Krieger, D. (1975). Therapeutic touch: The imprimatur of nursing. *American Journal of Nursing, 5,* 784–787.

Krieger, D., Peper, E., & Ancoli, S. (1979). Physiologic indices of therapeutic touch. *American Journal of Nursing, 4,* 660–662.

Kuhn, T. S. (1970). *The structure of scientific revolutions* (2nd ed.). Chicago: University of Chicago Press.

Laffrey, S. C. (1985). Health behavior choice as related to self-actualization and health conception. *Western Journal of Nursing Research, 7,* 279–294.

Laffrey, S. C. (1986). Development of a health conception scale. *Research in Nursing and Health, 9,* 107–114.

Malinski, V. M. (1980). *The relationship between hyperactivity in children and perception of short wavelength light: An investigation into the conceptual system proposed by Martha E. Rogers.* Unpublished doctoral dissertation, New York University, New York.

McDonald, S. F. (1981). A study of the relationship between visible lightwaves and the experience of pain. *Dissertation Abstracts International, 42,* 569B.

Monck, M. (1968). *The relationship between bio-electrical potential differences and suicidal behavior.* Unpublished doctoral dissertation, New York University, New York.

Neal, M. (1967). *Vestibular stimulation and developmental behavior of the small premature infant.* Nursing Research Report, New York: American Nurses Foundation, March 1968. Doctoral dissertation, New York University Division of Nurse Education.

Newman, M. A. (1972). Time estimation in relation to gait tempo. *Perceptual and Motor Skills, 34,* 359–366.

Newman, M. A. (1976). Movement tempo and the experience of time. *Nursing Research, 25,* 273–279.

Newman, M. A. (1982). Time as an index of expanding consciousness with age. *Nursing Research, 31,* 290–293.

Newman, M. A. (1983). Newman's health theory. In I. Clements & F. Roberts (Eds.), *Family health: A theoretical approach to nursing care* (pp. 161–175). New York: Wiley.

Newman, M. A. (1986). *Health as expanding consciousness.* St. Louis: Mosby.

Parse, R. R. (1981). *Man-living-health: A theory of nursing.* New York: Wiley.

Parse, R. R. (1987). *Nursing science: Major paradigms, theories, and critiques.* Philadelphia: Saunders.

Parsons, T. (1968). Professions. In *International encyclopedia of the social sciences* (Vol. 12, pp. 536–547). New York: Macmillan.

Popper, K. A. (1968). *Conjectures and refutations: The growth of scientific knowledge.* New York: Harper Torchbooks.

Quinn, J. F. (1982). An investigation of the effects of therapeutic touch done without physical contact on state anxiety of hospitalized cardiovascular patients (Doctoral dissertation, New York University, New York, NY, 1982). (University Microfilms No. DA 82-26788.) *Dissertation Abstracts International, 43,* 1797B.

Quinn, J. F. (1984). Therapeutic touch as energy exchange: Testing the theory. *Advances in Nursing Science, 6,* 42–49.

Raile, M. M. (1983). *The relationships of creativity, actualization, and empathy in unitary human development.* Unpublished doctoral dissertation, New York University, New York.

Ramey, I. (1968). The relationship between hemiplegia, muscle function, and bio-electric potential differences. Unpublished doctoral dissertation, New York University, New York.

Rawnsley, M. M. (1977). Perceptions of the speed of time in aging and in dying: An empirical investigation of the holistic theory of nursing proposed by Martha Rogers. *Dissertation Abstracts International, 38,* 1652B.

Reed, P. G. (1983). Implications of the life-span developmental framework for well-being in adulthood and aging. *Advances in Nursing Science, 6*(1), 18–25.

Reed, P. G. (1986a). Developmental resources and depression in the elderly. *Nursing Research, 35,* 368–374.

Reed, P. G. (1986b). Religiousness among terminally ill and healthy adults. *Research in Nursing and Health, 9*(1), 35–42.
Reed, P. G. (1987). Spirituality and well-being in terminally ill hospitalized adults. *Research in Nursing and Health, 10*(5), 335–344.
Rogers, M. E. (1961). *Educational revolution in nursing.* New York: Macmillan.
Rogers, M. E. (1964). *Reveille in nursing.* Philadelphia: Davis.
Rogers, M. E. (1970). *An introduction to the theoretical basis of nursing.* Philadelphia: Davis.
Rogers, M. E. (1980). Nursing: A science of unitary man. In J. P. Riehl & C. Roy (Eds.), *Conceptual models for nursing practice* (2nd ed.). New York: Appleton-Century-Crofts.
Rogers, M. E. (1986). Science of unitary human beings. In V. M. Malinski (Ed.), *Explorations on Martha Rogers' science of unitary human beings* (pp. 3–8). Norwalk, CT: Appleton-Century-Crofts.
Rogers, M. E. (1987). Rogers' science of unitary human beings. In R. R. Parse (Ed.), *Nursing science: Major paradigms, theories, and critiques* (pp. 139–146). Philadelphia: Saunders.
Schorr, J. A. (1983). Manifestations of consciousness and the developmental phenomenon of death. *Advances in Nursing Science, 6*(1), 26–35.
Smith, J. A. (1981). The idea of health: A philosophical inquiry. *Advances in Nursing Science, 3*(3), 42–60.
Smith, M. J. (1974). *An investigation of changes in judgement of duration with different patterns of auditory information for individuals confined to bed.* Unpublished doctoral dissertation, New York University, New York.
Smith, M. J. (1985). *An investigation of effects of different sound frequencies on vividness and creativity of imagery.* Unpublished doctoral dissertation, New York University, New York.
Whall, A. L. (1981). Nursing theory and the assessment of families. *Journal of Psychiatric Nursing and Mental Health Services, 19*(1), 30–36.

CHAPTER 57

Rogers' Contribution to Science at Large

John R. Phillips

Rogers is an avant garde scientist and scholar who has not been content with the acceptance of traditional views of the universe. She is committed to the development of knowledge, whereby it is impossible to use the old ideas that pervade much of science.

As a front-runner of contemporary science, she shows how these old views cannot be used to explain phenomena that do not fit into traditional paradigms of the universe. As a leader in the development of contemporary science, she advocates avidly the necessity of changing untenable views that do not conform to present knowledge. It was through her prescience of the universe and human beings that she created a Science of Unitary Human Beings, which foreshadowed the current developments in humankind.

A New Vision

The criticism that her model is too abstract is actually an attribute. Flores (1985) points out "that science develops by becoming more abstract" (p. 1). In keeping with Flores' ideas, it is through the abstractness of the concepts of Rogers' model that breakthroughs to new understanding of old problems and the evolution of human beings have emerged.

Rogers provides a vision of human evolution that gives breadth to human potentials. Crucial to an understanding of the change process of human evolution is the concept of energy field. Energy fields are of significance since the universe is energy.

Rogers' views of the dynamic nature of human beings as energy fields go beyond the world of the physical to the world of energy to get at the becoming rather than just the being of humans. Her concept of human energy field transcends the narrow views based on just the limited experiences of the physical body. In fact, within the perspective of human energy fields, the physical body is just one of the many manifestations of the pattern of the human field. As such, it is important to recognize that the unity of the pattern of the human energy field goes beyond direct observation of changes in the physical body. According to Rogers, an understanding of human evolution will be achieved through recognition and understanding of the human field pattern.

Since the physical body is a manifestation of the human energy field, there are conceptual, integral connections of the two phenomena. In other words, the changes we experience in the physical body are participating in the changing human field pattern. This change process participates in the growing diversity of human fields, which helps people to actualize their potentials. In other words, the creation of the physical body is one way the human energy field evolves a more diverse pattern.

Provides New Interpretations

Since we are dealing with the growing diversity of the human energy field, there is latitude for new interpretations of traditional views of human evolution that encompass the idea of reincarnation. Rather than the rebirth of the soul in a new body, it is actually the human energy field pattern that manifests another physical body. The creation of more than one physical body is one way the human energy field participates in the continous evolution of its diversity. As DeGregori (1985) indicates, "for more complex forms death is necessary to create the possibility for new life and the evolution of new life forms" (p. 7). However, we know that it is only the physical body that dies, not the human energy field.

Within such a view of the changing diversity of human beings, through the creation of physical bodies, there is need for a different perspective of people with multiple personalities. It is quite possible that the human field of people with multiple personalities is of such a high diversity that it can manifest its potentials in diverse ways through just one physical body. This is alluded to by Hale (1983), who points out that there is growing sentiment among multiples that fusion of the multiple personalities is not the answer. She states that fusion of the personalities could be a norm imposed by a one-personality world. She quotes one multiple as saying, "there are too many advantages to being multiple" (p. 106).

In the relative future, which in actuality is the relative present, there may be no need for a physical body. As has been stated, "Death is simply a shedding of the physical body, like the butterfly coming out of a cocoon . . . and the only thing you lose is something that you don't need anymore—your physical body" (Croissant & Dees, 1978, p. 71). The continued evolution of the human energy field may be as stated by George Bernard Shaw (1948) in his play *Back to Methuselah.*

> The day will come when there will be no people, only thought. And that will be life eternal. . . . None of us now believe that all this machinery of flesh and blood is necessary. It dies. It imprisons us on this petty planet and forbids us to range through the stars (pp. 253, 255).

This is not a ludicrous possibility when one considers Rogers' idea that the human energy field and the environmental energy field are infinite with the universe. In other words, human energy fields are everywhere in the universe. The idea of the infinite nature of human and environmental fields becomes important when emerging views of communication are examined.

Basis for New Health Modalities

The recognition of the integral nature of the physical body and the human energy field calls for a change in health modalities. Today, many of our intervention modalities focus on the physical body. These strategies are important for survival of the physical body; however, they do not get at the underlying pattern of the human energy field from which the physical body emerged. It is important to treat the physical body, but we need to help people to understand the changing pattern of the human field to help them optimize their health potentials. This is necessary since the so-called pathologies of the physical body are manifestations of the human energy field pattern.

The use of Rogers' model has been instrumental in the creation of or further refinement of health modalities related to the human energy field. One such modality is Therapeutic Touch, which I call human field touch, which helps people to participate in the patterning of the energy flow of the human field. It is through this energy patterning of the human field that the greatest amount of change in the physical body will occur, in contrast to those modalities that focus upon the physical body. It is through such strategies, and others to be developed, that prolongation of the living process of the physical body will take place. With further refinement of modalities such as visualization, meditation, imagery, and positive thinking, we can help people to move away from a focus on the physical body to participate knowingly in the patterning of the human field. Such strategies highlight the differences in pattern recognition of the physical body versus pattern recognition of the human energy field. Through greater knowledge of the pattern of the human energy field, we will gain insight into not only the joy and happiness of people, but also the pain and suffering manifest through the physical body. Understanding the rhythmical patterning processes of the human field in contrast to the rhythmical patterning processes of the physical body is mandated for optimum health care to people.

Such a view reflects Smith's (1983) models of health, especially the eudaimonistic model, which is concerned with the actualization of one's potentials. This is significant since meeting the responsibility of helping people achieve health, according to Keegan and Winstead-Fry (cited in Madrid & Winstead-Fry, 1986), will mean helping people participate in the life process by choosing and executing behaviors that lead to optimum fulfillment of their potentials. Such health care calls for synthesis and pattern recognition rather than looking at parts of the human field, especially the manifestation of the human field known as the physical body.

Enhances Pattern Recognition

The evolution of pattern recognition calls for a greater understanding of the pandimensionality of the universe—both human and environmental. Pattern recognition calls for a synthesis of space and time, which is what Rogers ("Eureka!", 1991) calls pandimensionality, "a nonlinear domain without spatial or temporal attributes" (p. 8).

When one uses pandimensional pattern recognition, there is awareness of energy flow and patterning of energy that is quite different from a three-dimensional perspective. Flores (1985) points out that the flow of energy from a three-dimensional perspective is related to opposition to gravity. However, with evolution and the structuring of energy, one is less subject to gravity. There is a conscious patterning of energy whereby there are parsimonious patterns of movement with increasing availability of energy. This indicates that the process of evolutionary change is toward more complex/parsimonious patterns of movement that make for increasing freedom from being subject to gravity.

This whole process of change Flores indicates is explained by Rogers' (1986) mutual human field and environmental field process which is helical in nature. From this perspective, one would agree with Flores (1985) that there is a "trend of evolution toward more and more non-physical movement across increasing dimensions of space and time" (p. 136).

At this point one needs to recall that a human being is an energy field and that the physical body is one manifestation of the field pattern. With this knowledge one can then understand how a person may manifest different types of movement. In paraphrasing Flores, there is evidence that certain complexities of the human field can move while the physical body resists movement.

Perception of Different Forms of Movement

Differences in these forms of movement can be illustrated through various forms of communication. There is no doubt that there is a growing diversity in the evolution of communication by human beings. This is evidenced through the advances in speech, writing, telephone, and satellite transmission. All of these modalities of communication, which involve some form of movement, can be explained by traditional science.

However, traditional science cannot explain the paranormal as a form of communication. There are no laws that explain what appears to be instantaneous communication over distance. It is thought to be impossible for anything to travel that fast.

This form of communication involves what Flores (1985) points out is "the transference or conveyance of information about events in space beyond the space occupied by the body itself" (p. 139). Flores goes on to say that this involves "an awareness that keeps expanding across ever increasing dimensions of space and time, awareness that continually reduces the necessity of actual physical movement across that space-time, the space-time that is the measure of evolutionary energy" (pp. 139–140).

Rogers' Science of Unitary Human Beings provides an elegant answer for the paranormal. Since the human energy field is pandimensional, and the environmental energy field is pandimensional, and both are infinite with the universe, and since the human field and the environmental field are integral with each other, then, there is no need for anything to go anywhere. Pandimensional pattern recognition enables one to perceive this paranormal form of communication anywhere in the universe, which in actuality is normal in Rogers' relative present, the infinite now.

Rogers' Scence of Unitary Human Beings provides a fuller answer for the paranormal than Sheldrake's (1981) concept of morphic resonance. In my estimation it provides clarification of the process delineated by Bohm's (1980) implicate order, which can be used to speculate about how the paranormal unfolds.

So, we can see that the present evolution of human beings involves various forms of communication, those related more to what we call the physical body and those we can relate to Rogers' human energy field. Rogers' principle of helicy indicates, as the past evolution of communication in human beings verifies, that there will be an increase in the diversity of communication, which involves greater pattern recognition.

Freedom of Movement

Essentially, one can agree with Flores (1985) that "increasing pattern awareness is part of the entire trend of evolution toward freedom from subjection to gravity . . . toward freedom of movement in space-time" (p. 141). The continued unfoldment of pandimensional pattern recognition will accelerate the evolution of human beings.

This acceleration is possible since Rogers' human energy field is infinite, where less energy is used since a pandimensional human being does not have to move through space-time. This is especially true since the integral nature of human and environmental fields mandates the use of less energy. With more diverse patterning of the human field accompanied with pandimensional pattern recognition, there will be more energy available to accelerate the growing diversity as indicated in the principle of helicy. In fact, Rogers (1980) says that "simple forms change less rapidly than complex ones" (p. 334). This is possible since one is dealing with energy of pattern rather than energy of parts.

Essentially, these differences in movement are what Ference (1986) was getting at when she derived her concept of human field motion, which deals with energy of field pattern, in contrast to physical motion, which requires greater expenditure of energy in dealing with parts. One could speculate also that this whole process involves Barrett's (1986) theory of power, where "power is the capacity to participate knowingly in the nature of change characterizing the continuous patterning of the human and environmental fields. Power is being aware of what one is choosing to do, feeling free to do it, and doing it intentionally" (p. 174).

Participation in Pattern Change

As Barrett points out in her theory of power, we need to emphasize how the environmental energy field participates in the change process of the human field pattern. The pattern of the human field evolves in concert with the unfolding of the environmental energy field pattern. A person cannot directly change the pattern of another person. The healing modalities mentioned earlier involve patterning the environmental field. Then, a person in mutual process with this environmental field pattern participates in changing his or her human field pattern. According to Barrett, this is enhancing a persons' power to participate knowingly in changes in their field pattern. As health care persons we provide various options from which people can choose, and we help them to achieve their choices through their own intent. Through such patterning of the environmental field, we help people to achieve their potentials through their own participation.

Understanding Changing Diversity of Environmental Field Pattern

Today, we hear about the doom or destructive aspects of advancements in technology, when in actuality technology is a source of diversity and creative potential that contributes to the evolution of humankind. Going back to Barrett's theory of power, the dynamics of technology provide choices that enhance one's ability to choose. Advances in technology give flexibility in the patterning of the environmental field so one can participate knowingly in the life process (DeGregori, 1985).

In this sense, technology is a means by which one patterns the environmental field to help human beings to participate in the growing diversity of the human field pattern. In a sense, a variety of technology provides greater possibility of exploration not only of the environmental field pattern but also of the human field pattern. In this exploration the patterns of the two fields will be accelerated, manifesting greater diversity through the principle of helicy.

Currently, it may seem that technology is more concerned with physical reality rather than helping people to understand the pandimensional universe. This perspective is highly questionable when one reads that scientists are working to create software for advanced pattern-seeing computer intelligence (Ferguson, 1983). Such an advancement is just one indicant of the potentials humans have within their own energy fields that have not been actualized.

There is no doubt that we live in a digital age with a variety of technology, which can be seen as a manifestation of the diverse pattern of the environmental field. We need to take cognizance of this technological change, especially since the digital age is seen as a possible next step in human evolution (Kalbacker, 1982). Computers can no longer be seen as number crunchers, but as imagination extenders where we can explore worlds that seem to not exist, bring our fantasies to life, and alert ourselves to our own creative acts (Dennett, 1982).

Changes in the environmental field pattern such as this will help to accelerate the paranormal potentials of human beings. This is especially true since it has been predicted that new technologies will be developed that will include programmerless computers, new types of human-machine relations that require no keyboarding, and even the making of mental telepathy (Kalbacker, 1982). These developments will help human beings to understand better the pandimensional universe postulated by Rogers. Technology will help unfold the paranormal in human beings. If this becomes a reality, then according to Toffler (1984), the changes are related to a "combustive mixture of diversity and accelerated change" (p. 42). This diversifying change in both the human and environmental fields certainly gives credence to Rogers' theory of accelerating change and her theory of the paranormal.

Conclusion

Rogers has made major contributions to science at large. However, it is more significant to recognize that she provides the direction science is taking. There is a resonating process to Rogers' ideas. Her ideas generate ideas in other people, who in turn help other people create new ideas about humans and their environments. This "spreading power" (DeGregori, 1985, p. 24) is only the beginning of a multitude of changes that will come about through use of her Science of Unitary Human Beings. As further understanding emerges, acceleration in the evolution of the potentials of human beings will occur.

There is a vast array of human potentials to be discovered in a pandimensional universe. As Barrett (1986) points out, it is possible for people to participate in their patterning process, and it will be Rogerian scientists and scholars who believe in a participatory universe who will help to accelerate the evolution of human beings.

References

Barrett, E. A. M. (1986). Investigation of the principle of helicy: The relationship of human field motion and power. In V. M. Malinski (Ed.), *Explorations on Martha Rogers' Science of Unitary Human Beings* (pp. 173–184). Norwalk, CT: Appleton-Century-Crofts.

Bohm, D. (1980). *Wholeness and the implicate order.* London: Routledge & Kegan Paul.

Croissant, K., & Dees, C. (1978). *Continuum: The immortality principle.* San Bernardino, CA: Franklin Press.

DeGregori, T. R. (1985). *A theory of technology: Continuity and change in human development.* Ames, IA: Iowa State University Press.

Dennett, D. C. (1982, December). The imagination extenders. *Psychology Today,* pp. 32–39.

Eureka! Four-dimensionality evolved into multidimensionality evolved into pandimensionality. (1991). *Rogerian Nursing Science News, 3*(3), 8.

Ference, H. M. (1986). The relationship of time experience, creativity traits, differentiation, and human field motion. In V. M. Malinski (Ed.), *Explorations on Martha Rogers' Science of Unitary Human Beings* (pp. 95–105). Norwalk, CT: Appleton-Century-Crofts.

Ferguson, M. (Ed.). (1983, September 12). Computer scientists work on software to mimic intuitive, pattern-seeing mind. *Brain/Mind Bulletin, 8*(15), 3.

Flores, K. (1985). *Relativity and consciousness: A new approach to evolution.* New York: Gordian Press.

Hale, E. (1983, April 17). Inside the divided mind. *The New York Times Magazine,* pp. 100–106.

Kalbacker, W. (1982, March). The digital age. *Science Digest,* pp. 66–70.

Madrid, M., & Winstead-Fry, P. (1986). Rogers's conceptual model. In P. Winstead-Fry (Ed.), *Case studies in nursing theory* (pp. 73–102). New York: National League for Nursing.

Rogers, M. E. (1980). Nursing: A science of unitary man. In J. P. Riehl & C. Roy (Eds.), *Conceptual models for nursing practice* (pp. 329–337). New York: Appleton-Century-Crofts.

Rogers, M. E. (1986). Science of Unitary Human Beings. In V. M. Malinski (Ed.), *Explorations on Martha Rogers' Science of Unitary Human Beings* (pp. 3–8). Norwalk, CT: Appleton-Century-Crofts.

Shaw, G. B. (1948). *Selected plays of Bernard Shaw* (Vol. 2). New York: Dodd, Mead.

Sheldrake, R. (1981). *A new science of life.* Boston: Tarcher.

Smith, J. A. (1983). *The idea of health: Implications for the nursing profession.* New York: Teachers College Press.

Toffler, A. (1984, October). The data deluge: Artificial intelligence. *Omni,* pp. 42, 166.

Epilogue

There is a future in nursing that stretches far beyond the dreams of Florence Nightingale whose vision prompted her to say, "May we hope that when we are all dead and gone, leaders will arise who will lead far beyond anything we have done." Tomorrow belongs to all of us. In meeting the challenge of today we are also preparing for an unknown tomorrow. (Rogers, 1962, p. 8)

Many have gratefully acknowledged the legacy of Martha E. Rogers' work for the profession and the discipline of nursing. This book is our attempt to express appreciation for that legacy by organizing some of Rogers' most memorable written work while simultaneously providing the reader with a glimpse of Rogers, the person and the nurse.

This book was born 4 years ago in a Greenwich Village restaurant while we were having dinner with Martha. We thank her for her wholehearted and continuous support and for providing us with access to her files. We hope the book will be useful not only for Rogerian scholars but for those who seek clear, unambiguous direction through creative ideas and thoughts on the difficulties facing the nursing world today and tomorrow. Many of Rogers' innovative ideas suggest a universality and a timeless quality. They hold as many creative potentials in the 1990s as they did in the 1960s, the 1970s, and the 1980s. Her ideas will carry us forward into the 21st century and beyond.

The past decade has witnessed considerable growth in application of Rogers' Science of Unitary Human Beings. Many schools other than New York University have adopted this science as the basis for their curriculum, including Washburn University School of Nursing in Topeka, Kansas, and the College of Mount Saint Vincent Department of Nursing in Riverdale, New York. Numerous schools have faculty sponsoring doctoral dissertations and master's theses based on Rogerian science. Nursing courses at the doctoral level have been offered at schools such as the Medical College of Georgia and the University of South Carolina. Nursing service organizations on a department-wide basis have implemented Rogerian science as the scientific paradigm for practice at the San Diego Veterans' Administration Hospital as well as at Children's Hospital Medical Center in Cincinnati, Ohio.

The Society of Rogerian Scholars, an international organization, is committed to fostering further development and use of the Science of Unitary Human Beings. The society has members across the world. You are invited to join by contacting the society at 1 (800) 474-9793.

Martha Rogers has actively participated in the development and implementation of the above endeavors. She continues with an active speaking, teaching, and consulting schedule. She has been awarded nine honorary doctorates. Rogers has presented scientific and professional papers to a wide range of interdisciplinary groups in 46 states and the territories of Puerto Rico and the Virgin Islands, as well as other countries, including Brazil, Canada, China, Columbia, Egypt, Japan, Mexico, Newfoundland, the Netherlands, Spain, and Germany.

There will be many ways that Rogers will be remembered. She helped to clear the fog of ignorance in nursing and lift the veil of ritualized tradition. Above all, one must not forget Rogers' commitment to the betterment of humankind and to the integral role nurses play in assisting people to optimize their potentials. This is best exemplified in the following, written by Rogers for *The Education Violet,* the N. Y. U. newspaper, in 1966:

> Nursing's story is a magnificent epic of service to mankind. It is about people: how they are born, and live and die; in health and in sickness; in joy and in sorrow. Its mission is the translation of knowledge into human service.
>
> Nursing is compassionate concern for human beings. It is the heart that understands and the hand that soothes. It is the intellect that synthesizes many learnings into meaningful ministrations.
>
> For students of nursing the future is a rich repository of far-flung opportunities around this planet and toward the further reaches of man's explorations of new worlds and new ideas. Theirs is the promise of deep satisfaction in a field long dedicated to serving the health needs of people.

At the Historical Salute held in 1989, Rogers was given a star in Ursa Major that bears her name. We know we'll meet with her there someday; you are all invited to join us!

— Violet M. Malinski and Elizabeth Ann Manhart Barrett

Reference

Rogers, M. E. (1962). *Nursing charts her course.* Paper presented at the Annual Lectureship, School of Nursing, Medical College of Georgia.

Bibliography

The great majority of the following citations were compiled by Jacqueline Fawcett, R.N., Ph.D., F.A.A.N., University of Pennsylvania School of Nursing. They are contained in the references for Rogers in her book, *Analysis and Evaluation of Conceptual Models of Nursing* (2nd ed.), published by F. A. Davis Company (1989), and in periodic addenda she has compiled since the book's publication.

Aggleton, P., & Chalmers, H. (1984). Rogers' unitary field model. *Nursing Times, 80*(50), 35–39.

Allanach, E. J. (1988). Perceived supportive behaviors and nursing occupational stress: An evolution of consciousness. *Advances in Nursing Science, 10*(2), 73–82.

Allen, E. K. (1990). Creativity as an index of unitary human development (Abstract of a master's thesis). *Rogerian Nursing Science News, II*(3), 5.

Allen, V. L. R. (1989). The relationship among time experience, human field motion, and clairvoyance: An investigation in the Rogerian conceptual system. *Dissertation Abstracts International, 50,* 121B.

Alligood, M. R. (1986). The relationship of creativity, actualization, and empathy in unitary human development. In V. M. Malinski (Ed.), *Explorations on Martha Rogers' science of unitary human beings* (pp. 145–154). Norwalk, CT: Appleton-Century-Crofts.

Alligood, M. R. (1989). Applying Rogers' model to nursing administration: Emphasis on environment, health. In B. Henry, C. Arndt, M. Di Vincenti, & A. Marriner-Tomey (Eds.), *Dimensions of nursing administration* (pp. 105–111). Boston: Blackwell Scientific Publications.

Alligood, M. R. (1990). Nursing care of the elderly: Futuristic projections. In E. A. M. Barrett (Ed.), *Visions of Rogers' science-based nursing* (pp. 129–142). New York: National League for Nursing.

Alligood, M. R. (1990). Rogers' theory: Research to practice. *Rogerian Nursing Science News, II*(3), 2–4.

Alligood, M. R. (1991). Guided reminiscence: A Rogers based intervention. *Rogerian Nursing Science News, III*(3), 1–4.

Alligood, M. R. (1991). Testing Rogers' theory of accelerating change: The relationships among creativity, actualization, and empathy in persons 18 to 92 years of age. *Western Journal of Nursing Research, 13,* 84–96.

Andersen, M. D., & Smereck, G. A. D. (1989). Personalized nursing LIGHT model. *Nursing Science Quarterly, 2,* 120–130.

Andersen, M. D., & Smereck, G. A. D. (1992). The consciousness rainbow: An explication of Rogerian field pattern manifestations. *Nursing Science Quarterly, 5,* 72–79.

Asay, M. K., & Ossler, C. C. (Eds.). (1984). Conceptual models of nursing: Applications in community health nursing. *Proceedings of the Eighth Annual Community Health Nursing Conference.* Chapel Hill: Department of Public Health Nursing, School of Public Health, University of North Carolina.

Atwood, J. R., & Gill-Rogers, B. (1984). Metatheory, methodology and practicality: Issues in research uses of Rogers' science of unitary man. *Nursing Research, 33,* 88–91.

Banonis, B. C. (1989). The lived experience of recovering from addiction: A phenomenological study. *Nursing Science Quarterly, 2,* 37–43.

Barber, H. R. K. (1987). Editorial: Trends in nursing: A model for emulation. *The Female Patient, 12*(3), 12, 14.

Barrett, E. A. M. (1986). Investigation of the principle of helicy: The relationship of human field motion and power. In V. M. Malinski (Ed.), *Explorations on Martha Rogers' science of unitary human beings* (pp. 173–184). Norwalk, CT: Appleton-Century-Crofts.

Barrett, E. A. M. (1988). Using Rogers' science of unitary human beings in nursing practice. *Nursing Science Quarterly, 1,* 50–51.

Barrett, E. A. M. (1989). A nursing theory of power for nursing practice: Derivation from Rogers' paradigm. In J. P. Riehl-Sisca (Ed.), *Conceptual models for nursing practice* (3rd ed., pp. 207–217). Norwalk, CT: Appleton-Century-Crofts.

Barrett, E. A. M. (1990). The continuing revolution of Rogers' science-based nursing education. In E. A. M. Barrett (Ed.), *Visions of Rogers' science-based nursing* (pp. 303–318). New York: National League for Nursing.

Barrett, E. A. M. (1990). Health patterning with clients in a private practice environment. In E. A. M. Barrett (Ed.), *Visions of Rogers' science-based practice* (pp. 105–116). New York: National League for Nursing.

Barrett, E. A. M. (1990). Rogerian patterns of scientific inquiry. In E. A. M. Barrett (Ed.), *Visions of Rogers' science-based nursing* (pp. 169–188). New York: National League for Nursing.

Barrett, E. A. M. (1990). Rogers' science-based nursing practice. In E. A. M. Barrett (Ed.), *Visions of Rogers' science-based nursing* (pp. 31–44). New York: National League for Nursing.

Barrett, E. A. M. (1990). Visions of Rogerian science in the future of humankind. In E. A. M. Barrett (Ed.), *Visions of Rogers' science-based nursing* (pp. 357–362). New York: National League for Nursing.

Barrett, E. A. M. (Ed.) (1990). *Visions of Rogers' science-based nursing.* New York: National League for Nursing.

Barrett, E. A. M. (1991). Space nursing. *Cutis, 48,* 299–303.

Barrett, E. A. M. (1992). Innovative imagery: A health-patterning modality for nursing practice. *Journal of Holistic Nursing, 10,* 154–166.

Barrett, E. A. M. (1993). Virtual reality: A health patterning modality for nursing in space. *Visions: The Journal of Rogerian Nursing Science,* Premiere Issue, 10–21.

Benedict, S. C., & Bunge, J. M. (1990). The relationship between human field motion and preferred visible wavelengths. *Nursing Science Quarterly, 3,* 73–80.

Biley, F. (1990). Rogers' model: An analysis. *Nursing (London), 4*(15), 31–33.

Biley, F. (1992). The perception of time as a factor in Rogers' science of unitary human beings: A literature review. *Journal of Advanced Nursing, 17,* 1141–1145.

Black, G., & Haight, B. K. (1992). Integrality as a holistic framework for the life-review process. *Holistic Nursing Practice, 7*(1), 7–15.

Blair, C. (1979). Hyperactivity in children: Viewed within the framework of synergistic man. *Nursing Forum, 18,* 293–303.

Boguslawski, M. (1990). Unitary human field practice modalities. In E. A. M. Barrett (Ed.), *Visions of Rogers' science-based nursing* (pp. 83–92). New York: National League for Nursing.

Boyd, C. (1985). Toward an understanding of mother-daughter identification using concept analysis. *Advances in Nursing Science, 7*(3), 78–86.

Boyd, C. (1990). Testing a model of mother-daughter identification. *Western Journal of Nursing Research, 12,* 448–468.

Bradley, D. B. (1987). Energy fields: Implications for nurses. *Journal of Holistic Nursing, 5*(1), 32–35.

Bramlett, M. H. (1991). Power, creativity and reminiscence in the elderly. *Dissertation Abstracts International, 51,* 3317B.

Bramlett, M. H., Gueldner, S. H., & Sowell, R. L. (1990). Consumer-centric advocacy: Its connection to nursing frameworks. *Nursing Science Quarterly, 3,* 156–161.

Bramlett, M. H., Gueldner, S. H., & Boettcher, J. H. (1993). Reflections on the science of unitary human beings in terms of Kuhn's requirement for explanatory power. *Visions: The Journal of Rogerian Science,* Premiere Issue, 22–35.

Branum, Q. K. (1986). Power as knowing participation in change: A model for nursing intervention. *Dissertation Abstracts International, 46,* 3780B.

Bray, J. D. (1990). The relationships of creativity, time experience and mystical experience. *Dissertation Abstracts International, 50,* 3394B.

Brouse, S. H. (1985). Effect of gender role identity on patterns of feminine and self-concept scores from late pregnancy to early postpartum. *Advances in Nursing Science, 7*(3), 32–48.

Buczny, B., Speirs, J., & Howard, J. R. (1989). Nursing care of a terminally ill client: Applying Martha Rogers' conceptual framework. *Home Healthcare Nurse, 7*(4), 13–18.

Butcher, H. K., & Forchuk, C. (1992). The overview effect: The impact of space exploration on the evolution of nursing science. *Nursing Science Quarterly, 5,* 118–123.

Butcher, H. K., & Parker, N. I. (1988). Guided imagery within Rogers' science of unitary human beings: An experimental study. *Nursing Science Quarterly, 1,* 103–110. [Reprinted in E. A. M. Barrett (Ed.), *Visions of Rogers' science-based nursing* (pp. 269–285). New York: National League for Nursing.]

Butcher, H. K., & Parker, N. I. (1990). Response to "Discussion of a study of pleasant guided imagery." In E. A. M. Barrett (Ed.), *Visions of Rogers' science-based nursing* (pp. 295–297). New York: National League for Nursing.

Butterfield, S. E. (1983). In search of commonalities: An analysis of two theoretical frameworks. *International Journal of Nursing Studies, 20,* 15–22.

Carboni, J. T. (1991). A Rogerian theoretical tapestry. *Nursing Science Quarterly, 4,* 130–136.

Carboni, J. T. (1992). Instrument development and the measurement of unitary constructs. *Nursing Science Quarterly, 5,* 134–142.

Caroselli-Dervan, C. (1990). Visionary opportunities for knowledge development in nursing administration. In E. A. M. Barrett (Ed.), *Visions of Rogers' science-based nursing* (pp. 151–158). New York: National League for Nursing.

Caroselli-Dervan, C. (1991). The relationship of power and feminism in female nurse executives in acute care hospitals. *Dissertation Abstracts International, 52,* 2990B.

Cerilli, K. (1989). An analysis of Martha Rogers' nursing as a science of unitary human beings. In J. P. Riehl-Sisca (Ed.), *Conceptual models for nursing practice* (3rd ed., pp. 189–195). Norwalk, CT: Appleton & Lange.

Chandler, G. E. (1987). The relationship of nursing work environment to empowerment and powerlessness. *Dissertation Abstracts International, 47,* 4822B.

Christenson, P., Sowell, R., & Gueldner, S. H. (1993). Nursing in space: Theoretical foundations and potential practice applications within Rogerian science. *Visions: The Journal of Rogerian Nursing Science,* Premiere Issue, 36–44.

Clarke, P. N. (1986). Theoretical and measurement issues in the study of field phenomena. *Advances in Nursing Science, 9*(1), 29–39.

Cody, W. K. (1991). Multidimensionality: Its meaning and significance. *Nursing Science Quarterly, 4,* 140–141.

Compton, M. A. (1989). A Rogerian view of drug abuse: Implications for nursing. *Nursing Science Quarterly, 2,* 98–105.

Conner, G. K. (1986). The manifestations of human field motion, creativity, and time experience patterns of female and male parents. *Dissertation Abstracts International, 47,* 1926B.

Cora, V. L. (1986). Family life process of intergenerational families with functionally dependent elders. *Dissertation Abstracts International, 47,* 568B.

Cowling, W. R., III. (1986). The relationship of mystical experience, differentiation, and creativity in college students. In V. M. Malinski (Ed.), *Explorations on Martha Rogers' science of unitary human beings* (pp. 131–141). Norwalk, CT: Appleton-Century-Crofts.

Cowling, W. R., III. (1986). The science of unitary human beings: Theoretical issues, methodological challenges, and research realities. In V. M. Malinski (Ed.), *Explorations on Martha Rogers' science of unitary human beings* (pp. 65–78). Norwalk, CT: Appleton-Century-Crofts.

Cowling, W. R., III. (1990). Chronological age as an anomalie of evolution. In E. A. M. Barrett (Ed.), *Visions of Rogers' science-based nursing* (pp. 143–150). New York: National League for Nursing.

Cowling, W. R., III. (1990). A template for unitary pattern-based nursing practice. In E. A. M. Barrett (Ed.), *Visions of Rogers' science-based nursing* (pp. 45–66). New York: National League for Nursing.

Cowling, W. R., III. (1993). Unitary knowing in nursing practice. *Nursing Science Quarterly, 6,* 201–207.

Crawford, G. (1982). The concept of pattern in nursing: Conceptual development and measurement. *Advances in Nursing Science, 5*(1), 1–6.

Crawford, G. (1985). A theoretical model of support network conflict experienced by new mothers. *Nursing Research, 34,* 100–102.

Daffron, J. M. (1989). Patterns of human field motion and human health. *Dissertation Abstracts International, 49,* 4229B.

Daily, J. S., Maupin, J. S., & Satterly, M. C. (1986). Martha E. Rogers: Unitary human beings. In A. Marriner (Ed.), *Nursing theorists and their work* (pp. 345–360). St. Louis: Mosby.

Davidson, A. W. (1992). Choice patterns: A theory of the human-environment relationship (Abstract). *Rogerian Nursing Science News, V*(1), 4–5.

Davidson, A. W., & Ray, M. A. (1991). Studying the human-environment phenomenon using the science of complexity. *Advances in Nursing Science, 14*(2), 73–87.

Davis, A. E. (1991). The relationship between the phenomenon of traumatic injury and the patterns of power, human field motion, esteem and risk taking (Abstract). *Rogerian Nursing Science News, III*(3), 8.

Decker, K. (1989). Theory in action: The geriatric assessment team. *Journal of Gerontological Nursing, 15*(10), 25–28.

DeFeo, D. J. (1990). Change: A central concern of nursing. *Nursing Science Quarterly, 3,* 88–94.

DeSevo, M. R. (1991). Temporal experience and the preference for musical sequence complexity: A study based on Martha Rogers' conceptual system. *Dissertation Abstracts International, 52,* 2992B.

Drake, M. L., Verhulst, D., & Fawcett, J. (1988). Physical and psychological symptoms experienced by Canadian women and their husbands during pregnancy and the postpartum. *Journal of Advanced Nursing, 13,* 436–440.

Dzurec, L. C. (1987). The nature of power experienced by individuals manifesting patterning labeled schizophrenic: An investigation of the principle of helicy. *Dissertation Abstracts International, 47,* 4467B.

Evans, B. A. (1991). The relationship among a pattern of influence in the organizational environment, power of the nurse, and the nurse's empathic attributes: A manifestation of integrality. *Dissertation Abstracts International, 51,* 5244B.

Falco, S. M., & Lobo, M. L. (1985). Martha E. Rogers. In Nursing Theories Conference Group (Ed.), *Nursing theories: The base for professional nursing practice* (2nd ed., pp. 214–234). Englewood Cliffs, NJ: Prentice-Hall.

Falco, S. M., & Lobo, M. L. (1990). Martha E. Rogers. In J. B. George (Ed.), *Nursing theories: The base for professional nursing practice* (3rd ed., pp. 211–230). Norwalk, CT: Appleton & Lange.

Fawcett, J. (1975). The family as a living open system: An emerging conceptual framework for nursing. *International Nursing Review, 22,* 113–116.

Fawcett, J. (1976). *The relationship between spouses' strength of identification and their patterns of change in perceived body space and articulation of body concept during and after pregnancy.* Unpublished doctoral dissertation, New York University, New York.

Fawcett, J. (1989). Spouses' experiences during pregnancy and the postpartum: A program of research and theory development. *Image: Journal of Nursing Scholarship, 21,* 149–152.

Fawcett, J. (1990). Response to letter to the editor. *Image: Journal of Nursing Scholarship, 22,* 197.

Fawcett, J., & Downs, F. S. (1986). *The relationship of theory and research.* Norwalk, CT: Appleton-Century-Crofts.

Fawcett, J., & York, R. (1986). Spouses' physical and psychological symptoms during pregnancy and the postpartum. *Nursing Research, 35,* 144–148.

Fawcett, J., & York, R. (1987). Spouses' strength of identification and reports of symptoms during pregnancy and the postpartum. *Florida Nursing Review, 2*(2), 1–10.

Feigenbaum, J. C. (1988). Historical trends in the role expectations of faculty in collegiate programs of professional nursing, 1901–1970. *Dissertation Abstracts International, 49,* 2125B.

Ference, H. M. (1986). Foundations of a nursing science and its evolution: A perspective. In V. M. Malinski (Ed.), *Explorations on Martha Rogers' science of unitary human beings* (pp. 35–44). Norwalk, CT: Appleton-Century-Crofts.

Ference, H. M. (1986). The relationship of time experience, creativity traits, differentiation, and human field motion. In V. M. Malinski (Ed.), *Explorations on Martha Rogers' science of unitary human beings* (pp. 95–105). Norwalk, CT: Appleton-Century-Crofts.

Ference, H. M. (1989). Comforting the dying: Nursing practice according to the Rogerian model. In J. P. Riehl-Sisca (Ed.), *Conceptual models for nursing practice* (3rd ed., pp. 197–205). Norwalk, CT: Appleton & Lange.

Ference, H. M. (1989). Nursing science theories and administration. In B. Henry, C. Arndt, M. Di Vincenti, & A. Marriner-Tomey (Eds.), *Dimensions of nursing administration* (pp. 121–131). Boston: Blackwell Scientific Publications.

Fisher, L. R., & Reichenbach, M. A. (1987/1988). From Tinkerbell to Rogers (How a fairy tale facilitated an understanding of Rogers' theory of unitary being). *Nursing Forum, 23,* 5–9.

Fitzpatrick, J. J. (1980). Patients' perceptions of time: Current research. *International Nursing Review, 27,* 148–153, 160.

Fitzpatrick, J. J. (1983). Life perspective rhythm model. In J. J. Fitzpatrick & A. L. Whall (Eds.), *Conceptual models of nursing: Analysis and evaluation* (pp. 295–302). Bowie, MD: Brady.

Fitzpatrick, J. J. (1988). Theory based on Rogers' conceptual model. *Journal of Gerontological Nursing, 14*(9), 14–19.

Fitzpatrick, J. J., & Donovan, M. J. (1978). Temporal experience and motor behavior among the aged. *Research in Nursing and Health, 1,* 60–68.

Fitzpatrick, J. J., Donovan, M. J., & Johnston, R. L. (1980). Experience of time during the crisis of cancer. *Cancer Nursing, 3,* 191–194.

Fitzpatrick, J. J., Whall, A. L., Johnston, R. L., & Floyd, J. A. (1982). *Nursing models and their psychiatric mental health applications.* Bowie, MD: Brady.

Floyd, J. A. (1983). Research using Rogers' conceptual system: Development of a testable theorem. *Advances in Nursing Science, 5*(2), 37–48.

Floyd, J. A. (1984). Interaction between personal sleep-wake rhythms and psychiatric hospital rest-activity schedule. *Nursing Research, 33,* 255–259.

Forker, J. E., & Billings, C. V. (1989). Nursing therapeutics in a group encounter. *Archives of Psychiatric Nursing, 3,* 108–112.

France, N. (1992). A phenomenological inquiry on the child's lived experience of perceiving the human energy field using therapeutic touch (Abstract). *Rogerian Nursing Science News, V*(1), 6.

Freda, M. C. (1989). A role model of leadership in and advocacy for nursing. *Nursing Forum, 24*(3–4), 9–13.

Fry, J. E. (1985). Reciprocity in mother-child interaction, correlates of attachment, and family environment in three-year-old children with congenital heart disease. *Dissertation Abstracts International, 46,* 113B.

Garon, M. (1991). Assessment and management of pain in the home care setting: Application of Rogers' science of unitary human beings. *Holistic Nursing Practice, 6*(1), 47–57.

Garon, M. (1992). Contributions of Martha Rogers to the development of nursing knowledge. *Nursing Outlook, 40,* 67–72.

Gaydos, L. S., & Farnham, R. (1988). Human-animal relationships within the context of Rogers' principle of integrality. *Advances in Nursing Science, 10*(4), 72–80.

Gill, B. P., & Atwood, J. R. (1981). Reciprocy and helicy used to relate mEGF and wound healing. *Nursing Research, 30,* 68–72.

Gioiella, E. (1989). Professionalizing nursing: A Rogers legacy. *Nursing Science Quarterly, 2,* 61–62.

Girardin, B. W. (1991). The relationship of lightwave frequency to sleep-wakefulness frequency in well, full-term Hispanic neonates. *Dissertation Abstracts International, 52,* 748B.

Goldberg, W. G., & Fitzpatrick, J. J. (1980). Movement therapy with the aged. *Nursing Research, 29,* 339–346.

Greiner, D. S. (1991). Rhythmicities. *Nursing Science Quarterly, 4,* 21–23.

Gueldner, S. H. (1986). The relationship between imposed motion and human field motion in elderly individuals living in nursing homes. In V. M. Malinski (Ed.), *Explorations on Martha Rogers' science of unitary human beings* (pp. 161–171). Norwalk, CT: Appleton-Century-Crofts.

Gueldner, S. H. (1989). Applying Rogers' model to nursing administration: Emphasis on client and nursing. In B. Henry, C. Arndt, M. Di Vincenti, & A. Marriner-Tomey (Eds.), *Dimensions of nursing administration* (pp. 113–119). Boston: Blackwell Scientific Publications.

Gulick, E. E., & Bugg, A. (1992). Holistic health patterning in multiple sclerosis. *Research in Nursing and Health, 15,* 175–185.

Guthrie, B. J. (1988). The relationships of tolerance of ambiguity, preference for processing information in the mixed mode to differentiation in female college students: An empirical investigation of the homeodynamic principle of helicy. *Dissertation Abstracts International, 49,* 74B.

Hanchett, E. S. (1988). *Nursing frameworks and community as client: Bridging the gap.* Norwalk, CT: Appleton & Lange.

Hanchett, E. S. (1990). Nursing models and community as client. *Nursing Science Quarterly, 3,* 67–72.

Hanchett, E. S. (1992). Concepts from eastern philosophy and Rogers' science of unitary human beings. *Nursing Science Quarterly, 5,* 164–170.

Hanley, M. A. (1990). Concept-integration: A board game as a learning tool. In E. A. M. Barrett (Ed.), *Visions of Rogers' science-based nursing* (pp. 335–344). New York: National League for Nursing.

Hardin, S. (1990). A caring community. In M. Leininger & J. Watson (Eds.), *The caring imperative in education* (pp. 217–225). New York: National League for Nursing.

Heggie, J. R., Schoenmehl, P. A., Chang, M. K., & Crieco, C. (1989). Selection and implementation of Dr. Martha Rogers' nursing conceptual model in an acute care setting. *Clinical Nurse Specialist, 3,* 143–147.

Heidt, P. R. (1990). Openness: A qualitative analysis of nurses' and patients' experiences of therapeutic touch. *Image: Journal of Nursing Scholarship, 22,* 180–186.

Hektor, L. M. (1989). Martha E. Rogers: A life history. *Nursing Science Quarterly, 2,* 63–73.

Huch, M. H. (1991). Perspectives on health. *Nursing Science Quarterly, 4,* 33–40.

Iveson-Iveson, J. (1982). The four dimensional nurse. *Nursing Mirror, 155*(22), 52.

Johnston, R. L. (1981). Temporality as a measure of unidirectionality with the Rogerian conceptual framework of nursing science. *Dissertation Abstracts International, 41,* 3740B.

Johnston, R. L. (1986). Approaching family intervention through Rogers' conceptual model. In A. L. Whall, *Family therapy theory for nursing: Four approaches* (pp. 11–32). Norwalk, CT: Appleton-Century-Crofts.

Johnston, R. L., Fitzpatrick, J. J., & Donovan, M. J. (1982). Developmental stage: Relationship to temporal dimensions (Abstract). *Nursing Research, 31,* 120.

Jones, D. A., Dunbar, C. F., & Jirovec, M. M. (1982). *Medical-surgical nursing: A conceptual approach.* New York: McGraw-Hill.

Joseph, L. (1990). Practical application of Rogers' theoretical framework for nursing. In M. E. Parker (Ed.), *Nursing theories in practice* (pp. 115–125). New York: National League for Nursing.

Jurgens, A., Meehan, T. C., & Wilson, H. L. (1987). Therapeutic touch as a nursing intervention. *Holistic Nursing Practice, 2*(1), 1–13.

Katch, M. P. (1983). A negentropic view of the aged. *Journal of Gerontological Nursing, 9,* 656–660.

Keller, E., & Bzdek, V. M. (1986). Effects of therapeutic touch on tension headache pain. *Nursing Research, 35,* 101–106.

Kim, H. S. (1983). Use of Rogers' conceptual system in research: Comments. *Nursing Research, 32,* 89–91.

Kodiath, M. F. (1991). A new view of the chronic pain patient. *Holistic Nursing Practice, 6*(1), 41–46.

Krieger, D. (1974). The relationship of touch, in intent to help or heal to subjects' in-vivo hemoglobin values: A study in personalized interaction. In American Nurses' Association, *Ninth Nursing Research Conference* (pp. 39–58). Kansas City, MO: American Nurses' Association.

Krieger, D. (1975). Therapeutic touch: The imprimatur of nursing. *American Journal of Nursing, 75,* 784–787.

Kutlenios, R. M. (1986). A comparison of holistic, mental and physical health nursing interventions with the elderly. *Dissertation Abstracts International, 47,* 995B.

Laffrey, S. C. (1985). Health behavior choice as related to self-actualization and health conception. *Western Journal of Nursing Research, 7,* 279–295.

Levine, N. H. (1976). A conceptual model for obstetric nursing. *Journal of Obstetric, Gynecologic, and Neonatal Nursing, 5*(2), 9–15.

Lindley, P. A. (1981). *An empirical study of the relationship of sensation seeking to the human energy field motion within Rogers' science of unitary human beings.* Unpublished master's thesis, University of Rochester, Rochester, NY.

Lothian, J. A. (1990). Continuing to breastfeed. *Dissertation Abstracts International, 51,* 665B.

Ludomirski-Kalmanson, B. (1985). The relationship between the environmental energy wave frequency pattern manifest in red light and blue light and human field motion in adult individuals with visual sensory perception and those with total blindness. *Dissertation Abstracts International, 45,* 2094B.

Lum, J. J., Chase, M., Cole, S. M., Johnson, A., Johnson, J. A., & Link, M. R. (1978). Nursing care of oncology patients receiving chemotherapy. *Nursing Research, 27,* 340–346.

Lutjens, L. R. J. (1991). *Martha Rogers: The science of unitary human beings.* Newbury Park, CA: Sage.

Macrae, J. A. (1983). A comparison between meditating subjects and non-meditating subjects on time experience and human field motion. *Dissertation Abstracts International, 43,* 3537B.

Madrid, M. (1990). The participating process of human field patterning in an acute-care environment. In E. A. M. Barrett (Ed.), *Visions of Rogers' science-based nursing* (pp. 93–104). New York: National League for Nursing.

Madrid, M., & Winstead-Fry, P. (1986). Rogers's conceptual model. In P. Winstead-Fry (Ed.), *Case studies in nursing theory* (pp. 73–102). New York: National League for Nursing.

Magan, S. J., Gibbon, E. J., & Mrozek, R. (1990). Nursing theory applications: A practice model. *Issues in Mental Health Nursing, 11,* 297–312.

Malinski, V. M. (1985). Martha E. Rogers' science of unitary human beings: Implications for cross-cultural nursing. In R. Wood & J. Kekahbah (Eds.), *Examining the cultural implications of Martha E. Rogers' science of unitary human beings* (pp. 27–42). Pawhuska, OK: Wood-Kekahbah Associates.

Malinski, V. M. (1986). Contemporary science and nursing: Parallels with Rogers. In V. M. Malinski (Ed.), *Explorations on Martha Rogers' science of unitary human beings* (pp. 15–24). Norwalk, CT: Appleton-Century-Crofts.

Malinski, V. M. (Ed.). (1986). *Explorations on Martha Rogers' science of unitary human beings.* Norwalk, CT: Appleton-Century-Crofts.

Malinski, V. M. (1986). Further ideas from Martha Rogers. In V. M. Malinski (Ed.), *Explorations on Martha Rogers' science of unitary human beings* (pp. 9–14). Norwalk, CT: Appleton-Century-Crofts.

Malinski, V. M. (1986). Nursing practice within the science of unitary human beings. In V. M. Malinski (Ed.), *Explorations on Martha Rogers' science of unitary human beings* (pp. 25–32). Norwalk, CT: Appleton-Century-Crofts.

Malinski, V. M. (1986). The relationship between hyperactivity in children and perception of short wavelength light. In V. M. Malinski (Ed.), *Explorations on Martha Rogers's science of unitary human beings* (pp. 107–117). Norwalk, CT: Appleton-Century-Crofts.

Malinski, V. (1989). Spirituality as integrality. *Rogerian Nursing Science News, II*(2), 4–5.

Malinski, V. M. (1990). The meaning of a progressive world view in nursing: Rogers' science of unitary human beings. In N. L. Chaska (Ed.), *The nursing profession: Turning points* (pp. 237–244). St. Louis: Mosby.

Malinski, V. M. (1990). The Rogerian science of unitary human beings as a knowledge base for nursing in space. In E. A. M. Barrett (Ed.), *Visions of Rogers' science-based nursing* (pp. 363–374). New York: National League for Nursing.

Malinski, V. M. (1991). The experience of laughing at oneself in older couples. *Nursing Science Quarterly, 4,* 69–75.

Malinski, V. M. (1991). Meditation as a health patterning modality. *Journal of Holistic Nursing, 9*(3), 41–47.

Malinski, V. M. (1991). Spirituality as integrality: A Rogerian perspective on the path of healing. *Journal of Holistic Nursing, 9*(1), 54–64.

Malinski, V. M. (1993). Therapeutic touch: The view from Rogerian nursing science. *Visions: The Journal of Rogerian Nursing Science,* Premiere Issue, 45–54.

Marriner, A. (1986). *Nursing theorists and their work.* St. Louis: Mosby.

Martin, M. L., Forchuk, C., Santopinto, M., & Butcher, H. K. (1992). Alternative approaches to nursing practice: Application of Peplau, Rogers, and Parse. *Nursing Science Quarterly, 5,* 80–85.

Mason, T., & Chandley, M. (1990). Nursing models in a special hospital: A critical analysis of efficacity. *Journal of Advanced Nursing, 15,* 667–673.

Mason, T., & Patterson, R. (1990). A critical review of the use of Rogers' model within a special hospital: A single case study. *Journal of Advanced Nursing, 15,* 130–141.

Mathwig, G. (1967). *Living open systems, reciprocal adaptations and the life process.* Unpublished doctoral dissertation, New York University, New York.

Mathwig, G. M., Young, A. A., & Pepper, J. M. (1990). Using Rogerian science in undergraduate and graduate nursing education. In E. A. M. Barrett (Ed.), *Visions of Rogers' science-based nursing* (pp. 319–334). New York: National League for Nursing.

McCanse, R. L. (1988). Healthy death readiness: Development of a measurement instrument. *Dissertation Abstracts International, 48,* 2606B.

McDonald, S. F. (1986). The relationship between visible lightwaves and the experience of pain. In V. M. Malinski (Ed.), *Explorations on Martha Rogers' science of unitary human beings* (pp. 119–127). Norwalk, CT: Appleton-Century-Crofts.

McEvoy, M. D. (1990). The relationships among the experience of dying, the experience of paranormal events, and creativity in adults. In E. A. M. Barrett (Ed.), *Visions of Rogers' science-based nursing* (pp. 209–228). New York: National League for Nursing.

McEvoy, M. D. (1990). Response to "Reflections on death as a process." In E. A. M. Barrett (Ed.), *Visions of Rogers' science-based nursing* (pp. 237–238). New York: National League for Nursing.

Meehan, T. C. (1990). The science of unitary human beings and theory-based practice: Therapeutic touch. In E. A. M. Barrett (Ed.), *Visions of Rogers' science-based nursing* (pp. 67–82). New York: National League for Nursing.

Meehan, T. C. (1990). Theory development. In E. A. M. Barrett (Ed.), *Visions of Rogers' science-based nursing* (pp. 197–208). New York: National League for Nursing.

Meehan, T. C. (1992). Professional nursing and Rogerian nursing science in New Zealand. *Rogerian Nursing Science News, IV*(3), 1–4.

Meehan, T. C. (1993). Therapeutic touch and postoperative pain: A Rogerian research study. *Nursing Science Quarterly, 6,* 69–78.

Meleis, A. I. (1985). *Theoretical nursing: Development and progress.* Philadelphia: Lippincott.

Miller, F. A. (1985). The relationship of sleep, wakefulness, and beyond waking experiences: A descriptive study of M. Rogers' concept of sleep-wake rhythm. *Dissertation Abstracts International, 46,* 116B.

Miller, L. A. (1979). An explanation of therapeutic touch using the science of unitary man. *Nursing Forum, 18,* 278–287.

Moccia, P. (1980). A study of the theory-practice dialectic: Towards a critique of the science of man. *Dissertation Abstracts International, 41,* 2560B.

Moccia, P. (1985). A further investigation of "Dialectical thinking as a means of understanding systems-in-development: Relevance to Rogers's principles." *Advances in Nursing Science, 7*(4), 33–38.

Moore, G. (1982). Perceptual complexity, memory and human duration experience. *Dissertation Abstracts International, 42,* 4363B.

Newman, M. A. (1972). Nursing's theoretical evolution. *Nursing Outlook, 20,* 449–453.

Newman, M. A. (1972). Time estimation in relation to gait tempo. *Perceptual and Motor Skills, 34,* 359–366.

Newman, M. A. (1976). Movement tempo and the experience of time. *Nursing Research, 25,* 273–279.

Newman, M. A. (1979). *Theory development in nursing.* Philadelphia: Davis.

Newshan, G. (1989). Therapeutic touch for symptom control in persons with AIDS. *Holistic Nursing Practice, 3*(4), 45–51.

Oliver, N. R. (1988). Processing unacceptable behaviors of coworkers: A naturalistic study of nurses at work. *Dissertation Abstracts International, 49,* 75B.

Paletta, J. L. (1990). The relationship of temporal experience to human time. In E. A. M. Barrett (Ed.), *Visions of Rogers' science-based nursing* (pp. 239–254). New York: National League for Nursing.

Paletta, J. L. (1990). Response to "What time is it?" In E. A. M. Barrett (Ed.), *Visions of Rogers' science-based nursing* (pp. 265–268). New York: National League for Nursing.

Parker, K. P. (1989). The theory of sentience evolution: A practice-level theory of sleeping, waking, and beyond waking patterns based on the science of unitary human beings. *Rogerian Nursing Science News, II*(1), 4–6.

Parse, R. R. (1981). *Man-living-health: A theory of nursing.* New York: Wiley.

Parse, R. R. (1987). *Nursing science: Major paradigms, theories, and critiques.* Philadelphia: Saunders.

Parse, R. R. (1989). Martha E. Rogers: A birthday celebration (Editorial). *Nursing Science Quarterly, 2,* 55.

Payne, M. B. (1989). The use of therapeutic touch with rehabilitation clients. *Rehabilitation Nursing, 14*(2), 69–72.

Phillips, J. R. (1989). Behold pattern. *Rogerian Nursing Science News, I*(3), 1, 5.

Phillips, J. R. (1989). Science of unitary human beings: Changing research perspectives. *Nursing Science Quarterly, 2,* 57–60.

Phillips, J. R. (1990). Changing human potentials and future visions of nursing: A human field image perspective. In E. A. M. Barrett (Ed.), *Visions of Rogers' science-based nursing* (pp. 13–25). New York: National League for Nursing.

Phillips, J. R. (1991). Human field research. *Nursing Science Quarterly, 4,* 142–143.

Porter, L. S. (1972). The impact of physical-physiological activity on infants' growth and development. *Nursing Research, 21,* 210–219.

Porter, L. S. (1972). Physical-physiological activity and infants' growth and development. In American Nurses' Association, *Seventh Nursing Research Conference* (pp. 1–43). New York: American Nurses' Association.

Quillin, S. I. M. (1984). Growth and development of infant and mother and mother-infant synchrony. *Dissertation Abstracts International, 44,* 3718B.

Quillin, S. I. M., & Runk, J. A. (1983). Martha Rogers' model. In J. J. Fitzpatrick & A. L. Whall (Eds.), *Conceptual models of nursing: Analysis of application* (pp. 245–261). Bowie, MD: Brady.

Quinn, A. A. (1989). Integrating a changing me: A grounded theory of the process of menopause for perimenopausal women. *Dissertation Abstracts International, 50,* 126B.

Quinn, J. F. (1984). Therapeutic touch as energy exchange: Testing the theory. *Advances in Nursing Science, 6*(2), 42–49.

Quinn, J. F. (1989). Therapeutic touch as energy exchange: Replication and extension. *Nursing Science Quarterly, 2,* 79–87.

Rankin, M. K. (1985). Effect of sound wave repatterning on symptoms of menopausal women. *Dissertation Abstracts International, 46,* 796B–797B.

Rapacz, K. (1989). Spirituality and the science of unitary human beings: A commentary. *Rogerian Nursing Science News, II*(2), 3–4.

Rapacz, K. E. (1990). The patterning of time experience and human field motion during the experience of pleasant guided imagery: A discussion. In E. A. M. Barrett (Ed.), *Visions of Rogers' science-based nursing* (pp. 287–294). New York: National League for Nursing.

Rapacz, K. E. (1991). *Human patterning and chronic pain.* Unpublished doctoral dissertation, Case Western Reserve University, Cleveland, OH.

Rapacz, K., & Reeder, F. (1990). Envisioning the future of Rogerian science (Abstract). *Rogerian Nursing Science News, III*(2), 7.

Rawnsley, M. (1985). H-E-A-L-T-H: A Rogerian perspective. *Journal of Holistic Nursing, 3*(1), 25–28.

Rawnsley, M. M. (1986). The relationship between the perception of the speed of time and the process of dying. In V. M. Malinski (Ed.), *Explorations on Martha Rogers' science of unitary human beings* (pp. 79–89). Norwalk, CT: Appleton-Century-Crofts.

Rawnsley, M. M. (1989). Response to "Empathy, diversity, and telepathy in mother-daughter dyads: An empirical investigation utilizing Rogers' conceptual framework." *Scholarly Inquiry for Nursing Practice, 3,* 45–51.

Rawnsley, M. M. (1990). Structuring the gap from conceptual system to research design within a Rogerian world view. In E. A. M. Barrett (Ed.), *Visions of Rogers' science-based nursing* (pp. 189–196). New York: National League for Nursing.

Rawnsley, M. M. (1990). What time is it? A response to a study of temporal experience. In E. A. M. Barrett (Ed.), *Visions of Rogers' science-based nursing* (pp. 265–268). New York: National League for Nursing.

Reed, P. G. (1986). The developmental conceptual framework: Nursing reformulations and applications for family therapy. In A. L. Whall (Ed.), *Family therapy theory for nursing: Four approaches* (pp. 69–91). Norwalk, CT: Appleton-Century-Crofts.

Reed, P. G. (1987). Spirituality and well-being in terminally ill hospitalized adults. *Research in Nursing and Health, 10,* 335–344.

Reed, P. G. (1989). Mental health of older adults. *Western Journal of Nursing Research, 11,* 143–163.

Reed, P. G. (1991). Toward a nursing theory of self-transcendence: Deductive reformulation using developmental theories. *Advances in Nursing Science, 13*(4), 64–77.

Reeder, F. (1984). Philosophical issues in the Rogerian science of unitary human beings. *Advances in Nursing Science, 6*(2), 14–23.

Reeder, F. (1985). Nursing research, holism and philosophies of science: Points of congruence between E. Husserl and M. E. Rogers. *Dissertation Abstracts International, 44,* 2498B–2499B.

Reeder, F. (1986). Basic theoretical research in the conceptual system of unitary human beings. In V. M. Malinski (Ed.), *Explorations on Martha Rogers' science of unitary human beings* (pp. 45–64). Norwalk, CT: Appleton-Century-Crofts.

Reeder, F. (1989). Relevance of spirituality/mysticism within the science of unitary human beings. *Rogerian Nursing Science News, II*(2), 2–3.

Reeder, F. (1993). The science of unitary human beings and interpretive human science. *Nursing Science Quarterly, 6,* 13–24.

Rigley, A. (1980). Martha Rogers—Challenging ideas for nursing. *The Lamp, 37*(2), 20–22.

Rizzo, J. A. (1990). Nursing service as an energy field: A response to "Visionary opportunities for knowledge development in nursing administration." In E. A. M. Barrett (Ed.), *Visions of Rogers' science-based nursing* (pp. 159–164). New York: National League for Nursing.

Rizzo, J. A. (1991). An investigation of the relationships of life satisfaction, purpose in life, and power in individuals sixty-five years and older. *Dissertation Abstracts International, 51,* 4280B.

Rogers, M. E. (1953). Responses to talks on menstrual health. *Nursing Outlook, 1,* 272–274.

Rogers, M. E. (1956). Public health nursing practice. In *The Yearbook of Modern Nursing—1956* (pp. 189–192). New York: Putnam's.

Rogers, M. E. (1957). Who speaks for nurses. *League Lines,* New York State League for Nursing, *3*(4).

Rogers, M. E. (1958). The associate degree graduate prepares for professional nursing practice at the baccalaureate degree level. In *The Yearbook of Modern Nursing—1957–1958* (pp. 275–279). New York: Putnam's.

Rogers, M. E. (1958). Foreword. In Hayt, Hayt, Groeschel, & McMullen, *Law of hospital and nurse.* New York: Hospital Textbook Company.

Rogers, M. E. (1958). The home visit. In *Selected papers: Workshop on army health nursing,* March 1956 and December 1957. Washington, DC.

Rogers, M. E. (1959). Nursing science. *League Lines,* New York State League for Nursing, *5*(1).

Rogers, M. E. (1959, September-December). The role of the university school of nursing in clinical specialization. *Bulletin of the College of Nurse Midwifery, 4*(3 & 4).

Rogers, M. E. (1959). Scope of professional nursing practice. *League Lines,* New York State League for Nursing, *5*(1).
Rogers, M. E. (1960). Excellence is where you find it. *Primed for Progress,* New York State League for Nursing, Reprint No. 1.
Rogers, M. E. (1961). *Educational revolution in nursing.* New York: Macmillan.
Rogers, M. E. (1961). Tomorrow belongs to you. *League Lines,* New York State League for Nursing, *7*(3).
Rogers, M. E. (1962). Viewpoints: Critical areas for nursing education in baccalaureate and higher degree programs. *NLN Publication No. 15-1041,* New York: National League for Nursing.
Rogers, M. E. (1963). Building a strong educational foundation. *American Journal of Nursing, 63*(6), 94–95.
Rogers, M. E. (1963, April-May). Some comments on the theoretical basis of nursing practice. *Nursing Science, 1.*
Rogers, M. E. (1963). Courage of their convictions. *Nursing Science, 1,* 44–47. (Wrote this column in Vol. 1, numbers 2, 3, & 4; Vol. 2, numbers 1, 2, 3, & 4; Vol. 3, number 1).
Rogers, M. E. (1963). Editorial. *Nursing Science, 1,* 40–43. (Wrote editorials in Vol. 1, numbers 2, 3, 5, & 6; Vol. 2, numbers 1, 2, 4, 5, & 6; Vol. 3, numbers 1, 3, 4, 5, & 6).
Rogers, M. E. (1963). Nursing quality for quantity. *Maryland Nursing News.* Maryland Nurses' Association.
Rogers, M. E. (1964). A philosophy of education basic to generic professional nursing programs. *Proceedings of the First Inter-University Faculty Work Conference.* New England Board of Higher Education.
Rogers, M. E. (1964). *Reveille in nursing.* Philadelphia: Davis.
Rogers, M. E. (1965, January). What the public demands of nursing today. *R.N.*
Rogers, M. E. (1966, January). Research in nursing. *Nursing Forum.*
Rogers, M. E. (1967, December). Professional commitment. *Image.*
Rogers, M. E. (1968). Nursing science: Research and researchers. *Teachers College Record, 69,* 469–476.
Rogers, M. E. (1968). For public safety: Higher education's responsibility for professional education in nursing. *Hartwick Review, 5*(1), 21–25.
Rogers, M. E. (1969). Nursing research: Relevant to practice. *Proceedings of the Fifth Nursing Research Conference.* New York: American Nurses' Association.
Rogers, M. E. (1969). Regional planning for graduate education in nursing. *Proceedings of the National Committee of Deans of Schools of Nursing Having Accredited Graduate Programs in Nursing.* New York: National League for Nursing.
Rogers, M. E. (1970). *An introduction to the theoretical basis of nursing.* Philadelphia: Davis.
Rogers, M. E. (1970). Yesterday a nurse—today a manager—what now. *Journal of the New York State Nurses' Association.*
Rogers, M. E. (1971). The PhD in nursing. *Proceedings of the NIH Conference on Doctoral Education for Nurses.*
Rogers, M. E. (1971). Predictive dimensions of nursing science. *Medical Service Digest.*
Rogers, M. E. (1972). Liberating nursing practice. *Challenge to Nursing Education.* New York: National League for Nursing.
Rogers, M. E. (1972, February). Nonsensical nomenclature that cons and coerces. *The Pennsylvania Nurse.*
Rogers, M. E. (1972). Nurses' expanding role and other euphemisms. *Journal of the New York State Nurses' Association, 3*(4), 5–10.
Rogers, M. E. (1972). Nursing: To be or not to be? *Nursing Outlook, 20,* 42–46.
Rogers, M. E. (1975). Euphemisms and nursing's future. *Image, 7*(2).
Rogers, M. E. (1975). Nursing is coming of age. *American Journal of Nursing, 75*(10).
Rogers, M. E. (1977). Nursing: To be or not to be. In B. Bullough & V. Bullough (Eds.), *Expanding horizons for nursing.* New York: Springer.
Rogers, M. E. (1978, December). *Application of theory in education and service* (Cassette Recording). Paper presented at Second Annual Nurse Educator Conference, New York.
Rogers, M. E. (1978). Emerging patterns in nursing education. In *Current perspectives in nursing education* (Vol. II, pp. 1–8). St. Louis: Mosby.
Rogers, M. E. (1978). Legislative and licensing problems in health care. *Nursing Administration Quarterly, 2*(3).
Rogers, M. E. (1978, January-February). A 1985 dissent. *Health/PAC Bulletin,* No. 80, 32–34.

Rogers, M. E. (1978, December). *Nursing science: A science of unitary man* (Cassette Recording). Paper presented at Second Annual Nurse Educator Conference, New York.

Rogers, M. E. (1980). Nursing: A science of unitary man. In J. P. Riehl & C. Roy (Eds.), *Conceptual models for nursing practice* (2nd ed., pp. 329–337). New York: Appleton-Century-Crofts.

Rogers, M. E. (1980). *Science of unitary man. Tape I. Unitary man and his world: A paradigm for nursing* (Cassette Recording). New York: Media for Nursing.

Rogers, M. E. (1980). *Science of unitary man. Tape II. Developing an organized abstract system: Synthesis of facts and ideas for a new product* (Cassette Recording). New York: Media for Nursing.

Rogers, M. E. (1980). *Science of unitary man. Tape III. Principles and theories: Directions for description, explanation and prediction* (Cassette Recording). New York: Media for Nursing.

Rogers, M. E. (1980). *Science of unitary man. Tape IV. Theories of accelerating evolution, paranormal phenomena and other events* (Cassette Recording). New York: Media for Nursing.

Rogers, M. E. (1980). *Science of unitary man. Tape V. Health and illness: New perspectives* (Cassette Recording). New York: Media for Nursing.

Rogers, M. E. (1980). *Science of unitary man. Tape VI. Interventive modalities: Translating theories into practice* (Cassette Recording). New York: Media for Nursing.

Rogers, M. E. (1981). Science of unitary man: A paradigm for nursing. In G. E. Lasker (Ed.), *Applied systems and cybernetics, Vol. 4. Systems research in health care, biocybernetics and ecology* (pp. 1719–1722). New York: Pergamon.

Rogers, M. E. (1983). The family coping with a surgical crisis: Analysis and application of Rogers' theory of nursing. In I. W. Clements & F. B. Roberts (Eds.), *Family health: A theoretical approach to nursing* (pp. 390–391). New York: Wiley.

Rogers, M. E. (1983). Science of unitary human beings: A paradigm for nursing. In I. W. Clements & F. B. Roberts (Eds.), *Family health: A theoretical approach to nursing care* (pp. 219–227). New York: Wiley.

Rogers, M. E. (1985). The nature and characteristics of professional education for nursing. *Journal of Professional Nursing, 1,* 381–383.

Rogers, M. E. (1985). The need for legislation for licensure to practice professional nursing. *Journal of Professional Nursing, 1,* 384.

Rogers, M. E. (1985). Nursing eduction: Preparation for the future. In *Patterns in education: The unfolding of nursing* (pp. 11–14). New York: National League for Nursing.

Rogers, M. E. (1985). *Panel discussion with theorists* (Cassette Recording). Discussion at Nurse Theorist Conference, Pittsburgh, PA.

Rogers, M. E. (1985). Science of unitary human beings: A paradigm for nursing. In R. Wood & J. Kekahbah (Eds.), *Examining the cultural implications of Martha E. Rogers' science of unitary human beings* (pp. 13–23). Pawhuska, OK: Wood-Kekahbah Associates.

Rogers, M. E. (1986). Science of unitary human beings. In V. M. Malinski (Ed.), *Explorations on Martha Rogers' science of unitary human beings* (pp. 3–8). Norwalk, CT: Appleton-Century-Crofts.

Rogers, M. E. (1987). Nursing research in the future. In J. Roode (Ed.), *Changing patterns in nursing education* (pp. 121–123). New York: National League for Nursing.

Rogers, M. E. (1987, May). *Rogers' framework* (Cassette Recording). Paper presented at Nurse Theorist Conference, Pittsburgh, PA.

Rogers, M. E. (1987). Rogers' science of unitary human beings. In R. R. Parse (Ed.), *Nursing science: Major paradigms, theories, and critiques* (pp. 139–146). Philadelphia: Saunders.

Rogers, M. E. (1987, May). *Small group D* (Cassette Recording). Discussion at Nurse Theorist Conference, Pittsburgh, PA.

Rogers, M. E. (1988). Nursing science and art: A prospective. *Nursing Science Quarterly, 1,* 99–102.

Rogers, M. E. (1989). Nursing: A science of unitary human beings. In J. P. Riehl-Sisca (Ed.), *Conceptual models for nursing practice* (3rd ed., pp. 181–188). Norwalk, CT: Appleton and Lange.

Rogers, M. E. (1990). Nursing: Science of unitary, irreducible, human beings: Update 1990. In E. A. M. Barrett (Ed.), *Visions of Rogers' science-based nursing* (pp. 5–11). New York: National League for Nursing.

Rogers, M. E. (1990). Space-age paradigm for new frontiers in nursing. In M. E. Parker (Ed.), *Nursing theories in practice* (pp. 105–113). New York: National League for Nursing.

Rogers, M. E. (1992). Nightingale's *Notes on Nursing:* Prelude to the 21st century. In F. N. Nightingale, *Notes on nursing: What it is, and what it is not* (Commemorative edition, pp. 58–62). Philadelphia: Lippincott. (Originally published in 1854).

Rogers, M. E. (1992). Nursing science and the space age. *Nursing Science Quarterly, 5,* 27–34.

Rogers, M. E., Doyle, M. B., Racolin, A., & Walsh, P. C. (1990). A conversation with Martha Rogers on nursing in space. In E. A. M. Barrett (Ed.), *Visions of Rogers' science-based nursing* (pp. 375–386). New York: National League for Nursing.

Rogers, M. E., Meehan, T. C., & Malinski, V. (1988). Rogerian practice perspectives: Excerpts from transcripts of dialogues among Martha E. Rogers, Therese Connell Meehan, & Violet Malinski. *Rogerian Nursing Science News, I*(1), 4–5, 8.

Safier, G. (1977). *Contemporary American leaders: An oral history.* New York: McGraw-Hill.

Sanchez, R. (1989). Empathy, diversity, and telepathy in mother-daughter dyads: An empirical investigation utilizing Rogers' conceptual framework. *Scholarly Inquiry for Nursing Practice, 3,* 45–51.

Sarter, B. (1987). Evolutionary idealism: A philosophical foundation for holistic nursing theory. *Advances in Nursing Science, 9*(2), 1–9.

Sarter, B. (1988). Philosophical sources of nursing theory. *Nursing Science Quarterly, 1,* 52–59.

Sarter, B. (1988). *The stream of becoming: A study of Martha Rogers' theory.* New York: National League for Nursing.

Sarter, B. (1989). Some philosophical issues in the science of unitary human beings. *Nursing Science Quarterly, 2,* 74–78.

Scandrett-Hibdon, S. L. (1990). The endogenous healing process in adult black women. *Journal of Holistic Nursing, 8*(1), 47–62.

Schodt, C. M. (1989). Parental-fetal attachment and couvade: A study of pattern of human-environment integrality. *Nursing Science Quarterly, 2,* 88–97.

Schorr, J. A. (1983). Manifestations of consciousness and the developmental phenomenon of death. *Advances in Nursing Science, 6*(1), 26–35.

Schroeder, C. (1990). Rogers' science of unitary human beings and Jonas' philosophy of organism. *Rogerian Nursing Science News, III*(2), 3–4.

Schroeder, C., & Smith, M. C. (1991). Nursing conceptual frameworks arising from field theory: A critique of the body as manifestation of underlying field. Commentary: Disembodiment or "Where's the body in field theory?" (Schroeder). Response: Affirming the unitary perspective (Smith). *Nursing Science Quarterly, 4,* 146–152.

Sellers, S. C. (1991). A philosophical analysis of conceptual models of nursing. *Dissertation Abstracts International, 52,* 1937B.

Silva, M. C. (1987). Conceptual models of nursing. In J. J. Fitzpatrick & R. L. Taunton (Eds.), *Annual Review of Nursing Research* (Vol. 5, pp. 229–246). New York: Springer.

Silva, M. C., & Sorrell, J. M. (1987, April). *Doctoral dissertation research based on five nursing models: A select bibliography: January 1952 through February 1987.* (Available from M. C. Silva, George Mason University School of Nursing, Fairfax, VA).

Skillman, L (1991). A challenge to our current methods for studying and understanding human mutual processing. *Rogerian Nursing Science News, III*(3), 4–7.

Smith, C. T. (1991). The lived experience of staying healthy in rural black families. *Dissertation Abstracts International, 50,* 3925B.

Smith, D. W. (1990). *Power and spirituality among polio survivors.* Unpublished doctoral dissertation, New York University, New York.

Smith, L. (1983). A conceptual model of families incorporating an adolescent mother and child into the household. *Advances in Nursing Science, 6*(1), 45–60.

Smith, M. C. (1987). An investigation of the effects of different sound frequencies on vividness and creativity of imagery. *Dissertation Abstracts International, 47,* 3708B.

Smith, M. C. (1988). Testing propositions derived from Rogers' conceptual system. *Nursing Science Quarterly, 1,* 60–67.

Smith, M. C. (1990). Pattern in nursing practice. *Nursing Science Quarterly, 3,* 57–59.

Smith, M. J. (1975). Changes in judgement of duration with different patterns of auditory information for individuals confined to bed. *Nursing Research, 24,* 93–98.

Smith, M. J. (1979). Duration experience for bed-confined subjects: A replication and refinement. *Nursing Research, 28,* 139–144.

Smith, M. J. (1984). Temporal experience and bed rest: Replication and refinement. *Nursing Research, 33,* 298–302.

Smith, M. J. (1986). Human-environment process: A test of Rogers' principle of integrality. *Advances in Nursing Science, 9*(1), 21–28.

Smith, M. J. (1988). Perspectives on nursing science. *Nursing Science Quarterly, 1,* 80–85.

Smith, M. J. (1989). Four dimensionality: Where to go with it. *Nursing Science Quarterly, 2,* 56.

Stevens, B. J. (1984). *Nursing theory: Analysis, application, evaluation* (2nd ed.). Boston: Little, Brown.

Swanson, A. R. (1990). Issues in dissertation proposal development. In E. A. M. Barrett (Ed.), *Visions of Rogers' science-based nursing* (pp. 345–351). New York: National League for Nursing.

Takahashi, T. (1992). Perspectives on nursing knowledge. *Nursing Science Quarterly, 5,* 86–91.

Thomas, S. D. (1990). Intentionality in the human-environment encounter in an ambulatory care environment. In E. A. M. Barrett (Ed.), *Visions of Rogers' science-based nursing* (pp. 117–128). New York: National League for Nursing.

Thompson, J. E. (1990). Finding the borderline's border: Can Martha Rogers help? *Perspectives in Psychiatric Care, 26*(4), 7–10.

Thompson, L. S., & Hindle, J. S. (1990). Assessment of the unitary human being: One clinician's dilemma. *Rogerian Nursing Science News, III*(2), 4–5.

Trangenstein, P. A. (1989). Relationships of power and job diversity to job satisfaction and job involvement: An empirical investigation of Rogers' principle of integrality. *Dissertation Abstracts International, 49,* 3110B–3111B.

Tuyn, L. K. (1992). Solution-oriented therapy and Rogerian nursing science: An integrated approach. *Archives of Psychiatric Nursing, VI,* 83–89.

Uys, L. R. (1987). Foundational studies in nursing. *Journal of Advanced Nursing, 12,* 275–280.

Whall, A. L. (1981). Nursing theory and the assessment of families. *Journal of Psychiatric Nursing and Mental Health Services, 19*(1), 30–36.

Whall, A. L. (1987). A critique of Rogers' framework. In R. R. Parse (Ed.), *Nursing science: Major paradigms, theories, and critiques* (pp. 147–158). Philadelphia: Saunders.

Whelton, B. J. (1979). An operationalization of Martha Rogers' theory throughout the nursing process. *International Journal of Nursing Studies, 16,* 7–20.

Wilson, L. M., & Fitzpatrick, J. J. (1984). Dialectic thinking as a means of understanding systems-in-development: Relevance to Rogers' principles. *Advances in Nursing Science, 6*(2), 24–41.

Winstead-Fry, P. (1990). Reflections on death as a dying process: A response to a study of the experience of dying. In E. A. M. Barrett (Ed.), *Visions of Rogers' science-based nursing* (pp. 229–236). New York: National League for Nursing.

Wood, R., & Kekahbah, J. (Eds.). (1985). *Examining the cultural implications of Martha E. Rogers' science of unitary human beings.* Pawhuska, OK: Wood-Kekahbah Associates.

Wright, S. M. (1991). Validity of the human energy field assessment form. *Western Journal of Nursing Research, 13,* 635–647.

Yarcheski, A., & Mahon, N. E. (1991). An empirical test of Rogers' original and revised theory of correlates in adolescents. *Research in Nursing and Health, 14,* 447–455.

Yaros, P. S. (1986). The relationship of maternal rhythmic behavior and infant interactional attention. *Dissertation Abstracts International, 47,* 136B.

Young, A. A. (1985). The Rogerian conceptual system: A framework for nursing education and service. In R. Wood & J. Kekahbah (Eds.), *Examining the cultural implications of Martha E. Rogers' science of unitary human beings* (pp. 53–69). Pawhuska, OK: Wood-Kekahbah Associates.

Young, A. A., & Keil, C. (1981). The Washburn nursing curriculum: Interpreting Martha Rogers in the land of Oz. *The Kansas Nurse, 56*(4), 7–9, 23.

Zadinsky, J. K. (1990). Knowing participation in the parent-infant mutual process. *Rogerian Nursing Science News, III*(2), 5–6.

Computer-Assisted Literature Searches: Helpful Hints from Dr. Fawcett

Cumulative Index to Nursing and Allied Health Literature (*CINAHL*)

CD-ROM: Use Science of Unitary Human Beings

BRS-COLLEAGUE: Use Unitary Human Beings

Dissertation Abstracts International (Includes *Master's Abstracts International*)

BRS-COLLEAGUE: Use Life Process Model.ab.
Unitary Human Beings.ab.
Martha Rogers.ab.

Note 1: Do not confuse Martha E. Rogers, author of the Science of Unitary Human Beings, with Martha E. Rogers, a nurse consultant from Toronto, Canada. The Canadian Martha is the author of several articles dealing with conceptual models.

Note 2: Dissertations since 1989 also are available via CINAHL.

Medline

Use Models, Nursing
Nursing Theory

(These subject headings will yield citations for various nursing models and theories, including the Science of Unitary Human Beings. It seems to be the most effective search strategy on Medline.)

GLOSSARY

Nursing Science: A Science of Unitary Human Beings*

Martha E. Rogers, RN; ScD; FAAN

Learned Profession: A science and an art.

Science: An organized body of abstract knowledge. A synthesis of facts and ideas. A new product.

Art: The imaginative and creative use of knowledge.

Negentropy: Increasing heterogeneity, differentiation, diversity of field pattern.

Energy Field: The fundamental unit of the living and the nonliving. Field is a unifying concept. Energy signifies the dynamic nature of the field. Energy fields are infinite.

Pattern: The distinguishing characteristic of an energy field perceived as a single wave.

Pandimensional: A nonlinear domain without spatial or temporal attributes.

Unitary Human Being (human field): An irreducible, pandimensional energy field identified by pattern and manifesting characteristics that are specific to the whole and which cannot be predicted from knowledge of the parts.

Environment (environmental field): An irreducible, pandimensional energy field identified by pattern and integral with the human field.

*Updated 9/1/90.

APPENDIX A

Genealogy as Provided by Laura Wilhite, Family Historian

Martha Elizabeth Rogers was born May 12, 1914, to Bruce Taylor Rogers and Lucy Mulholland Keener Rogers. She was named after her paternal grandmother, Martha Elizabeth Luttrell Rogers. On the Luttrell side, the Rogers family traces its lineage to Sir Geoffrey Luttrell, who died circa 1216. The Luttrells inhabited Dunster Castle in Somerset, England, inherited from Lady Elizabeth Luttrell. In Saxon times the castle was an important frontier fortress guarding against invasion by the Northmen and Celts. As inheritance was through the first-born son, the second son, James Luttrell, born circa 1630, emigrated to Maryland around 1667, married, and raised a family. Martha's paternal great-grandfather, James Luttrell, was a descendent of this Luttrell on his father's side. On his mother's side, James Luttrell was a descendant of William Witt, a French Huguenot who fled from the persecutions of King Louis XIV of France. Together with other members of the colony that left South Hampton, England, in 1699, William Witt helped to found the Huguenot colony of Manakin, Pawhatan County, Virginia. His grandson, John Witt, Jr., fought in the American Revolution.

Martha's maternal grandmother, Laura Janette Brownlee, was a descendant (father's side) of Thomas Brownlee, Laird of Torfoot, who resided near Strathaven, Lanarkshire, Scotland. Through the Brownlee family, the Rogerses trace a distant connection to William McKinley, 25th President of the United States. On her mother's side, Laura Brownlee was a descendent of the Reverend John Mulholland, born in County Atrim near Belfast, Ireland. He and his sons worked in Mulholland Linen Mills, mentioned by Charles Dickens in one of his novels. The Reverend Mulholland also preached a series of sermons before Charles I of England. A number of maternal ancestors were ministers, primarily Presbyterians, while ministers on the paternal side tended to be Methodist. Martha's niece, Nancy Jane Wilhite, is a Methodist minister at the Harriman, Tennessee, Methodist Church.

Dunster Castle is now part of the National Trust. The site on which it stands has been occupied for over 1000 years, but the oldest surviving feature of the present castle dates only to the 13th century. It was sold in 1376 to Lady

Elizabeth Luttrell. The Luttrell family remodeled and added to the castle over the centuries. They gave the castle and surrounding park to the National Trust in 1976. Laura Wilhite described the castle as a beautiful, breathtaking sight with magnificent plaster ceilings and walls, preserved antique furnishings, an art gallery with large paintings done on leather, and lovely gardens. Dunster Castle is a site Martha Rogers and members of her family enjoy visiting.

APPENDIX B

Selecting Your Career in Nursing

Nursing is exciting, challenging, and satisfying. The various careers in nursing provide many opportunities for persons with different interests, abilities, and goals. Numerous and varied employment openings are available.

What Kind of Nursing Do You Want to Do? There Are Three Kinds of General Practitioners in Nursing

Each practitioner is an important part of the nursing team. Your ability, interest, and goals will help you in deciding whether you want to prepare for:

1. Professional Registered Nurse practice,
2. Technical Registered Nurse practice, or
3. Licensed Practical Nurse practice.

What Kind of Programs Prepare for These Different Kinds of Nursing Practice?

Professional Registered Nurse Programs

Professional education in nursing is offered only in colleges and universities. Programs are 4 to 5 years in length, and lead to a baccalaureate degree with an upper division major in nursing. These programs prepare for the broad scope of nursing practice and require substantial knowledge in the liberal arts; biological, physical, and social sciences; and upper division nursing theory with its related laboratory study. Students in nursing are integral parts of the total student body throughout their entire educational program. Courses in nursing are taught by qualified college faculty in nursing and are dependent on prerequisites in general education and the basic sciences for their comprehension. Nursing courses represent only a portion of the courses taught at a senior college level. Laboratory study in nursing represents regularly scheduled

Excerpted with permission from *Nursing Science, 1,* 77–84, June-July, 1963. Copyright 1963, F. A. Davis Company.

courses. Many community resources such as hospitals, public health agencies, and schools provide the settings for laboratory study.

Graduates are prepared to assume professional responsibility for promotion of health and prevention of disease, and for nursing diagnosis, therapy, and rehabilitation. They assume increasing responsibility for themselves and for appropriate guidance of Registered Nurse graduates of associate degree and hospital school programs, practical nurses, and auxiliary personnel. They work in a peer relationship with professional personnel in other disciplines. These programs provide the foundation for nurses who wish to go on for Master's and Doctoral study in nursing. Graduates are qualified for examination for licensure as Registered Nurses and for professional practice in nursing.

Technical Registered Nurse Programs

There are several different kinds of programs that prepare for technical Registered Nurse practice. These programs range in length from 2 to 5 years, but all prepare for the same kind of nursing practice.

Associate Degree Programs

These are college programs. They are 2 years in length and are located in and entirely controlled by junior and community colleges. Students in nursing are college students just as are other students in the educational institution. Courses in nursing are taught by qualified college faculty in nursing. These programs include both liberal arts courses and instruction and experience in clinical areas. Local hospitals and other agencies are used as laboratories for the students. Graduates are qualified for examination for licensure as Registered Nurses. If possible you should select this type of program if you wish to prepare for technical Registered Nurse practice.

Hospital Programs

These are non-collegiate programs. They are generally 3 calendar years in length and are owned and controlled by hospitals. Graduates are qualified for examination for licensure as Registered Nurses. Graduates of these programs should not expect to get college credit for the hospital school program.

Practical Nurse Programs

Programs that prepare for practical nursing are vocational in nature. Students develop general and specific skills in the care of sick people. Their responsibilities are carried out in cooperation with and under the guidance of technical and professional nurses. These programs are generally 1 year in length and are generally located in the vocational educational system. Graduates are qualified for examination for licensure as Licensed Practical Nurses.

Regardless of the kind of program you select it is important that you like people, that you want to do things for people and with people.

The brochure from which this material is excerpted ends with questions students can ask themselves in deciding which career in nursing is right for them, information about financial assistance, and a note about the importance of attending a program accredited by the National League for Nursing, with the League's address.

Index

Abstract system, science as, 245. *See also* Nursing science; Science
Accelerating evolution
  freedom of movement and, 334
  nursing in space and, 297–299
  theory of, 223–224, 229–230, 263–264, 294–295
Accountability, 30–31, 128–132. *See also* Responsibility
Accreditation, problems with, 165–166
Acquired immunodeficiency syndrome. *See* AIDS
Administrative positions, shortage of nursing personnel for, 153
Aging process. *See also* Life process
  longevity and, 264, 294
  Science of Unitary Man and, 231
  theoretical basis of nursing and, 223
AHA. *See* American Hospital Association
AIDS, 242–243
  nosophobia and, 302
Albany, March on (1970), 117*f*
American Hospital Association (AHA)
  legislation and, 79
  unionization and, 164
American Journal of Nursing, 120
American Medical Association, nurse-practitioner movement and, 121–122
American Nurses Association (ANA), 69, 71
  Economic Security Program of, 164
  Facts About Nursing (1967), 86
  position statement on nursing education (1965), 121, 136
American Nurses Foundation, 71
ANA. *See* American Nurses Association
Anti-educationism. *See also* Nursing education
  doing syndrome and, 179–180
  unification model and, 175–178
Applied research, 45–46, 110, 115. *See also* Research
Arizona, Rogers' work in, 15, 17–18
Art. *See also* Nursing, art of
  defined, 241, 352
"Associate Degree Graduate Prepares for Professional Nursing Practice at the Baccalaureate Level," 120
Associate degree programs, 356. *See also* Technical education
Audiotapes, documenting Rogers' thoughts, 10
Authority, nursing identity and, 141–142
Autonomy
  future of nursing and, 266, 272–273, 281
  nurse-practitioner movement and, 121–122
  nursing and medicine and, 184
Baccalaureate degree education. *See also* Nursing education
  accountability and, 131
  changes instituted in 1960s, 40
  NYU
    evolution of, 41–43
    graduate study and, 91, 96
  Rogers' editorials on, 30
Barrett, Elizabeth Ann Manhart, 273, 334
Basic research, 45, 115. *See also* Research
  defined, 108
  need for, in science of nursing, 111
Becker, Howard S., 82
Bishop, William, 71
Boundaries, explicit, scientific models and, 325
Brakebill, Laura Keener, 4*f*
Bridgman, Margaret, 69, 89, 315
Brown, Esther Lucile, 38, 69–70, 89, 314
Brownlee, Laura Janette, 353
Brownlee, Lucy M., 1*f*
Brownlee, Thomas, 353
Bureau of Competition, FTC, 165
"Business Roundtable," 164

California, nursing education in, 65
Caring
  "high touch" and, 290
  nursing practice and, 266
Causality
  illusion of, 229
  open systems versus, 241
Certification. *See* Licensure
Change
  accelerating evolution and, 223–224, 229–230
  "expanding role" of nursing and, 134
  expected, nursing in space and, 304
  future. *See* Future of nursing
  health field and, 163–164
  nursing implications of, Rogers' editorials on, 30
  pattern, participation in, 334
  research on nature of, 238
  rhythmical correlates of, 230–231
  synchrony of, 216–217
Chaos theory, 301
Chaska, Norma, 25, 27
Cheema, Sheila, 273
Children's Hospital Medical Center, Cincinnati, 337
"Clinical research," Rogers' objection to term of, 45–46, 110, 115
Coalition for Alternatives in Nutrition and Health Care, 252
Coleman, Jane Rogers, 3, 4*f*, 5–6

Collaboration
  nursing/medicine, 184
  team, physicians' assistants and, 159–160
Colleagueship, principle of, 326
College of Mount Saint Vincent, 337
Colleges. *See also* Education
  responsibility of, for professional education in nursing, 80–88
Collegiate Education in Nursing, 89
Columbia University, Teachers College, 70
  Rogers' attendance at, 15, 16
Committee for the Study of Nursing Education, 69
Committee on the Function of Nursing, 70
Committee on the Future of the National League for Nursing, 71
Committee on the Grading of Nursing Schools, 69
Communality, principle of, 326
Communication
  of concepts, 212
  paranormal as form of, 333–334
Community-based, meaning of, 243
Community services
  future of nursing and, 286
  "health services" versus "sick services," 130–131. *See also* Health services
Competition, principle of, 326
Complementarity, 199, 235. *See also* Integrality
  unitary man and, 228
Complexification, wholeness and, 300–301
Concept Formalization in Nursing, 316
Concepts, communication of, 212
Conceptual Models for Nursing Practice, 202
Conceptual system
  defined, 241
  of nursing, 210–213, 220–224
    principles and, 214, 228–229
  significance of, 326
  theories and, 205–206
Conferences, international, 273
Confirmation, principle of, 326
Continuity, principle of, 326
"Cop-Out Compromises," 120
Cost accounting, 165
Costs. *See* Financial considerations
Council of Baccalaureate and Higher Degree Programs, National League for Nursing, 89–90
Credentialing, 166. *See also* Licensure
Curriculum, nursing. *See* Nursing education
Cybernation: The Silent Conquest (Michael), 50

Death and dying
  concern with, 295
  interpretations of, 331
Deception, health system and, 164
Desacralization of science, 208
Descriptive principles, 214
Developmental patterns
  increasing diversity of, 294–295
  synchrony and, 216
Diagnosis related groups (DRGs), 290
Diagnostic process, nursing practice and, 64
Disease. *See also specific disease*
  dread of, 301–304
"Divide and conquer" approach, nursing identity and, 145–146
Dock, Lavinia, 123
Doctoral education, 97–102. *See also* Nursing education
  importance of, 86–87
  NYU, evolution of, 41–43
  research and, 45
  Rogers' views on, 29–30, 38
Doing syndrome, 179–180
"Doing syndrome," 43
Domains, scientific, 325
DRGs (diagnosis related groups), 290
Dying. *See* Death and dying

Economic considerations. *See* Financial considerations
Economic Security Program, ANA, 164
Editorials, *Nursing Science,* 30–31, 59–60, 69–72, 74–79
Educating the Nurse for the Future, 61–68
Education. *See also* Anti-educationism; Nursing education
  Rogers'
    early, 12–14
    graduate, 15, 16
Education beyond the High School, 71
Education for the Health Professions, 71
Educational Revolution in Nursing, 28–29, 39, 197–198, 315, 321
Empirical evidence, scientific models and, 325
Employment practices, 153
  future technology and, 290
Energy fields, 226, 234–235, 252, 293. *See also* Field patterning; Human-environment relationship
  continuous motion of, 246–247
  defined, 241, 245*t*, 260*t*, 352
  paranormal events and, 333
  resonancy principle and, 218–219
  scientific developments related to, 323
  vision of humans as, 330–331
    health modalities related to, 332
    implications for physical body, 331
Environment
  defined, 228, 241, 245*t*, 253, 260*t*, 352
  human relationship to. *See* Human-environment relationship
Environmental field pattern. *See* Field patterning
Ethical issues, 166
Eudaimonistic model of health, 332
Euphemisms, 167. *See also specific euphemisms*
  future of nursing and, 155–162, 285–286
  nursing science and, 144
  role of nursing and, 133–138
Evaluative process, nursing practice and, 64
Evolution
  accelerating, 223–224, 229–230, 263–264, 294–295
    freedom of movement and, 334

nursing in space and, 297–299
Rogers' view of, 330–331
new interpretations of traditional views and, 331
Excellence, 126–127
"Expanded role," euphemism of, 131–132, 133–138, 144, 148, 167
Experience, knowledge versus, 63
Explanatory principles, 214
Explicit boundaries, scientific models and, 325
"Extending the Scope of Nursing Practice: A Report of the Secretary's Committee to Study Extended Roles for Nurses," 135

Facts About Nursing (ANA; 1967), 86
Faculty
professional education and, 43
responsiveness of, graduate-level nursing education and, 93–94
"Faculty Practice," 179
Family Health: A Theoretical Approach to Nursing, 201
Family health practice, initiation of, 150
Family health practitioners, 144
Family of Martha E. Rogers, 1*f*, 3–9, 4*f*
philosophical influences of, 317–319
Rogers' recollections of, 12–13
Federal Council on Wage and Price Stability, 165
Federal government. *See also specific agencies, programs, or regulations*
nursing education and, 66, 78–79
Federal Trade Commission (FTC), Bureau of Competition of, 165
Fernandez, Ruben D., 123
Fetus, mother and, as one field versus two, 247
Field concept, 234, 241. *See also* Energy fields
Field patterning, 246–247
accelerating evolution and, 264
change process and, participation in, 334
diversity in
changing, 335
relative, 202–203
manifestations of, in unitary human beings, 247*t*, 253, 262*t*
pandimensional pattern recognition and, 332–333
worldview and, 262–263
Financial considerations
cost containment and, 290–291
future of nursing and, 277
euphemisms in, 156–157
graduate-level nursing education and, NYU, 92–93
Forum on Doctoral Education (1989), 326
Four-dimensionality. *See also* Pandimensionality
defined, 241
human-environment relationship and, 227*f*, 227–228, 235
Freeman, Ruth, 19, 31, 315
FTC. *See* Federal Trade Commission

Future of nursing, 276–279
euphemisms in, 155–162
high-tech, high touch in, 288–291
legislative and licensing problems and, 168–169
nursing science and art and, 239–243
preparation for, nursing education and, 103–106
research in, 114–116
Rogers' views of, 26, 271–275, 282–286, 296–304
scenario for nursing in 2001 A.D., 280–281
Science of Unitary, Irreducible Human Beings and, 244
space-age paradigm for, 250–255. *See also* Space age
Future Shock, 91, 229

Genealogy, 353–354. *See also* Family of Martha E. Rogers
Generality, scientific models and, 326
Ginsberg, Eli, 70, 89, 314
Goal-directedness, helicy and, 217
Goldmark, Josephine, 69
Gorman, M. Leah, 122, 123
Government, federal. *See* Federal government
Groups, Science of Unitary Beings applied to, 247
"Guidelines for Master's Degree Programs in Nursing," 89–90

Hartford, CT, Visiting Nurse Association of, Hartford, CT, 16
Hassenplug, Lulu Wolf, 30
Health care crisis, future of nursing and, euphemisms in, 157
Health care field
changing, 163–164
legislative and licensing problems in, 163–169
medical monopoly on, 277, 286
new modalities in, Rogers' model as basis for, 332
Health credentialing, 166
HEALTH PAC, 169
Health-Pac Bulletin, 120
Rogers' peer review dissent in, 170–172
Health services
leadership in, 132
public demands for, 140
"sick services" versus, 130–131
"Health Status, Health Resources, and Consolidated Structural Parameters: Implications for Health Care Policy," 277
Health system, problems in, 164–167
Helene Fuld Institutional Award, 10
Helicy, 199, 217–218, 218*f*, 246*t*, 253, 262*t*
future of nursing and, 294
nursing science and, 235, 242
pattern recognition and, 333
scientific developments related to, 324
unitary man and, 228

Herrick, C. Judson, 111
Historical Salute to Martha E. Rogers on the Occasion of Her 75th Birthday, 308, 338
Hoexter, Joan, 11, 19, 21–22, 122, 123
Hoffman, C.A., 157
Holism, 260
"Holistic"
"integral" versus, 203
"unitary" versus, 234
Homeodynamics, 242, 246, 246*t*, 253, 262*t*, 294–295
conceptual model of nursing and, 223
nursing science and, 199, 214–219
Science of Unitary Human Beings and, 235–236
Science of Unitary Man and, 228–229
Homeokinesis, 235
Homeostasis, 235
Homo spacialis, 247, 248
Homo spatialis, 203
Homo spatialis, 256, 257, 298
Hospital care, declining quality of, 167
Hospital profits, 291
Hospital registered nurse programs, 356. *See also* Technical education
Human beings, unitary. *See* Science of Unitary Human Beings
Human development. *See also* evolution
study of, science of nursing as, 96
Human-environment relationship, 207
accelerating evolution of. *See* Accelerating evolution
conceptual model of nursing and, 211, 223–224
helicy and, 217–218, 218*f*
pattern change and, 334
reciprocy and, 215–216
resonancy and, 218–219
synchrony and, 216–217
unitary man and, 226–231. *See also* Science of Unitary Human Beings
Human field. *See also* Energy fields
defined, 241, 245*t*, 352
rhythms of
change and, 230–231, 264, 294
helicy principle and, 217
Human field motion, 334
Human field touch (therapeutic touch), 237, 243, 248, 295, 332
Human potentials, pandimensionality and, 336
Hutchin, Robert, 91
Hyperactivity, Science of Unitary Man and, 231
Hypertension, Science of Unitary Man and, 231
Hypothesis generation, scientific models and, 326

Illness. *See also specific type*
dread of, 301–304
Image: The Journal of Nursing Scholarship, 120
"Impact of Technological Change," 92
Independent nurse, registered nurse versus, 182–184
Independent nursing, requirements for, SAIN proposal to amend New York State Education Law, 185–191
Innovation, helicy and, 218
Institutional licensure, 166. *See also* Licensure
Instructive Nursing Association of Boston, 159
"Integral," "holistic" versus, 203
Integrality, 246*t*, 253, 262*t*. *See also* Complementarity
future of nursing and, 294
nursing science and, 235, 242
scientific developments related to, 324
Intellectual discipline, science as, 325
International conferences (1982–1992), 273
Interpersonal Relations in Nursing, 314
Interventive process, nursing practice and, 64
Introduction to the Theoretical Basis of Nursing, 198, 321
impact of, 24
writing and publication of, 22–23
reactions to, 23–24
"Intuitive nursing," professional nursing versus, 28–29

Job frontier, technology and, 290
Johns Hopkins University, Rogers' studies at, 15, 18
Joint Appointments, Rogers' position on, 43, 179–180

Keener, Laura B., 1*f*
Kemble, Elizabeth L., 30, 55, 233
Kennedy-Mills proposal, 165
King, Imogene, 31
Knowledge. *See also* Education
experience versus, 63
nursing, 143
role of nurse in space and, 299–300
Science of Unitary Human Beings and, 234
use of knowledge versus, 45, 208
Knowledge base of nursing, development of, 39, 40–41
"Knowledgeable compassion," 29–30, 32
"Knowledgeable intervention," 32
Knowledgeable nursing, Rogers' views on, 39
Knoxville, TN, Rogers' childhood and early education in, 12–14
Knoxville General Hospital, Rogers' nursing education at, 13–14
Kohnke, Mary P., 122
Krieger, Dolores, 31

Language. *See* Terminology
Leadership, responsibility for, 132
Learned profession, 32
defined, 241, 352
Learning Society, The, 91

Legislation
licensure and, 192–193
nursing education and, 78–79
problems relating to, 163–169
Levine, Myra, 31
Liaison Committee on Medical Education, 165
Licensed nursing personnel. *See also* Licensure; Nurse(s)
employed in nursing, 149, 149*t*
Licensure
entry levels and, nursing education and, 104, 285
focus of, loss of, 166–167
future of nursing and, 277–278
importance of, 151–153
legislation needed for, 192–193
problems relating to, 163–169
SAIN proposal on, 44
"umbrella" that isn't, 173–174
Life history of Martha E. Rogers
childhood and early education (1914–1937), 12–14
family recollections of, 3–9
following NYU years (1976–present), 24–27
New York University years (1954–1975), 19–24
Rogers' reflections on, 10–27
years of work and study (1938–1953), 15–18
Life process. *See also* Aging process
evolution of, 213
homeodynamic nature of, 215. *See also* Homeodynamics
as spiral, 212, 212*f*
helicy principle and, 217–218, 218*f*
Literature, *Nursing Science* recommendations for nurses, 31
Longevity, increasing, 264, 294
Lundy, Katherine, 3, 7–8, 11, 22
Luttrell, James, 353
Luttrell, Lady Elizabeth, 353–354
Luttrell, Sir Geoffrey, 3, 353

Malinski, Violet M., 273
March on Albany (1970), 117*f*
Master's degree education. *See also* Nursing education
NYU, 89–96
evolution of, 41–43
Rogers', 15, 16
Rogers' views on, 38
Matheney, Ruth V., 30
Mathwig, Gean, 11, 21, 24, 25, 122
McGriff, Erline P., 122, 123
McKinley, William, 353
McManus, R. Louise, 38
Media for Nursing, Inc., 10
Medical College of Georgia, 337
Medicare, overcharges to, 291
Medicine
monopoly on health care, 277, 286
nursing and, autonomous/collaborative careers in, 184
Meehan, Thérése Connell, 273
Meetings Internationale, 10
Michael, Donald, 50
Michigan, Rogers' years as public health nurse in, 15–16
Michigan League for Nursing, 119–120
Moccia, Patricia A., 122
Montag, Mildred, 70, 148
Mother, fetus and, as one field versus two, 247
Movement
different forms of, perception of, 333–334
freedom of, 334
Mulholland, Rev. John, 353
Multidimensional. *See also* Four-dimensionality; Pandimensional
defined, 245*t*, 253
Rogers' use of term, 202
Multiple personalities, 331
Murphy, Marion, 30

National Education Association, Department of Higher Education, 70
National Institute of Mental Health, 168
National Leadership Conference on America's Health Policy (1976), 166
National League for Nursing, 10, 39, 69, 72, 356
accreditation and, 165
Committee on the Future of, 71
"Guidelines for Master's Degree Programs in Nursing," 89–90
organizational structure of, 71
National Manpower Training and Development Act, 66
National Nursing Council, 69
National Science Foundation, basic research definition of, 108
National unity, nursing identity and, 146
"Nature of a Profession" (Becker), 82
Negentropy, defined, 241, 352
New York City, Rogers' graduate education in, 15, 16
New York State, nursing education in, 65
New York State Governor's Commission, 71
New York State League for Nursing (NYSLN), 39, 48–49
Rogers' professional politics and, 119
New York State League Lines, 51, 120, 126–127
New York State Nurse Practice Act
Education Law of, SAIN proposal for amendment of, 185–191
revision of, 121
March on Albany for (1970), 117*f*
New York State Nurses Association (NYSNA), "1985 proposal" of, 121
New York State Office of Public Health Nursing, 62
New York University (NYU)
nursing education at
doctoral level, 97–102
evolution of, 41–43
master's level, 89–96

New York University (NYU)—*Continued*
Rogers' years at, 19–24
nursing context during, 314–315
revolution in nursing education and, 37–38
Nightingale, Florence, 150, 158, 286
Non-invasive therapeutic modalities, 237, 243, 248
Normal, defined, 230
Nosophobia, 301–304
NP programs, 168. *See also* Nurse-practitioner movement
Nurse(s)
baccalaureate degree education for, Rogers' editorials on, 30
careers available for, 355–356
"expanded role" of, 131–132, 133–138, 144, 148, 167
licensed, employment figures on, 149, 149*t*
myth of similarity of, types of programs and, 173–174
power structure threatened by, 168
purpose of, 114
role in space, body of nursing knowledge and, 299–300
shortage of, 131
myth of, 178
study of, study of nursing versus, 115
Nurse Practice Act, New York State. *See* New York State Nurse Practice Act
Nurse-practitioner movement, 147–154. *See also* NP programs; Physicians' assistants
politics of, 121–122, 142
Nurse-scientist doctoral programs, Rogers' position on, 42–43
Nurses for a Growing Nation, 71
Nursing
art of, science and, 114, 239–243
career selection in, 355–356
characteristics of, as learned profession, 109
conceptual model of. *See* Conceptual system, of nursing
differentiating careers in, 39, 182–184, 355–356
euphemisms relating to, 133–138
evolution as science. *See also* Nursing science
research and, 114
future of. *See* Future of nursing
identity of, 140–146
future of nursing and, 285–286
as science, 245
knowledge base of, development of, 39, 40–41
licensed nursing personnel employed in, 149, 149*t*. *See also* Licensure
medicine and, autonomous/collaborative careers in, 184
problems in, 167–168
profession of
Rogers' impact on, 123–124
social ends of, 109
psychodynamic, 314
purpose of, 265–266
Rogers' understanding of, 313–314
Rogers' early views on, 28–32
in space. *See* Space age
study of, study of nurses versus, 115
survival of, autonomy and, 272–273
theoretical basis of, 220–224
Rogers' early views on, 29
uniqueness of, 114, 244–245, 285
Nursing and Nursing Education in the United States (Goldmark), 69
Nursing Charts Her Course, 54–57
Nursing context, Rogers' development of ideas and, 313–316
Nursing Development Conference Group, 316
Nursing education. *See also* Education
accountability and, 131
continuing relevance of Rogers' ideas on, 43–44
doctoral, 97–102
entry levels and, 104, 285
excellence and, 126–127
federal government and, 66, 78–79
future of nursing and, 277
nosophobia implications for, 301–304
Nursing Science editorials on, 30, 59–60, 69–72
NYU
evolution of, 41–43
graduate, 89–96
papers presented by Rogers on
Educating the Nurse for the Future, 61–68
Nursing Charts Her Course, 54–57
Williamsburg (1962), 48–53
politics of, 121
euphemisms and, 133–138
practical nurse programs in, 65–66
preparation for future and, 103–106
professional
public safety and, 80–88
technical versus, 66–67, 85–86, 355–356
research and, 45, 76–77
responsibility for, 62
revolution in, 37–44
Rogers' early views on, 28–29
SAIN proposal for amendment to New York State Education Law, 185–191
Science of Unitary Human Beings in, 337
scientific knowledge in, 208
space-age paradigm and, 254–255
technical
need for, 85
professional versus, 66–67, 85–86, 355–356
types of programs in, 355–356
myth of similarity of nurses and, 173–174
Nursing for the Future, 38, 69–70, 89
Nursing knowledge, 143. *See also* Knowledge
role of nurse in space and, 299–300
Nursing Outlook, 72
Nursing practice
nursing science and, 64
Reveille in Nursing definition of, 41
science and art of, space age and, 265–266

Science of Unitary Man and, 231–232
space-age paradigm and, 254–255, 265–266
types of, 355–356
Nursing Profession: A Time to Speak (Chaska), Rogers' chapter in, 25, 27
Nursing research. *See* Research
Nursing Science, 30–31
editorials from, 30–31, 59–60, 69–72, 74–79
Nursing science, 142–144. *See also* Science of Unitary Human Beings
aims of, 205–208
art of nursing and, 114
definitions of, 325–326
euphemisms and, 134
evolution of
highlights in, 197–204
nursing identity and, 140–146
future of nursing and, 239–243
humanistic nature of, 208
key definitions specific to, 245*t*, 260*t*
nursing practice and, 64
principles of, 199, 214–219
reciprocy, 215–216
synchrony, 216–217
research and, 107–113
future of, 114–116
Reveille in Nursing definition of, 41
Rogers' contributions to development of, 322–327
Rogers' views on, 27
development of, 41
early, 29–30
nursing education and, 63–64
space age and, 256–266
paradigm of, 252–253
terminology used in, 352
"Nursing Science," 120
Nursing Science Quarterly, 26, 202
Nursing students. *See also* Nursing education
Rogers' interactions with, 44
NYSLN. *See* New York State League for Nursing
NYSNA. *See* New York State Nurses Association

Obsolescence, doing syndrome and, 179–180
Occupational certification. *See* Licensure
O'Neal, Daniel J. III, 123
Openness
causality versus, 241
human-environment relationship and, 227, 235, 246
scientific developments related to, 323
Organization, patterns and. *See* Pattern(s)
Overexpansion, health system and, 165

Pandimensional. *See also* Multidimensional
defined, 260*t*, 352
Pandimensionality, 263
freedom of movement and, 334
human potentials and, 336
nature of reality and, 264
paranormal events and, 333
pattern recognition and, 332–333
scientific developments related to, 323–324
worldview and, 260–261
Paranormal events, 230, 264, 295
changing environmental field pattern and, 335
different forms of movement and, 333–334
Parsimony, scientific models and, 326
Pattern(s)
defined, 241, 245*t*, 252, 260*t*, 352
human-environment relationship and, 227, 235, 236
resonancy and, 218–219
nursing science worldview and, 261–262
recognition of
enhancement through Rogers' model, 332–333
freedom of movement and, 334
scientific developments related to, 323
Patterning. *See also* Field patterning
relative diversity in, manifestations of, 202
Peer review, 170–172
Perception
of different forms of movement, 333–334
reality and, 229
Personalities, multiple, 331
Personnel. *See* Professional personnel; *specific type*
Ph.D.. *See* Doctoral education
Phillips, John R., 273
Philosophical context, Rogers' development of ideas and, 317–321
Phoenix, AZ, Rogers' work in, 15, 17–18
"Physician extender," 167
Physicians' assistants, 131. *See also* Nurse-practitioner movement
economic value of, to M.D.'s, 156
future of nursing and, 156–162
Pitel, Martha, 30
Politics. *See also specific political issues*
professional, Rogers', 119–124
Power
Barrett's theory of, 334
cost accounting for, 165
Power structure, nurses' threat to, 168
Practical nurse programs, 65–66, 356
Practical nursing, requirements for, SAIN proposal to amend New York State Education Law, 185–191
Practitioner movement. *See* Nurse-practitioner movement
Predictive principles, 214
President's Commission on Higher Education (1947), 70–71
Price, Donald, 50
Price, Pamela, 122
Professional autonomy. *See* Autonomy
Professional education, 355–356. *See also* Nursing education
future and, 104–105
technical education versus, 66–67, 85–86

Professional personnel. *See also* Nurse(s)
active
distribution with degrees in nursing, 152*t*
numbers of, 149, 149*t*, 150, 150*t*
Professional politics. *See also specific political issues*
Rogers', 119–124
Professional standards, *Nursing Science* editorial on, 74–75
Professional standards review organizations (PSROs), 167
Profit(s)
cost accounting for, 165
hospitals and, 291
PSROs, 167
"Psychodynamic nursing," 314
Public demands
for health services, 140, 277
for participation, 132
Public health, nursing education and, graduate-level, 92
Public safety, nursing education and, responsibility for, 80–88
Publications. *See also specific publications*
Rogers' professional politics expressed in, 120
Purpose of nursing, Rogers' early views on, 29

Quality of hospital care, declining, 167
Quality of nursing, education and, 66–68

Reality
pandimensional nature of, 264
perception and, 229
Reciprocy, 199, 215–216
Registered nurses. *See also* Nurse(s)
independent nurses versus, 182–184
licensure of, 151–152. *See also* Licensure
programs for, 355–356
Registered nursing, requirements for, SAIN proposal to amend New York State Education Law, 185–191
Reincarnation, 331
Relationships, research as study of, 115
Report of the New York State Governor's Commission on Education for the Health Professions, 65
Research
doctoral education and, 101
future of, 114–116
on nature of change, 238
potential for, identification of, 111
preparation for, 112
presented in *Nursing Science,* 31
researchers and, nursing science and, 107–113
revolution in, 44–46
Rogers' editorials on, 30, 76–77
Research Institute of America, 288
Resolution on Licensure for Entry Levels to Practice in Nursing, SAIN, 181
Resonancy, 199, 218–219, 246*t*, 262*t*
future of nursing and, 253, 294
nursing science and, 235, 242
scientific developments related to, 324
unitary man and, 228
Responsibility. *See also* Accountability
of graduates, 64
for nursing education, 62
public safety and, 80–88
nursing science and, 143
for professional standards, 74–75
Reveille in Nursing, 29–30, 40, 198, 321
definitions in, 40–41
Revised Nurse Practice Act of New York State, March on Albany for (1970), 117*f*
Rhythms
change and, 230–231, 264, 294
helicy principle and, 217
Robert Wood Johnson Foundation, 168
Robinson, Shirley M., 123
Rogerian nursing science. *See* Nursing science; Science of Unitary Human Beings
Rogerian Nursing Science News, 201, 203
Rogers, Bruce Taylor, 3, 353
Rogers, Jane. *See* Coleman, Jane Rogers
Rogers, Laura. *See* Wilhite, Laura Rogers
Rogers, Lucy K. (Lucy Mulholland Keener), 1*f*, 3, 353
Rogers, Martha E., 1*f*, 4*f*, 35*f*, 117*f*, 195*f*, 269*f*, 307*f*
charismatic leadership of, 120
continuing legacy of, 337–338
contribution to science at large, 330–336
early views of, 28–32
editorials written by, 30–31, 59–60, 69–72, 74–79
family of, 1*f*, 3–9, 4*f*
genealogy, 353–354
philosophical influences of, 317–319
Rogers' recollections of, 12–13
"fundamental project" of, 27
historical salute to, 308
ideas about nursing in space, 296–304
ideas developed by
nursing context and, 313–316
philosophical context and, 317–321
social context and, 309–312
impact on profession of nursing, 123–124
life history of
family recollections of, 3–9
Rogers' reflections on, 10–27
nursing science perspective of, 27
papers presented by
Educating the Nurse for the Future, 61–68
Nursing Charts Her Course, 54–57
at Williamsburg (1962), 48–53
personal attributes of, 26–27
professional politics of, 119–124
Society of Rogerian Scholars and, 273
status in scholarly community of nursing, 326–327
temporal consistency in ideas of, 32
theory of. *See* Science of Unitary Human Beings
views on future of nursing, 26, 271–279, 282–286, 296–304
Rogers, Martha Elizabeth Luttrell, 3, 353

Safety, public, nursing education and, 80–88
SAIN. *See* Society for Advancement in Nursing
San Diego Veterans' Administration Hospital, 337
Science
characteristics of, 324–326
defined, 241, 245, 352
desacralization of, 208
development of, process of, 326–327
nursing as. *See also* Nursing science
Rogers' contributions to development of, 322–327
nursing identity as, 245
Rogers' contribution to, 330–336
Science of Unitary, Irreducible Human Beings, 244–248, 245*t*–247*t*
Science of Unitary Human Beings, 3, 10, 233–238. *See also* Nursing science
applications of, growth in, 337
basic assumptions of, 198
basic research in, 45. *See also* Research
emergence of, 197–204
field patterning and. *See* Field patterning
homeodynamics and, 219
idea of, during Rogers' years at NYU, 20
paranormal events and, 230, 264, 295, 333–334
properties of unitary man and, 130
space age and, 259–263, 260*t*–262*t*
terminology used in, 352
theoretical basis of, 220–224
theories in, 263–265
update (1990), 244–248, 245*t*–247*t*
Science of Unitary Man, 225–232. *See also* Science of Unitary Human Beings
environment and, conceptual system for, 226–231
practical implications of, 231–232
Science of Unitary Man: A Paradigm for Nursing, 200–201
Scientific principles, 214–219
Scientific terminology. *See also* Terminology
evolution of, 207
"Scope of Professional Nursing Practice," 120
"Sick services," "health services" versus, 130–131
Sigma Theta Tau, 10
Simplicity, scientific models and, 326
Simultaneity paradigm, 10, 200–201. *See also* Science of Unitary Human Beings
Sister Charles Marie (Frank), 30, 62, 72
"Slinky" example of life process, 212, 212*f*
Social context, Rogers' development of ideas and, 309–312
Social Security Act, 148
Society, goals of, nursing profession and, 109
Society for Advancement in Nursing (SAIN), 122–123
newsletter of, 120
perspective of, 182–184
proposed act to amend the Education Law in relation to requirements in New York State, 185–191
Resolution on Licensure for Entry Levels to Practice in Nursing, 181
unification model of, myth versus reality, 175–178
Society for Advancement in Nursing (SAIN) proposal, 44, 121
Society of Rogerian Scholars, 273–274, 337
Space age. *See also* Future of nursing
nursing in space and, conversation with Rogers on, 296–304
nursing science and, 256–266
paradigm of, 250–255
Rogers' interest in, 272
worldview and, 292–295
Space-time continuum
freedom of movement in, 334
synchrony and, 216–217
theoretical basis of nursing and, 222
Spiral of life, helicy principle and, 217–218, 218*f*
Standards. *See also* Licensure
PSROs and, 167
Status, nursing identity and, 141–142
Stewart, Isabel, 123
Students, Rogers' interactions with, 44
Surgeon General's Consultant Group in Nursing, 69, 72
Synchrony, 199, 216–217
Synthesis, worldview of, 260

Teachers College, Columbia University, 70
Rogers' attendance at, 15, 16
Team approach, physicians' assistants and, 159–160
Technical education. *See also* Nursing education
need for, 85, 131
professional education versus, 66–67, 85–86, 355–356
Technology
changing diversity of environmental field pattern and, 335
future and, 288–291. *See also* Future of nursing
perspective on, 144–145
professional education and
preparation for future and, 105–106
responsibility for, 83
Terminology
conceptual system and, 235
defined in *Reveille in Nursing,* 40–41
euphemistic. *See* Euphemisms
evolution of, in Science of Unitary Human Beings, 197–204
glossary of, 352
Rogers' selection of, beliefs revealed by, 32
scientific, evolution of, 207
specific to science of nursing, 245*t*, 260*t*
Theoretical basis of nursing, 220–224
Rogers' early views on, 29
Theoretical research. *See* Basic research; Research
Theories
conceptual systems and, 205–206
nursing science and, 245
in Science of Unitary Human Beings, 263–265

Theory of Martha E. Rogers. *See* Science of Unitary Human Beings
Therapeutic touch, 237, 243, 248, 295, 332
Time and space. *See* Space-time continuum
Toffler, Alvin, 91, 229
Touch
  high-tech future and, 288–291
  therapeutic, 237, 243, 248, 332
Transcendent unity, 296–297
Truth, methods of discovering, scientific approach and, 208
Twenty Thousand Nurses Tell Their Story, 71

Undergraduate education. *See* Baccalaureate degree education
Unification Model, Rogers' position on, 43, 175–178, 179–180, 286
Unionization, 164
"Unitary," "holistic" versus, 234
Unitary human being. *See also* Science of Unitary Human Beings
  defined, 235, 241, 245*t*, 260*t*, 352
Unitary man, 225–232
  defined, 228
Unitary person, defined, 253
Unity
  nursing identity and, 146
  transcendent, 296–297
Universities. *See also* Education
  responsibility of, for professional education in nursing, 80–88
"University and Professional Education," 93
University of South Carolina, 337
University of Tennessee, Rogers' attendance at, 13
U.S. Medicine, 157
U.S. Public Health Service, health credentialing and, 166

Videotapes, documenting Rogers' thoughts, 10, 11
Visiting Nurse Association, Hartford, CT, Rogers' position at, 16
Visiting Nurse Service, Rogers' establishment of, in Arizona, 15, 17
Visiting Nursing, establishment of, 159
Vocational programs, 65–66, 356

Wagoner, Elizabeth, 123
Warner, Beverly A., 123
Washburn University School of Nursing, 337
Waves, energy. *See also* Energy field
  resonancy principle and, 218–219
"Well-being," Rogers' focus on, 32
"Who Speaks for Nurses?," 120
Wholeness of man. *See also* Science of Unitary Human Beings
  complexification and, 300–301
  conceptual model of nursing and, 212–213
Wilhite, James, 3, 7
Wilhite, Laura Rogers, 3, 4*f*, 4–5, 354
  genealogy provided by, 353–354
Wilhite, Mel B., 3, 4, 6–7
Wilhite, Rev. Nancy J., 3, 7, 353
Witt, John Jr., 353
Witt, William, 353
Worldviews
  nursing science and, 245, 257–259
  older versus newer, 261*t*
  philosophical context of Rogers' ideas and, 317–321
  space age and, 292–295